~~KEY TEXT~~
REFERENCE

D1426663

SPORTING BODIES, DAMAGED SELVES:

SOCIOLOGICAL STUDIES OF SPORTS-RELATED INJURY

RESEARCH IN THE SOCIOLOGY OF SPORT

Series Editor: Kevin Young

Volume 1:   *Theory, Sport & Society*
            Edited by Joseph Maguire and Kevin Young, 2002

RESEARCH IN THE SOCIOLOGY OF SPORT   VOLUME 2

SPORTING BODIES, DAMAGED SELVES:

SOCIOLOGICAL STUDIES OF SPORTS-RELATED INJURY

EDITED BY

KEVIN YOUNG

Department of Sociology, University of Calgary, Alberta, Canada

2004

ELSEVIER
JAI

Amsterdam – Boston – Heidelberg – London – New York – Oxford
Paris – San Diego – San Francisco – Singapore – Sydney – Tokyo

ELSEVIER B.V.	ELSEVIER Inc.	**ELSEVIER Ltd**	ELSEVIER Ltd
Radarweg 29	525 B Street, Suite 1900	**The Boulevard, Langford**	84 Theobalds Road
P.O. Box 211	San Diego	**Lane, Kidlington**	London
1000 AE Amsterdam	CA 92101-4495	**Oxford OX5 1GB**	WC1X 8RR
The Netherlands	USA	**UK**	UK

First edition 2004

Library of Congress Cataloging in Publication Data
A catalog record is available from the Library of Congress.

British Library Cataloguing in Publication Data
A catalogue record is available from the British Library.

ISBN: 0-7623-0884-2
ISSN: 1476-2854 (Series)

♾ The paper used in this publication meets the requirements of ANSI/NISO Z39.48-1992 (Permanence of Paper). Printed in The Netherlands.

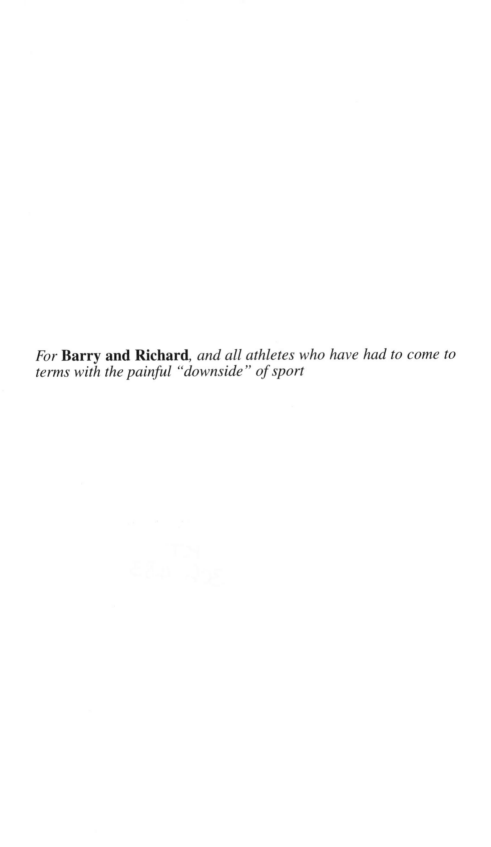

For **Barry and Richard***, and all athletes who have had to come to terms with the painful "downside" of sport*

Contents

Preface

One of the most common assumptions made about sport is that being an athlete is beneficial for both body and mind, and that sport is practised by healthy bodies experiencing healthy outcomes. While the world of sport is populated by persons on and off the field who wish that this were true, anyone who has played, coached, administered or simply watched from the sidelines will attest that this view is, at least in part, a misconception, often forwarded by those unwilling to acknowledge what Messner and Sabo have called the "very limiting, often painful downside of sport" (1990: 14). The potentially healthful benefits of sport and exercise have been well-documented (Berger & Owen 1988; Biddle & Fox 1989; Curtis & Russell 1997; Sargeant & Siddons 1998), but the less healthy, injurious consequences of sport have been far less widely researched, certainly by sociologists. In many sports and at many levels, sport is also about learning to live with pain and hurt and, for a disconcertingly large number of athletes, injury and even disablement that can last well beyond the playing years. Of the sundry badly kept secrets from the world of sport, this is surely among the worst. Everyone knows that it is almost impossible to play sport without experiencing pain; every athlete has a story to tell about injury.

Countless athletes and former athletes have spoken about pain and injury, some extremely eloquently,[1] and about the relationship between the requirements of

---

[1] While many high level athletes have addressed their pain and injury experiences thoughtfully, comments made by former National Hockey League player, Eric Nesterenko are among the most considered. Quoted in Terkel's (1974) provocative book *Working*, Nesterenko made the following observations on the use of cynicism toward coaches and owners as a means of coping with exploitive employer attitudes to injury:

> I became disillusioned with the game not being the pure thing it was earlier in my life. I began to see the exploitation of the players by the owners. You realize owners don't really care for you. You're a piece of property. They try to get as much out of you as they can. I remember once I had a torn shoulder. It was well in the process of healing. But I knew it wasn't right yet. They brought the doctor in. He said, "You can play." I played and ripped it completely. I was laid up. So I look at the owner. He shrugs his shoulders, walks away. He doesn't really hate me. He's impersonal (1974: 501).

sport and dealing with physical hurt. But few have done this more austerely than former British World Champion boxer, Barry McGuigan:

> As a boxer, you build up tolerance to pain. In fact, your immune system learns how to deal with it. The hardest I was ever hit was by Juan Laporte. I was never hit so hard again. It was an incredible experience. I threw a lazy left and he beat me to the punch with a right over the top, on to the left side of my jaw beneath the cheekbone. It snapped my head round in a circle. I got what Ali used to describe as "blue flashes" — like an explosion inside. Normally, all you can do is hope your head clears quickly and that you can pretend that you're not hurt. But this punch brought on a huge blue flash and the sensation of pins and needles on the *inside* of my body, down the left side, right down to the ground. When I looked at Laporte, it was as if he'd got into a car in the rain and the windows were all steamed up. I couldn't see him at all. But gradually the fan began to work and slowly he got clearer and clearer. I held onto him like a vice and let go only when my vision cleared. And all the while I had these pins and needles on the inside, trying to worm their way out. Pain is defined in boxing by how it affects your ability to function. A boxer *knows* when an opponent is hurt and, like a dog sensing a badger's desperation, he turns up the heat. So disguising pain is imperative. It becomes instinctive. Boxing *is* the acceptance of pain (*The Independent on Sunday*, February 15, 2004: 16).

McGuigan's comments are chilling, but they raise fascinating questions about the sorts of coping strategies athletes must adopt if they are to continue to play — these are addressed at length in a variety of ways and from a variety of national settings in this volume.

Of course, not all athletes are involved in such brutal and brutalising pursuits as boxers, or at such elite levels as McGuigan. But this is not to say that McGuigan's account is unfamiliar to less qualified athletes in either similarly violent or other, less combative, sports. For example, in a study of Canadian male athletes participating in a range of sports including football, soccer, rugby, ice hockey, climbing, squash, downhill skiing and track and field conducted a decade ago, Philip White, William McTeer and I collated our respondents' accounts of pain and injury in the following manner:

> . . . all of the men had experienced an injury serious enough to have altered the course of their lives or to have resulted in some form

> of disablement... All had experienced very painful injuries, and most had incurred multiple injuries. The aggregate picture... read like an emergency room nightmare... fractures to most bones, a ruptured spleen, concussions, a lacerated kidney, a punctured testicle, shoulder and other joint dislocations, torn ligaments, heart attack, and a stroke. Long-term results of these injuries included carpal tunnel syndrome, chronic pain variously located, a removed kidney, partial paralysis, tendinitis, arthritis, and body parts kept in place with braces, plates, pins and other devices (Young *et al.* 1994: 179).

Despite their disturbing commentaries on pain, all but two of the athletes in the study returned enthusiastically to relatively or very high-risk sports; the two who did not expressed a desire to return but were physically unable to. Both reported that "injuring out" of sport was, as one of them put it, "fully devastating."

And then there's Stephen's story. A young, British man in his mid-twenties, Stephen[2] has never played professional sport, but might have in either rugby or soccer had circumstances, and his body, allowed. From his early teens, repeated cycles of injury have resulted in numerous surgeries and other medical "interventions," thousands of pounds in medical costs, over 100 stitches and a severely scarred body. Figure 1 summarises some of Stephen's injury experiences, his age at the point they occurred, the sorts of surgical attention necessary, and his reflections on his extensive injury encounters. It is clear that Stephen's injuries are outcomes of numerous things — the nature of his preferred sports and the value systems that pervade them, the way in which he has chosen to play his sports, and sheer bad luck. Since the chapters in this volume deal directly with the full panorama of injury from causation to medical treatment to narratives of reflection to financial implications, in a sense, Stephen's tale is representative of a "dimensions, problems, and issues" theme that runs through the book as a whole. Figure 1 is not an easy read, but its contents will be all too familiar to many readers. As numbing as the injury biography of this "ordinary" athlete is, the point is that Stephen is not alone; like others, he may even be lucky not to have fared worse (see Chapter 18). Again, not all athletes will be able to report such unsettling sports histories, but many can — it is certainly the case that almost every athlete knows another athlete who can.

---

[2] "Stephen" is a pseudonym, but the summary account of this young man's injury "chronicles" provided here is real.

Date & age	Injury	Playing context	Medical costs	Level of pain / injury	Thoughts on treatment	Overall reflections
1992 (14)	Small tear on left knee meniscus; required shaving	Tackle in school football	£1,000	Minimal pain but locking sensation and swelling	Very good treatment; back playing within a couple of weeks	Felt like a 'regular' muscle strain that required small surgical procedure
1994 (16)	Felt snapping in left knee and heard loud 'pop'; continued to play for 15 minutes but knee kept giving way	Football – foot stuck in dry rut and knee twisted	£1,000	Loud pop scared me; as day went on, swelling was extreme	Good, but surgeon was blunt informing me of ACL rupture; very upsetting	Had visions of never being able to play sport again
1994 (17)	Full ACL reconstruction following previous injury. Meniscus also repaired following tear	See above	£5,000	Recall bad 'post op' pain; awoke to find knee on a 'continual motion machine'; pain subsided after 12 hours	Thorough; doctors very aggressive with pre- and post-op; made to walk within 24 hrs	Awoke to bad post op pain; happy when surgeon informed me all went well; keen to get up and about and running
1995 (17)	Dislocation of right thumb	Final of National Rugby '7's; was being cocky trying to take a quick '22 drop out' and opponent kicked and damaged hand	Free - NHS	Massive pain; distressing as thumb was perpendicular to back of hand by fourth knuckle; felt queasy to look at it	Good treatment from a young Scottish rugby player doctor who appreciated that I was anxious to get it fixed without surgery	Huge pain; anxious not to have surgery; as soon as thumb was put back, pain disappeared; removed cast 3 weeks early to play again; no repercussions
1996 (19)	Torn right knee medial meniscus	Rugby; fell awkwardly after tackle	£1,000	Very painful; massive swelling	Great treatment; precise explanations. Was back home 24 hours after op	Was relieved as I was convinced I had ruptured ACL
1997 (19)	Torn right knee medial meniscus	Rugby; tackled as I kicked ball	£1,000	Minimal pain, but obvious what I had done.	As 1996	Felt down; fully aware of what had happened
1997 (20)	Torn right knee medial meniscus	Rugby tackle	£1,000	See above	See above	

Figure 1: Stephen's injury chronicles.

Year (Age)	Injury	Cause	Cost	Pain	Treatment / physio experience	Feelings
1998 (20)	Torn right knee medial meniscus		£1,000	See above	See above	
1999 (22)	Prolapsed disc	Rugby weight training on day after match; was very fatigued and felt twinge while doing seated rows; twinge got worse over next 48 hours until I couldn't stand up straight	£1,500	Minimal pain at first; got gradually worse for 48 hours until it peaked and then it died off to nothing	Very poor physio experience telling me it was muscular problem; changed physio; referred to back specialist who MRI'd me; epidural followed	Pain free and was pleased to get it over with; running within 3 weeks of epidural
2000 (22)	Arthroscopy following knee injury	Rugby; heard loud snap and thought I had broken leg while training; no contact involved; I twisted and my foot stuck in a rut	£1,000	Very painful when snap occurred; when it became obvious leg was not broken, knew what had happened	Happy with treatment, but frustrated; knew what was wrong but had to endure MRI scan and x-rays, etc.	Painful, but was keen to get operation over as I felt I knew prognosis. Felt very down for first 24 hours
2000 (22)	Full ACL reconstruction of right knee following above injury	See above	£7,000	Painful, but much less distressing than previous ACL; had much more confidence in the procedure to succeed	Impressed with advice pertaining to rehabilitation & with explanations about procedures	Again painful, but as with previous ACL reconstruction I was very keen on getting back to running, etc.
2002 (24)	Torn right medial meniscus	Rugby; heavy contact training session; I was 'manning' a tackle shield and was hit from the side just above knee	£1,000	Minimal pain, but as with previous cartilage tears I felt I recognised the problem immediately	Good treatment as with other times; if anything even better this time as I felt surgeon was more 'sport aware'	Keen to get back to things, but meniscus was removed rather than repaired; thus longer recuperation time

Figure 1: (*Continued*)

For my part, and as the American sociologist C. Wright Mills (1959) might have predicted, the research fascination that spawns this volume has an inevitably biographical component. As with all contributors to this volume, I have acquired my knowledge of sport injury and pain both *directly* as a former athlete and *indirectly* as a social scientist. As a former rugby and soccer player at English and Canadian schools and universities with subsequent experiences in other sports, I have had my fill of injuries, frustratingly long rehabilitation programmes, and lasting aches and pains. For close to 2 decades I have sufffered from a lower back problem that began when I played university rugby in Canada, and that has familiarised me with the world of anti-inflammatory drugs and so-called "painkillers." Among other injuries, I have also experienced a broken finger, 3 broken noses, and ligamental damage to both knees and both ankles. In the bigger scheme of sporting things, these are relatively minor injury episodes and, again, one might even say that I, too, have been "lucky," given the risks that I have taken in sports such as (for many years) rugby and soccer, and (more occasionally) skydiving, windsurfing, climbing and barefoot water skiing to have *only* been injured in these ways.

Over the years, I have discovered that there is an intriguing twist to speaking about injury with "legitimacy" in sport circles that is likely tied up with the sorts of bravado and macho credentialism that so many scholars have shown to underpin dominant sport culture (cf. Burstyn 1999; Messner & Sabo 1990). Specifically, as injury-research colleague Philip White and I wrote in 1999:

> ... when we have raised issues about violence, aggression, and sport, a common illogical response by some people (predominantly men) who seem to be threatened by such challenges [to the dominant ways of playing and thinking about sport] are questions such as, "Oh yeah, have *you* ever played contact sport. Have *you* ever been injured?" Fortunately (and unfortunately) for both of us, the answer to both of these questions is 'Yes' and 'Yes'. Both of us had prolonged and active careers in soccer and rugby, and we have both been hospitalized with serious injuries suffered when younger (White & Young 1999: 70).

Personally and intellectually, the telling point is that as we reflected on it more seriously over the years, it:

> ... became evident that we were ambivalent about the physical damage incurred during our athletic careers. On the one hand, we both derived a great deal of enjoyment and satisfaction from

playing sports like rugby — the thrills and spills, the competition, the comraderie, and (dare we say it) the affirmation of our masculinity. On the other hand, there was always a side of us that suspected we had caved in to the types of pressure put on many young men (and increasingly women) to expose their bodies to levels of risk that could be considered excessive (Young & White 1999: 204).

Of course, in relating such biographical observations, I am acutely aware that some readers will have lives that are far more pervaded by sports-related pain and injury encounters than mine. Regardless, for me, editing this volume has been an exercise in becoming more fully aware of the diverse articulations of the sport injury phenomena around me. In my case, these include, but are not limited to: the hundreds of students who have stories of broken bodies to tell; family members whose athletic victories are soured by the negative impact of those successes on their ageing bodies; the coaches I know who, while responsible and fair off the field of play, make no excuses for their lack of empathy for their injured players on it, especially during games; the Kinesiological/performance model colleagues and sports medicine practitioners who simply take injury and pain for granted and seem rarely to have critically reflected on where it comes from or what it might mean; a son whose miscellaneous injuries may force him to change his preferred sports altogether; the myriad media outlets all around us which hawk athletic hurt in the form of lurid "Plays of the Day," "Hits of the Week" or front cover fist-fights to meet a certain component of audience demand and reap profit (Young 1990, 1991); and, by the discouraging fact that the academy has pandered to corporate opportunism ever before it wholly understands what sport injury is or what its full range of implications are.[3] In each of these ways and more, it is clear to me that if one is engaged in sport, one is likely also engaged in the acknowledgement of pain.

---

[3] A perfect illustration of this occurred at the 2000 Pre-Olympic Congress in Brisbane, Australia. In addition to a very slick exhibit promoting hundreds of gadgets for fixing body parts broken or hurt by sport, the registration package included a range of exotic medications, information on how to "kill" pain and even an instructional CD advising how to ease back pain (for a cost), but no acknowledgement that sports-related injury and pain might also be reduced by changing the way that sport is played or the norms around it. The contradiction is obvious — the academy, and especially the cluster of bio-sciences of sport, have been complicit in forging partnerships with the pharmaceutical and drug industry, which has clear interests in not wanting sport injury to go away any time soon, at the same time as professing to deal with the huge human and financial costs of sport injury in a meaningful and athlete-friendly way.

This is the first volume in the *Research in the Sociology of Sport* series with a substantive focus, and it is fitting that this focus represents one of the most burgeoning areas of research within the contemporary sociology of sport field. As I go on to explain in the *Introduction* that follows, sociology has not been fast out of the blocks in attending to matters of injury and pain in sport, but an impressive literature is developing, and the time seems right to review and assemble a sample of that work in this forum. Indeed, to my knowledge, this volume represents the first collection of studies dedicated entirely to sports-related pain and injury research conducted by sociologists. In brief, this, then, is a book that begins to explore the multiple and varied dimensions of how pain and injury are embedded within sports cultures.

It is enormously exciting to bring together cutting-edge work from a developing field but, given the nature of the research topic, this excitement is inevitably tempered by a sense of regret that there is a *need* for this work to be undertaken at all. My sense of this need comes not only from my own work in the area and the growing literature I refer to, but from experiences teaching Sociology of Sport classes at universities on both sides of the Atlantic. Student responses to sociological studies of sport injury have been extremely enlightening. On the one hand, students absorb the material eagerly, but often do not know how to react. Some of the most assertive responses come from student athletes whose core selves are likely interwoven with their sporting ventures, and whose athletic identities might have been assembled on the very basis of how they have met with and negotiated injury, in their own eyes, as well as in the eyes of others such as teammates and coaches. For these students, it is apparently heretical to ever question what Don Sabo calls "the Pain Principle" (1994) of sport. As one student observed matter-of-factly recently in class, injury just *is*! Over the years, the perplexing ways that people seem willing to leap to the defence of such "problems" in sport has led to lively class discussions in which I have been accused, despite my generally pro-sport proclivities, of taking the dubious journey from scholar-to-muckraker-to-Judas — how dare I betray "innocent" sport and its "unintended" outcomes in such a way!

On the other hand, and since so many of my sociology of sport students have themselves been injured and can empathise personally with the materials, I have been surprised at how many of them describe the readings I allocate on the topic as helpful, even moving; as though it is a relief for them to read other people telling *their* stories. Here, reading and teaching intersect uneasily with a crude form of therapy as injured students identify themselves vicariously in documented accounts and discover that injury has been challenging, isolating and devastating for others, too. In large part, this book is for all such students who have shared, or simply reflected seriously upon, their versions of sports pain. I thank them all for sharing their ordeals and their reflections, and it is my hope that they will find this collection of readings illuminating intellectually and privately helpful.

Following a brief review of the rapidly developing literature on pain and injury in sport conducted by sociologists in the *Introduction*, the book is divided into three main sections. Entitled *Pain Cultures*, Part I offers five readings that address the varied structures and processes dominant in sport that result in the normalisation of risk, and sport being played in such a way that renders injury likely and pain inevitable. Here, the focus is on such matters as the biological, psychological and sociological genesis of risk (Donnelly), power structures in sport that culminate in athletes "getting hooked on hurt" (Sabo), the complex and wide-ranging networks of social relationships connected to sport that promote risk (Nixon), the quality and quantity of health care delivery to athletes (Kotarba), and how institutionally tolerated conventions within certain sport cultures can lead to pathological forms of weight management (Johns).

Part II shifts attention to substantive case studies, or *Pain Zones*. Here, we have eight empirical offerings which, for the most part, represent smaller snapshots of larger research endeavours. In this section, the over-arching trend is on the ways that athletes injured and/or in pain have interpreted their own experiences in their own terms and categories and using their own sense-making techniques, as we saw Barry McGuigan, "Stephen" and other athletes do earlier. Male and female athlete cultures under investigation here include soccer (Roderick), rowing (Pike), rodeo and football (Frey et al.), cycling (Albert), handball (Thing), basketball (Singer), rugby (Howe), along with a selection of others (Charlesworth and Young).

The focus in the final section of the volume, Part III, is on the implications and aftereffects of pain and injury in sport, or what I call *Pain Parameters*. In this section, the role of the medical and athletic therapy industry that attends to athletes in pain (Walk and Safai), the implications of sport injury for public health and social policy (Waddington), the financial and other "costs" associated with sport injury (White), and the legal ramifications of injury cases (Young) are among matters considered in some depth.

Overall, this book represents cutting-edge work on sports-related injury being conducted by male and female scholars from a number of countries and from a number of points of view. Because pain and injury in sport are being studied using diverse explanatory and technical tools, no one theoretical or methodological approach is prioritised over others, though the varied contributions are in every sense "critical" and "sociological." It is my hope that in *Sporting Bodies, Damaged Selves* readers will find an accessible sample of the heterogeneous and vibrant work that is being undertaken in one of the fastest growing fields of the subdiscipline. This volume may well be the first such collection of readings in this field but, given the current fascination of sociologists of sport with the subject matter, a swelling literature and the voracious pace of its development, it is unlikely to be the last.

References

Are you sitting comfortably? (2004, February 15). *The Independent on Sunday* (pp. 16–17).

Berger, B., & Owen, D. (1988). Stress reduction and mood enhancement in four exercise modes: Swimming, body conditioning, hatha yoga, and fencing. *Research Quarterly for Exercise and Sport, 59,* 148–159.

Biddle, S. J. H., & Fox, K. R. (1989). Exercise and health psychology: Emerging relationships. *British Journal of Medical Psychology, 62,* 205–216.

Burstyn, V. (1999). *The rites of men: Manhood, politics, and the culture of sport.* Toronto: University of Toronto Press.

Curtis, J., & Russell, S. (Eds) (1997). *Physical activity in human experience: Interdisciplinary perspectives.* Champaign, IL: Human Kinetics.

Messner, M., & Sabo, D. (1990). *Sport, men and the gender order: Critical feminist perspectives.* Champaign, IL: Human Kinetics.

Mills, C. W. (1959). *The sociological imagination.* New York: Oxford University Press.

Sabo, D. (1994). The body politics of sports injury: Culture, power and the pain principle. Paper presented at the National Athletic Trainers Association, Dallas, TX, November 6.

Sargeant, A., & Siddons, H. (1998). From community health to elite sport. In: *Proceedings of the Third Annual Congress of the European College of Sport Science.* Manchester and Liverpool, UK: Centre for Health Care Development.

Terkel, S. (1974). *Working.* New York: Avon.

White, P., & Young, K. (1999). Is sport injury gendered? In: P. White, & K. Young (Eds), *Sport and gender in Canada* (pp. 69–84). Don Mills, Ont.: Oxford University Press.

Young, K. (1990). Treatment of sports violence by the Canadian mass media. *Report to Sport Canada's Applied Sport Research Program.* Government of Canada, August (pp. 65).

Young, K. (1991). *Writers, rimmers, and slotters: Privileging violence in the construction of the sports page.* North American Society for the Sociology of Sport, Milwaukee, WI, November 6–9.

Young, K., & White, P. (1999). Threats to sport careers: Elite athletes talk about injury and pain. In: J. Coakley, & P. Donnelly (Eds), *Inside sports* (pp. 203–213). London: Routledge.

Young, K., White, P., & McTeer, W. (1994). Body talk: Male athletes reflect on sport, injury, and pain. *Sociology of Sport Journal, 11*(2), 175–195.

Acknowledgements

Sincere thanks to the many people who have helped in the preparation and assembly of this second volume of *Research in the Sociology of Sport*. To the contributors, thank you for being willing to participate in one of the first book-length sociological examinations of sports-related pain and injury — a burgeoning sub-field of inquiry in the sociology of sport. The staff at Elsevier deserve special thanks for their dedication and enthusiasm for this project. In particular, I would like to thank Geraldine Billingham, Ann Corney, Ann Marie Davenport and Lesley Roberts for their involvement, support and guidance at various stages of the work. The book is dedicated to athletes everywhere whose painful sporting encounters, whether through intent or sheer bad luck, have led to damaged bodies and questioned selves.

Introduction

Sports-Related Pain and Injury: Sociological Notes

Kevin Young

The subject of pain and injury in sport has generated a great deal of public debate but surprisingly little research from a sociological point of view. Indeed, in contrast to other disciplines such as biomechanics, physiology or psychology, a sociological literature on sports-related pain and injury is just beginning to develop. A partial explanation may be found in the fact that sociological attention paid to injury and pain in sport has consistently been subsumed under the more general umbrella classification of "sports violence" rather than viewed as an area of study unto itself. In Canada, for instance, initial sociological inquiry was pioneered in the 1980s and 1990s by Michael Smith (1983, 1987, 1991) who posed preliminary questions about the social, physical and legal dimensions of injury and pain. While certainly recognising the significance of injury research and laying the foundation for future work, Smith mainly approached injury as the downside to aggressive sport and sport played aggressively rather than as an autonomous field of research per se.

Since the 1980s, and likely in step with a broader turn to "body" studies in the parent discipline (cf. Featherstone *et al.* 1991; Frank 1991; Freund 1991; Lupton 1995; Shilling 1993), a number of sociologists of sport (mainly based in Britain and North America, but also increasingly from continental European countries, as well as Australasia and Asia), have taken a different view and have examined sport injury more closely. Indeed, the literature on pain, injury and — relatedly — physicality in sport has expanded rapidly; this expansion is ongoing. Aspects of injury which have been examined so far by sociologists include causes and contexts

Sporting Bodies, Damaged Selves
Research in the Sociology of Sport, Volume 2, 1–25
© 2004 Published by Elsevier Ltd.
ISSN: 1476-2854/doi:10.1016/S1476-2854(04)02023-0

(in this volume, these are called *Pain Cultures*), injury rates and explanations of how injury is directly 'lived' and reflected upon by athletes themselves (*Pain Zones*), as well as social responses to injury such as how the media treat it, how medical and legal organizations have responded to injury episodes, and the implications of injury for health and social policy (*Pain Parameters*).

The literature is already impressively diverse. For example: Howard Nixon (1992, 1993, 1994a, b, 1996), who has probably written more consistently on the topic of sports-related injury than any other sociologist of sport over the past 15 years, has placed pain and injury in the context of "cultures of risk" that characterise sport, as well as the socially stratified "sportsnets" (or networks of social relationships) that athletes belong to; Don Sabo (1986, 1994) has examined the gendered underpinnings of sports injury and the philosophical codes many athletes adopt to approach pain; Robert Hughes and Jay Coakley (1991) have drawn from deviancy theory to explain violence and injury in sport as outcomes of over-conformity to a "sport ethic" that pervades much of modern sport and that prioritises risk over well-being; Curry (1993), Donnelly & Young (1988) and Holmes & Frey (1990) have shown how athletes who shy away from pain and injury are seldom attributed status as "real athletes" in sport groups; Martin Roderick *et al.* (2000), Parissa Safai (2001), David Howe (2001) and Stephan Walk (1997) have explored the role and complicity of the medical industry in sports injury; Nancy Theberge (1997), Elizabeth Pike (2000) and Hannah Charlesworth (2004) are among the first female sociologists examining the experience of pain and injury in the lives of female athletes; and, accompanied by colleagues and singly, I have investigated: (a) how risk has social, subcultural and economic/occupational dimensions (Young 1993); (b) the various sense-making strategies male and female athletes use to play through pain and that allow them to return to play even when at risk of further injury (Young 1997; Young *et al.* 1994; Young & White 1995); as well as (c) how consent and liability issues are interpreted by the courts when sports injury has been litigated (Young 1993; Young & Wamsley 1996). But, for all its richness and diversity, this is only a partial picture of the variety of work on the subject that is currently being undertaken and compiled by sociologists.

Because this field has mushroomed so rapidly, the time seems right to take stock of what sociologists are telling us regarding the central dimensions and implications of athletic "pain zones" — to examine what has been done on sports-related pain and injury, what themes are being pursued and how, what problems are emerging, what gaps exist and how they might be filled. As such, Figure 1 offers a convenient tabular summary of the existing themes in sociological pain and injury research. Its framework and contents, now elucidated in terms of a review of the

1. Contextualizing Injury	2. Injury Exposed
Kotarba (1983) Sabo (1986; 1994) Hughes & Coakley (1991) Morris (1991) Messner (1990; 1992) Nixon (1992) Young (1993)	Smith (1983) Adams *et al.* (1987) Sports Council (1991) Caine *et al.* (1996) Larson *et al.* (1996) Mueller *et al.* (1996) McCutcheon *et al.* (1997)
3. Anticipating, Living with & Recovering from Injury	**4. Injury Costs**
Snyder (1990) Young *et al.* (1994) Sparkes (1996; 1999) Pike (2000) Charlesworth (2004)	Sorensen & Sonne-holm (1980) Sports Council (1991) Hume & Marshall (1994) Mueller *et al.* (1996) Young & White (2000)
5. Injury as Spectacle	**6. Injury, Health, and Public Policy**
Young (1990; 1991) Nixon (1993) Gillett *et al.* (1996)	Fuller (1995) Hawkins & Fuller (1998) Waddington (2000)
7. Punishing Injury: Legal Reactions	**8. Injury Under-Exposed**
Horrow (1980; 1982) Smith (1983; 1987; 1991) Watson & MacLellan (1986) Barnes (1988) Young & Wamsley (1996)	Nixon (1993) Theberge (1997) Walk (1997) Waddington (2000) Donnelly (2003)

Figure 1: Sports-related pain zones: Central dimensions (and select references).

literature,[1] cumulatively capture the principal curiosities of sociologists of sport to date.

---

[1] Because so many of the contributions that follow offer some version of a review of the literature in the context of their specific work, and in the interests of avoiding repetition, this review of the literature will be relatively brief and restricted to the 8-cell typology offered here (see Figure 1).

While by no means exhaustive, the respective cells in the table reflect these main themes. Cell 1 acknowledges the multiple and varied causes of sport injury but, more germane for our purposes, raises macro sociological questions in establishing a wider *social context* for injury; cells 2 and 3 deal with issues of *becoming injured, experiencing injury,* and *moving beyond it* (which might include simply learning how to live *with* it); and cells 4–7 tackle the question of *social responses to sport injury.* Finally, cell 8 addresses potential problem areas in the literature where far more research and clarity are needed.

1. Contextualising Injury

Among the most important questions any student of sport must ask when examining sports-related pain and injury are "what causes it?" and "where does it come from?" Clearly, there is a range of appropriate answers and, unsurprisingly, these answers are striated along disciplinary lines.

Physiologically, one can point to a number of causal factors such as the basic technical requirements of sport and the various stresses and strains placed on bones, joints and muscles. For example, in Britain, the Football Association's Head of Sports Medicine, Alan Hodson, has recently remarked that "...58% of injuries in football [soccer] are non-contact, arising from things like turning, landing, slowing down and sprinting... that is the nature of the game..." (*The Independent,* January 26, 2001: 28). Some subdisciplines within the sport sciences such as sports medicine and exercise physiology have produced copious volumes of epidemiological research (cf. Adams *et al.* 1987; Caine *et al.* 1996; Harries *et al.* 1996; Mueller *et al.* 1996; Vinger & Hoerner 1981) on the link between specific athletic endeavours and, for instance, acute, chronic or catastrophic injuries to particular body parts of general athlete populations as well as more narrowly defined groups such as "growing" (paediatric) athletes (Hyndman 1996), ageing athletes (Menard 1996), and athletes with disabilities (Booth 1996). Similarly extensive literatures on injury are available for athletes in most sports.

Though obviously significant in and of themselves, sociologists are less concerned with these "nature-of-the-game" sorts of factors than they are with the kinds of micro and macro contexts (sport-related cultures, structures, processes and mores) that represent the settings and circumstances in which sports injury occurs. In this respect, sports injury can indeed be seen to result from the nature of sport itself, but also from the way it is played, administered and managed.

Several sociologists such as Frey (1991), Hughes & Coakley (1991) and Nixon (1992) have suggested that sport occurs in a cultural context which normalises and glorifies risk, pain and injury, and amid an institutional network of social relationships ("sportsnets") that pressures athletes to play with pain. This is the context for the creation of the so-called "sport ethic," a value embodied in many sporting subcultures which encourages athletes to strive for distinction, make sacrifices, play through pain and accept few limits in their quest for success, team spirit and status. Nixon calls this overall setting a "culture of risk"; here, athletes accept the probability of minor injury and the possibility of major injury. For Hughes and Coakley and Nixon, it is "over-conformity" to the norms of the sport ethic that produces in athletes a willingness to play through pain, return hastily from injury, and vilify other athletes who refuse to conform to the same set of expectations.

A focus on how pain and injury are routinely normalised in sport can also be found in other work. In their study of elite amateur wrestling, Curry & Strauss (1994) show that the social organisation of college sport in the USA widely accepts injury as an expected feature of sport, so much so that athletes "who demonstrate the least amount of reaction to pain and injury are then glorified as good examples" (p. 197). Roderick *et al.* (2000) found similar justification techniques and institutional pressures in their interview-based study of professional soccer players in England. Importantly, Roderick *et al.* demonstrate how pain normalisation emerges out of both externally-imposed institutional settings as well as self-imposed values athletes learn to accept as participants early on. In their words:

> Playing with pain or when injured is a central aspect of the culture of professional football. Young players quickly learn that one of the characteristics which football club managers look for in a player is that he should have what, in professional football, is regarded as a 'good attitude'. One way in which players can demonstrate to their manager that they have such an attitude is by being prepared to play with pain or when injured (2000: 71).

Such normalisation processes and value systems which make themselves known to many recreational and amateur athletes as *choices* becomes systematised as *pre-requisites* at the professional level. As I argued in an earlier paper assessing injury in some professional sports as a form of workplace victimisation and organisational neglect:

> By any measure, professional sport is a violent and hazardous workplace, replete with its own unique forms of "industrial disease." No other single milieu, including the risky and labour-intensive settings of miners, oil drillers, or construction site workers can compare with the routine injuries of team sports

such as football, ice hockey, soccer, rugby and the like . . . Athletic injury results from the nature of forceful sports work itself but also . . . from its organization (ownership, management) and supervision (coaching) in a venal occupational culture designed to produce profit. Over-training, playing while injured, and improper coaching or tackling/hitting techniques, all of which are usually avoidable, represent examples of the conventional hazards of sports workplaces (Young 1993: 373, 377).

At the professional level at least, injury may thus be understood as the outcome of intricate relationships which involve levels of both player consent and compliance as well as employee exploitation, victimisation and abuse.

While socialisation into specific sports realms with specific traditions and cultures is thus seen as a key to understanding sports-related pain and injury, the sociological literature also underscores the primacy of gendered roles and identities in these athletic settings. For instance, much of the literature which has tackled the experience of male athletes in North America and Britain has linked the acceptance of pain and the tolerance of risk to dominant notions of masculinity pervading sport in those societies (cf. Messner 1990, 1992; Sabo 1986; Young 1993). Sport now becomes viewed as a context for the expression and reproduction of hegemonic forms of masculinity where violence, pain and injury are legitimate and, indeed, "make sense." Male athletes unwilling to conform to such standards of "manliness" may become mocked, ostracised or even drop out altogether (Young *et al.* 1994).

In this connection, where the use of force by and injuries for male athletes are concerned, there is a striking parallel between athletes and military personnel — that is, in their ordinary pursuits, they become injured, maimed, or sometimes killed and go on to receive commendations such as awards and special tributes for their dedication and sacrifice. Recognition of this kind serves not just to honour the hurt individual but to rationalise any doubts one might have as to the merits of the act, and consolidate it as admirable and "manly." In this sense, male tolerance of risk and injury becomes reframed as masculinising and meaningful. In turn, this message then pervades sport at many levels and in many forms, and becomes a kind of standard for young and aspiring athletes to try to replicate and model.

When one factors together what the victimisation and the gender literature has to say about professional male athletes, we can begin to grasp how many male athletes feel that they are locked into an occupational trap. While acknowledging that playing at risk and with injuries can lead to permanent physical damage, most athletes are aware that their work setting is largely intolerant to injury. Under further pressure to display a particular brand of tough masculinity and not to complain about being hurt, the professional athlete falls prey to both legally binding professional obligations ("play or don't get paid") *and* to the revered values of his own work culture ("play hurt and show that you can take the pain like a man"). Unsurprisingly, this 'double-jeopardy' is especially true of heavy contact team sports such as "gridiron" football, rugby and ice hockey, where styles of speaking about injury are often telling. For instance, in the ultra-macho culture of North American football, the phrase "you play unless the bone sticks through meat" has become so pervasive that this author found the very same rationales and discourses being used at far lower levels of the game in Western Canadian universities (Young *et al.* 1994).

But what do such masculinist value systems tell us about female participants, if anything? Very recently, there has been a growth in the number of studies of physicality, pain and injury in the lives of female athletes (Charlesworth 2004; Halbert 1997; Johns 1998; Pike 2000; Rail 1992; Snyder 1990; Theberge 1997; Young 1997; Young & White 1995). While this literature has clearly indicated that female athletes may also accept risk-tolerant sports cultures in the pursuit of sports commitment and athletic identity, the degree to which they "over-conform" to the conventions of the so-called sport ethic and cultures of risk relative to their male counterparts is less clear.

An extensive review of the literature on gender differences in sport injury in Young & White (2000: 117–122) shows that there is some persuasive evidence from a number of countries that female athletes in certain sports are injured far less than their male counterparts. This is true, for instance, for some U.S. high school sports, for serious and catastrophic sport injuries in winter sports (such as ice hockey), water sports (such as swimming, diving, boating), and motor sports (such as snow-mobiling) in Canada, as well as for young Finnish athletes in sports such as soccer, volleyball and basketball. It is apparent, then, that gender is *some sort of determinant* of sport injury, though we are uncertain as to the exact nature of this relationship. What is also unclear from the data is why males tend to incur more severe injuries than do females, but the weight of the evidence that exists so far seems to point once again to the way that sport is played, and to the already well-studied link between sports-related aggression and risk-taking in the process of masculinisation.

Undoubtedly, the contextual origins of sports-related pain and injury are neither homogeneous nor limited in type. In addition to value systems that represent the playing and subcultural sides of sport as well as "nature of the game" issues discussed above, pain and injury may be linked to a constellation of factors such as: the positional requirements of a given sport; over-training; playing while injured; improper coaching or tackling/hitting techniques; reckless styles of play; outdated, faulty or dangerous equipment or facilities; the violent conduct or intentions of opponents; irresponsible medical advice; poor or negligent officiating; the taking of expected risks and the taking of risks that cannot reasonably be expected; and, innumerable other factors, all of which are, again, usually avoidable. Indeed, one of the only factors that injured athletes and the groups that assemble and administer them cannot fully control is bad luck, though even this can be anticipated responsibly. For the most part, however, sociologists have been concerned with placing injury in the sport settings that encourage/facilitate/champion pain and injury in the first instance. As such, the literature suggests that the two major sociological causes of sport injury are socialisation into specific sport cultures where risk is widely tolerated, and socialisation into gendered identities strongly linked to these cultures.

2. Injury Exposed

If there is any such thing as an abundance of information on sports injury, it is on the different types, rates and levels of injury in the varied micro-settings of sport. While this information has not always been brought together or made publicly accessible as systematically as it might have been, many leagues, sports organisations, and teams have collected data on injuries in their respective sports. To date, and as already noted, far more of this collation work has been completed by sports administrators, medically-oriented sport scientists, physiologists and psychologists (e.g. Larson *et al.* 1996; Mueller *et al.* 1996; Sports Council 1991) than by sociologists (e.g. McCutcheon *et al.* (1997) is an excellent exception to this rule). While not necessarily sociological or theoretically driven, this is, in my view, important work; we simply need to know basic "extent," "rate" and "nature of" data before proceeding to explanatory and interpretational levels of analysis.

As one small example, it seems reasonable to assert that it would be difficult to find a sport setting more routinely injurious than North American football. Here, we have an injury culture that casts the sport in an unambiguously bad light. In an earlier study, I collated data from diverse disciplinary sources as well as media commentaries to report that "football injuries may include arthritis, concussion, fractures, and, most catastrophically, blindness, paralysis and even death" (Young 1993: 377). Larson *et al.* (1996), Mueller *et al.* (1996) and many others have shown similar evidence of disturbingly severe injury records in football. More recently, risks related to the weight and size requirements, training protocols and other subcultural norms of the game have been brought into sharp relief by the collapse and/or deaths of several top-flight players. This includes the case of 27-year old Minnesota Vikings "All-Pro" lineman Korey Stringer, who died in 2001 from heat stroke following practice on what has been described as one of the hottest days of the year in Makato, Minnesota (*Time*, August 13, 2001: 54).[2]

Using such rate and extent data as are available, however varied in their derivation, nature and scope, it now becomes possible to probe such sports to examine factors such as the traditions, common practices and subcultural value systems — that is, dimensions of more interest to sociologists. The fact of the matter is that rate and extent data *are* available for most sports, including non-contact and non-team sports. It seems reasonable to argue that better use of them could be made by sociologists, at least as a basis for more sophisticated explanatory work.

3. Anticipating, Living with and Recovering from Injury

Given arguments made in the Preface and in the preceding section, it is clear that learning to live with pain and injury is simply a requirement of many sports. The message is plain enough — pain and injury "come with the territory" as it were; it is expected in the very fabric of almost all sport settings. Once again, it is almost impossible to play sport without experiencing pain; every athlete has a story to tell about injury.

Perhaps representing the broadest strand of sociological research on pain and injury so far available, a number of interpretive qualitative studies undertaken on a range of sports participants and from a range of theoretical points of view have uncovered the varied ways in which risk, pain and injury are directly experienced. This growing body of work includes studies of pain "lived" by participants in a wide spectrum of sports, such as rowers (Pike 2000), cyclists (Albert 1999), wrestlers (Curry 1993), bodybuilders (E. Smith, 1989), runners (Ewald & Jiobu 1985), wreck divers (Hunt 1996), rugby players (Howe 2001; Malcolm & Sheard 2002), and rodeo participants and football players (Frey *et al.* 1997), as well as studies of injury experiences from miscellaneous clusters of sports (Charlesworth 2004; Young 1997; Young & White 1995).

In a study of the role that physicality plays in the construction of masculinity and men's health, and using data from Canadian university athletes (see Figure 2), Young *et al.* (1994) discovered that male athletes use a range of interpretive strategies to make sense of pain which amount to what Mills (1959) might call "vocabularies of motive" and Sykes and Matza might call "techniques of

---

[2] According to *Newsweek* magazine, Stringer's death followed 19 other deaths of high school and college football players in the USA since 1995 (August 13, 2001: 53).

1. Hidden Pain	2. Disrespected Pain
Participants go out of their way to ignore pain, to pretend it is not there:	An attitude of irreverence to 'everyday pain'. Differentiate pain from injury:
"I came straight down on my shoulders and . . . I heard a pop. A very, very audible pop and it hurt like hell. And I thought, well, it might only hurt when I land so I'll give it another whirl . . . I got up and I jumped again and I actually jumped another six or so times and I recall afterwards basically being doubled over and not being able to do anything because it didn't hurt until I hit the mat. . . I generally would go through a real state of denial" (Track and field athlete)	*"Last year I ripped my 'trap' and separated my shoulder . . . Every now and again it flares up and then I take a bunch of Tylenols and forget about that pain. That's probably the most pain I have. But is that injury? (Football player)*
"Then, I responded the same way that I responded with the present injury because I would just try to hide it" (Hockey player)	*"We have this term in football. People refer to it as a difference between Pain and Injury. If you can walk or you can run to any degree, you know, they look at your injury in terms of percentages . . . So, you tend to take a couple of pain killers and tape her up nice and tight and ice before you play, and away you go" (Football player)*
3. Unwelcomed Pain	**4. Depersonalized Pain**
Pain is poorly received by teammates, coaches, and others. Displaying pain is described as a 'demoralizer' and may be punished:	A way of thinking and speaking about injury that emphasizes that it is the body not the self that has given out:
"There's always that pressure because . . . you don't want to tell your quarterback you're injured because he'll have reservations about getting you the ball . . . Plus it puts more pressure on him because he's got more on his mind. It's a matter of just don't tell anybody else about yourself and just do your job, basically" (Football player)	*"It's like it's not a part of you. Like it's a totally different portion or something" (Soccer player)*
With my femur . . . all I felt was my left leg wrapping around my right leg. Then I fell down. I tried not to show pain and lay there on the ice. I was trying to get up and I remember just falling back down again. And then I remember the coach coming up and trying to help me up and he said "Come on you can get up." "You're tough," or whatever, but there was no way. I remember my Dad even giving me shit" (Hockey player)	*"As a result of these ways of knowing injury, body damage itself is often articulated through the use of impersonal and techno-rational discourse. Legs become 'iced', knees 'scoped', ankles 'strapped', aches and pains 'killed', and mechanical glitches (pulls, strains, tears, breaks) simply 'fixed', often artificially. Remarkably, J____ noted that the pain from his ruptured spleen was "just like squeezing an orange," except rather than juice "a little bit of blood came out." Referring to a skiing accident which resulted in him "actually living on half a kidney . . . one kidney was totally ripped open and the other was lacerated," G____ described his injury as "the equivalent of dropping two eggs on the floor — one cracked one smashed""* *(Young et al., 1994: 186).*

Figure 2:   Athlete strategies for making sense of pain. *Source:* Adapted from Young *et al.* (1994: 182–186).

neutralization" (1989). These include: going out of one's way to ignore pain (1. *Hidden Pain*); adopting an attitude of irreverence to it and prioritising certain kinds of pain over others (2. *Disrespected Pain*); understanding that it may be poorly received by team-mates, coaches and others and that acknowledging it may lead to sanctions or Garfinkel-esque "degradation ceremonies" (1967) (3. *Unwelcomed Pain*); and, adopting a particular way of thinking and speaking about pain that allows one's sense on invulnerability to persist (4. *Depersonalized Pain*). Brief examples of these four key strategies, all of which centre on suppressing affect and rationalising pain, are highlighted in Figure 2. Beyond these examples, the same study further uncovered common techniques used by athletes to "reframe" injury in positive ways in order to allow them to return to play, even while at risk of prolonging, or even exacerbating, pain and suffering.

Similar investigations into the meanings and narratives of embodied pain in diverse sport settings have been offered by Kotarba (1983), Theberge (1997), Thomas & Rintala (1989), Snyder (1990), Roderick *et al.* (2000), Pike (2000) and Charlesworth (2004), among others. Importantly, such work has started to uncover close parallels in the ways in which male and female athletes understand pain and injury, in the ways they rationalise it, and use its symptoms and its effects to judge character and role in sports groups (cf. Charlesworth 2004; Pike 2000; Young 1997; Young & White 1995). Indeed, so strikingly similar have been the results of their interview-based studies conducted with Canadian male and female athletes, that Young and White have contended that:

> Both female and male discourses of sport were replete with the language of conquest (performance orientations and achievement principles). Female athletes were as willing as men to expose themselves to physical risk, and women *and* men were relatively unreflexive on matters such as being pressured to perform aggressively [and] to play with injury (pp. 55–56).

While their data lead Young and White (1995) to argue that "If there is a difference between the way male and female athletes in our projects appear to understand pain and injury, it is only a matter of degree" (p. 51), they also cautiously recommend more research on the ways that female athletes appear to be colonising traditionally male-exclusive spaces in sport before conclusions regarding the implications of that colonisation, including approaches to pain and injury within it, can confidently be made. It certainly seems likely that as female sport expands, and as sport opportunity for girls and women increases, female experiences of sport injury will also amplify. Understanding the full ramifications of these experiences will require more consistent research efforts by sociologists of sport.

Finally, the interpretive sociological literature on anticipating and living with pain and recovering from injury features a growing collection of biographical and "self-reflexive" studies. Apparently compelled by Millsian (1959) notions of the importance of biography in sociological ventures, and by Frank's claim that "the beginning of theorizing about the body . . . lies in our own embodiment as theorists" (1996: 57), several sport researchers have explained pain in their own athletic lives using techniques of "narrative reconstruction" (Frank 1991). These studies include Sparkes' (1996, 1999) fascinating "auto-ethnographical" explorations of encounters with pain and body "disruptions," Collinson's (2003) precisely recorded "temporal" account of the frustrations of both running-related injuries and often unreliable and unsympathetic medical practitioners, and Charlesworth's (2004) thorough examination of the physical and emotional dimensions of female athlete pain interpreted from the perspective of an author familiar with chronic illness.

4. Injury Costs

Defined economically, the costs of sports injury are startling. Injury represents a massive imposition for national, regional and local governments, as well as sports and health organizations every year in many countries around the world.

Collating the existing research (very little of which is sociological) on health care costs from a number of national contexts, Young & White (2000) found the literature to be dated but nevertheless telling. Their review cites evidence that:

> In the United Kingdom . . . 7% of sports injuries resulted in participants taking time off work, resulting in a total of 11.5 million working days lost annually in England and Wales, at a cost of 575 million pounds in production value . . . In Denmark . . . the annual cost of treating "acute sports injuries" was 2.3 million pounds. A Swiss study . . . estimated that the total direct and indirect costs of sport accidents in 1976 [was] 400 million pounds . . . [and] From New Zealand . . . [it was] reported that 15% of the treatments received at the Dunedin Hospital Emergency Department were for sports injuries and that sport accounted for 17% of all injuries compensated by the Accident Compensation Corporation (p. 122).

A 1990 report on sports injuries to the Australian National Better Health Program noted that the medical treatment of sport injury in Australia cost an estimated $330–$400 million in 1987–1988, and a further $400 million lost through worker absenteeism (Centre for Health Promotion and Research 1990). Kirkby (1995) reports that sport injuries cost Germany more than $US 2500 million per year, and that, in the USA, "the yearly cost to the economy of roller skating accidents alone was [in 1983] $100 million" (p. 456). Similarly astounding figures can be provided for most countries where sports participation is common. In Western societies, at least, the proliferation of sports injuries has given rise to enormously successful treatment industries such as sports medicine, sports massage, physiotherapy, and chiropractic medicine, whose success — ironically — depends on there being a cost to heal sport injury in the first place.

In addition to the toll that injury takes on states and governments, the financial cost of injuries is also a critical factor in the everyday business of professional sport where injury "losses" can be huge. A recent illustration comes from England, where player injuries — that is to say, the number of athletes unavailable to train and play each week due to injury — have been reported to cost English soccer clubs £40 million every year (*The Independent*, January 26, 2001: 28). Clearly, this example underscores the capitalist dimensions of elite sport, where athlete labour is but one aspect of any given club's business plan (Young 1993).

Needless to say, the "costs" associated with sport injury go well beyond matters of finance. As Mueller *et al.* (1996: 99) have remarked with respect to catastrophic sport injury in young athletes, "injury is devastating not only to the injured athlete, but also the athlete's family, school and community." While it may be true that sociologists have not played a central role in examining the economic impact of injury, there is certainly work available on the human costs. This work comes in a variety of forms, which includes examinations of how injuries may leave athletes with a compromised or destroyed sense of self-worth, or even suicidal (Charlesworth 2004; Pike 2000; Young *et al.* 1994). Touching on each of these varied interpretations of the phenomena, Philip White's contribution to this volume (see Chapter 17) adds significantly to what we know about the assorted "costs" of injury.

5. Injury as Spectacle

Though most people interested in sport, such as the readers of this book, will know from first hand experience what sports-related pain and injury *feel like* in a sensory or tactile way, it is nevertheless the case that sports injury reaches most people indirectly as a set of images transmitted by the mass media. In many ways, the contemporary emphasis placed on competition and winning at all costs and the omnipresence of the sports media means that professional and elite sport have become mediated, and often celebrated, worlds of hurt and disability. The roaming television lens captures and replays the writhing athletic body in "super slo-mo," while commentators and well-known media personalities respond using discourses of approval and rationalisation (Gillett *et al.* 1996; Young 1991). Meanwhile, the carefully selected and edited tabloid photograph freezes the injurious moment, as humorous and "punny" captions belie the actual agony behind the contact in focus. Combined, visual and verbal media messages serve to marginalise pain, and to re-present the now commodified sports moment not as hurt per se, but as a routine (Morse (1983) argues artistic and even sensual) sign of athletic commitment. In the process, injured athletes become lionised as heroes exposing themselves to danger, and showing willingness, in the vernacular of North American televised football and ice hockey, to "pay the price" (Nixon 1993; Young 1990, 1991). Numerous examples could be provided, but (from a different sport and with a female athlete) perhaps one of the most recognisable is the case of American gymnast Kerri Strugg who completed a vault at the 1996 Olympic Games with two freshly torn ankle ligaments and became internationally lauded for being "courageous" and "heroic" (*Sports Illustrated*, August 5, 1996: 58–65).

A further aspect of sport injury as spectacle that has so far received scant sociological attention may be found in sport advertising. Here, too, pain and injury are both trivialised and made to appear normal and unthreatening. Complementing wider ideologies throughout North American sport (witness, for example, sport stadia known to local fans as the "House of Pain," or the seemingly ubiquitous attitude/rationale "No Pain, No Gain" in gyms across the continent), the sport magazine industry is replete with examples of well-known sports companies using snappy (but often literally untrue) catch-phrases to sell their products: "Own the Pain and you will Own the Game" (Adidas); "Pain is Weakness Leaving the Body" (Adidas); "Rubber, Chains and Pain. You'll Love It!" (Carrera). Needless to say, these mediated codes only add to an already pervasive culture of risk in sport.

Relatively few sociologists have looked at mediated pain and injury. One of the most interesting, if modest, studies can be found in Nixon (1993) who conducted research on what he calls the "mediated cultural influences of playing hurt," and who similarly concludes that the sports media frequently "convey the messages of the culture of risk" (p. 190). This includes, for him, the way in which these messages encourage a "kind of self-abusive addiction" (p. 189) in athletes. However, Nixon goes on to comment thoughtfully about the fact that media messages do not become wholly or uncritically absorbed into social practice by "unthinking" players. He writes: "we should not conclude . . . that athletes are so effectively socialized or strongly influenced that they cannot see behind the messages and pressures to play with pain and injuries or that they cannot make their own decisions about these matters" (p. 188). In these respects, Nixon's arguments regarding the power and influence of the culture of risk he describes so convincingly in his numerous other studies parallel the work of others, such as Young's (1993) discussion of the consent/manipulation paradox in some professional sport settings, and Stebbins' (1987) study of Canadian football players, both of which show that athletes may be quite aware of their own subjugation and exploitation at the hands of ownership as well as the media industry.

In brief, the media play an active and participatory role in popular impressions of pain and injury in sport. As Young & Smith (1988/1989) wrote about related codes of injury-producing violence: "The media frequently convey the idea that violence is accepted, even desirable behaviour and ... violence doers are to be admired." The relationship between the media and pain and injury in sport may be examined in a number of ways as suggested here, but more research would help us better understand this relationship.

6. Injury, Health and Public Policy

While sport is often assumed to be intertwined with health, it is quite clear from the literature, then, that participation in many sports at many levels is accompanied by common and often serious health risks. Working from this position, and acknowledging that it is not fair, realistic or helpful to generalise about all sports in this connection, it seems reasonable on the basis of what we know so far to assert that more could be done to better understand the origins of risk, and make particular sports safer in particular ways. As such, research on the policy implications of risk, pain and injury for individual and community health is very much needed; so far, this work is in short supply, at least as it applies to sociology.

Predictably, the disruption caused by pain and injury in sport to individuals and those around them has prompted a considerable literature on the prevention of sports injuries. As Kirkby (1995: 469) has written:

> Whether it is viewed from the perspective of the financial cost of sport injuries to society, the personal and social distress and disruption caused by sport injuries at all levels of competition, or their effects on domestic and international success in elite sport, there is no doubting the importance of the prevention of sport injuries and rehabilitation to sport.

Much of this prevention work has been amassed by psychologists of sport who have focussed on "coping and social support" issues (Kirkby 1995: 468). This sort of work is important enough, though critics of this approach might raise questions regarding how sport and its participants can be made safer, and unreasonable risks removed, by making fundamental changes in the structure and nature of sport itself. Given the cultural resonance of sport in so many societies, this, it seems, is hard to do — witness, for instance, calls to ban boxing or to make headgear mandatory, to decrease the speed car racers drive at and to make their vehicles more robust, to reduce eye and facial injuries in ice hockey by requiring visors, and the like. Recommendations such as these have all been met with considerable opposition from groups who quite clearly define risk differently or, just as likely, simply revere risk.

It is true, however, that player safety and individual/public health is a matter on the radar screens of many sport organisations and bodies. These "matters" have been studied by social scientists, including sociologists: Hawkins & Fuller (1998) have studied the health regulatory practices of soccer clubs in England and Wales using a public health/socio-legal perspective; Waddington (2000) has examined the health implications of a sportsworld immersed in drug use and cheating; Fuller (1995) has looked at health and safety legislation for a cluster of professional sports in Britain; and, Young (1993) has explored the need for regulatory laws to reduce the number of "white collar crimes" he argues take place in many of the self-policing sport bodies of North America.

Of course, this brief selection of sources and the public health interests they represent has been complemented by national survey work conducted by states and governments in a number of countries, both with adult and child participants, as well as by the controlling bodies of individual sports (see Chapters 16 and 17). However, since so many sport cultures define sport and athletic success in terms of pushing the frontiers of human performance, which renders risk inevitable, it remains to be seen how effective such work might be. When one adds the drive toward corporate profit in the administration of many of our most popular sports, and the health risks we know that this implies, it is difficult to remain optimistic about the interventions well-meaning policy-makers might have on dominant sports models.

7. Punishing Injury: Legal Reactions

While the volume of case law on prosecuted sports violence/sports injury cases is enormous (it is often difficult to distinguish between the two since injuries that become litigated are often the outcomes of violent play), the amount of sociological attention paid to legal reactions is still relatively small. It is also difficult to generalise about sport injury litigation because the legal process can be extremely culture-specific, but in most jurisdictions, it seems clear that the courts have preferred to avoid litigating sport injury, principally because the nature of many athletic activities requires risk and force used, directly or indirectly, against another person, and a certain amount of physical harm being incurred. However, the research that has been conducted has indicated that sport injury cases have been prosecuted for some time in several countries, though not consistently, and not without contradiction.

Injurious cases resulting in charges of, for example, assault formally being laid have often been returned by court justices to sports leagues and organisations to deal with "in-house" where, so the argument goes, there is a nuanced familiarity with the "wrongness" of the act in question. This has not normally included acts which are so obviously outside the rules of the given sport and the law of the land that they have required criminal intervention from the outset, but even these sorts of cases have not been dealt with by the courts easily or consistently (Young & Wamsley 1996). Complicating all such cases is the issue of consent. In the make-up of many sports, especially team contact sports, athletes express or imply a degree of consent to the use of force done by and against them. Underlying notions of voluntary assumption of risk have led to innumerable legal struggles in violence/injury cases.

Britain, America and Canada lead the sociological research on how sport injury has been dealt with and punished legally. For example, in Britain, anyone interested in examining the relationship between sports and law might begin with Grayson (1988), although the more comprehensive and recent compendium by Gardiner *et al.* (1998) is far more relevant for our purposes. Good, but early and now outdated, socio-legal definitional work on how sense is made of various violent/injurious acts may be found in Smith (1983), and in an excellent general review of sports law in Barnes (1988). Horrow (1980, 1982) and Hechter (1976/1977) offer incisive examinations of the role of the criminal law in sport violence/sport injury cases, and Young (1993) reviews the ways that the North American courts have dealt with various grievances related to sport injury, as well as the sorts of legal defenses that have served to protect injurious athletes over the years. In Canada, most of the work that has been done on criminalised sports cases has examined the case of ice hockey. Watson & MacLellan (1986), Reasons (1992) and Young & Wamsley (1996) are all cases in point.

As Chapter 18 indicates, legal intervention into sport violence/sport injury cases has not been linear, uncontested or entirely successful. There appears to be some Trans-Atlantic evidence that civil and criminal charges against athletes causing injury to opponents are on the rise but, once again, more systematic research from a number of sports jurisdictions is required.

8. Injury Under-Exposed

That some of the central dimensions of "pain zones" have been "exposed" and that our knowledge and understanding of sports-related pain and injury are growing should not lead us to think that we know all there is to know; far from it. On the overall trajectory of understanding the social dimensions of sports-related pain and injury, we are just beginning. Certain aspects of injury that are of clear significance both to sociology and to society have been "under-exposed," and our knowledge of these factors remains vague.

The contributions to this volume in general go some way to addressing such lacunae. However, to be realistic about extant knowledge, we need to juxtapose the gains sociologists of sport have made on the subject of late against remaining gaps in knowledge. Addressing these gaps would most certainly improve the status of that knowledge. The following points are salient, but certainly not exhaustive, in this connection:

(i)   most pain and injury studies have dealt with the experiences of male athletes and, despite gradual shifts in the gender focus of injury work, have neglected or under-emphasised those of females;

(ii) despite the fact that sports injury is clearly not restricted to adult participation, the physically and emotionally painful ramifications of injury for young and child athletes, and the extent to which sport might be abusive to children's bodies, has been almost entirely ignored (Donnelly 2003);

(iii) the bulk of our knowledge of sports-related injury and pain derives from surveys and other quantitative techniques conducted in the other sports sciences and by the sport industry itself which, while again useful in its own way, does not normally illuminate key matters such as how pain and injury are lived, reflected upon or resolved at various levels;

(iv) we still have relatively little knowledge of how pain and injury are responded to by the media, though (more extensive) evidence from the sports violence literature strongly suggests that the media at times choreograph and exploit sports injury in the pursuit of sales and profit;

(v)   with only a few exceptions, much of the research is limited to injured elite participants (Brock & Kleiber 1994; Howe 2001; Young & White 1995), despite the fact that the majority of athletes who play or who have been injured are not and never will be involved at the highest levels of their sport;

(vi) despite much conjecture, the links between injury and practices known to be common in certain sports such as eating disorders (Ryan 1996) and steroid use (Courson 1991) remain unclear;

(vii) we have some knowledge about the way sport injury disrupts lives and interferes with notions of self-concept in a temporary sense, but less knowledge about the long-term effects of injury for individual physical and mental health and well-being. This has only been touched on by a small handful of sociologists (cf. Messner 1990; Roderick *et al.* 2000);[3]

(viii) despite enormous potential given the fundamentally physical, social and emotional nature of the problem, sociologists seem reluctant to approach their work in an interdisciplinary way and to take advantage of the considerable and very developed clinical literatures in the "harder" sports science disciplines such as biomechanics, physiology as well as psychology;

(ix) and, finally, despite definitional efforts in the mainstream (Kotarba 1983; Morris 1991) and some modest efforts in the sociology of sport literature to have athletes differentiate between pain and injury using their own terms and categories (e.g. Young *et al.* 1994), definitional work on what constitutes "pain" and "injury" remains to be undertaken with the same sort of rigour with which, for instance, Lyng (1990) has defined risky "edgework,"[4] as at least two philosophers of sport have correctly noted (McNamee 2004; Parry 2004).

As fresh and welcome as the growing body of sociological work on sports-related pain and injury is, it is equally clear that gaps in knowledge such as these exist and that far more research is needed.

Summary

Injury in sport is so ubiquitous that it has been described, with some justification in my view, as an "unthwarted epidemic" (Vinger & Hoerner 1981). Where its study is concerned, sociologists of sport have made impressive and encouraging advances, despite coming to the area relatively late. These advances have taken

---

[3] In this respect, sociologists could benefit from a more thoughtful use of media or biographical accounts of the long-term injury problems encountered by former athletes. Three recent cases from English soccer stand out. First, former Charlton Athletic player Garry Nelson has noted that "Injuries are a player's way of life" (1996: 246); second, former "hardman" and captain of Liverpool Football Club, Tommy Smith, now in his 50s, is 40% disabled by osteoarthritis and lives with constant pain (*The Independent*, October 3, 2000: 11); and third, a 2002 inquest into the death of former West Bromwich Albion striker Jeff Astle disclosed that Astle, known in his playing years as one of the hardest headers of the ball in the game, died from illnesses brought on by his repeated heading of heavy leather-encased soccer balls. Interestingly, the coroner in the case recorded a verdict of "death by industrial disease" (*The Guardian*, November 12, 2002: 5).

[4] The concept of "edgework" is used by Lyng (1990) to refer to the experience of participants in dangerous and high-risk activities.

us beyond the uncritical and rather limiting explanatory borders of the bulk of the early epidemiological work on the subject. It is clear from what we know so far that sport can lead to injurious outcomes not only due to the nature of athletic activity per se, but also because of the way that sport activity is planned, organised, managed and practised. This volume contains hundreds of illustrated cases of sport injury; a considerable number of them will have as much to do with the way sport is played and administered (i.e. with what is expected of athletes to succeed, and what, concomitantly, athletes are taught to expect of themselves) as the nature of the game itself. More than any other, it is this fact that renders a *sociology* of "pain cultures," "pain zones" and "pain parameters" necessary.

References

Adams, S., Adrian, M., & M. Bayless (Eds) (1987). *Catastrophic injuries in sport: Avoidance strategies*. Indianapolis: Benchmark.

Albert, E. (1999). Dealing with danger: The normalization of risk in cycling. *International Review for the Sociology of Sport, 34*(2), 157–171.

Barnes, J. (1988). *Sports and the law in Canada*. Toronto: Butterworths.

Booth, D. (1996). Athletes with disabilities. In: M. Harries, C. Williams, W. Stanish, & L. Micheli (Eds), *Oxford textbook of sports medicine* (pp. 634–645). New York: Oxford University Press.

Brock, S. C., & Kleiber, D. A. (1994). Narrative in medicine: The stories of elite college athletes' career-ending injuries. *Qualitative Health Research, 4*, 411–430.

Caine, D. J., Caine, C. G., & Lindner, K. J. (Eds) (1996). *Epidemiology of sports injuries*. Champaign, IL: Human Kinetics.

Centre for Health Promotion and Research (1990). *Sports injuries in Australia: Causes, costs, and prevention*. A Report to the National Better Health Program. Sydney: National Better Health Program.

Charlesworth, H. (2004). *Sports-related injury, risk, and pain: The experiences of English female university athletes*. Unpublished Doctoral Dissertation, Loughborough University, UK.

Collinson, J. A. (2003). Running into injury: Distance running and temporality. *Sociology of Sport Journal, 20*(4), 331–351.

Courson, S. (1991). *False glory*. Stamford, CT: Longmeadow.

Curry, T. (1993). A little pain never hurt anyone: Athletic career socialization and the normalization of sports injury. *Symbolic Interaction, 16*, 273–290.

Curry, T., & Strauss, R. (1994). A little pain never hurt anybody: A photo-essay on the normalization of sport injuries. *Sociology of Sport Journal, 11*, 195–208.

Donnelly, P. (2003). Marching out of step: Sport, social order and the case of child labour. Keynote Address, Second World Congress of Sociology of Sport, Cologne, Germany, June 18–21.

Donnelly, P., & Young, K. (1988). The construction and confirmation of identity in sport subcultures. *Sociology of Sport Journal, 5,* 223–240.

Ewald, K., & Jiobu, R. M. (1985). Explaining positive deviance: Becker's model and the case of runners and bodybuilders. *Sociology of Sport Journal, 2,* 144–156.

Featherstone, M., Hepworth, M., & Turner, B. S. (Eds) (1991). *The body: Social processes and cultural theory.* London: Sage.

Frank, A. (1991). For a sociology of the body: An analytic review. In: M. Featherstone, M. Hepworth, & B. S. Turner (Eds), *The body: Social processes and cultural theory* (pp. 36–102). London: Sage.

Frank, A. (1996). Reconciliatory alchemy: Bodies, narratives, and power. *Body and Society, 2*(3), 53–71.

Freund, P. E. S. (1991). *Health, illness, and the social body: A critical sociology.* London: Prentice-Hall.

Frey, J. (1991). Social risk and the meaning of sport. *Sociology of Sport Journal, 8,* 136–145.

Frey, J., Preston, F. W., & Bernhard, B. (1997). Risk and injury: A comparison of football and rodeo subcultures. Paper presented at the North American Society for the Sociology of Sport, Toronto, November 5–8.

Fuller, C. (1995). Implications of health and safety legislation for the professional sportsperson. *British Journal of Sports Medicine, 29,* 5–9.

Gardiner, S., Felix, A., James, M., Welch, R., & O'Leary, J. (1998). *Sports law.* London: Cavendish.

Garfinkel, H. (1967). Conditions of successful degradation ceremonies. In: J. Manis, & B. Meltzer (Eds), *Symbolic interaction: A reader in social psychology* (pp. 205–213). Boston, MA: Allyn & Bacon.

Gillett, J., White, P., & Young, K. (1996). 'The prime minister of saturday night': Don Cherry, the CBC, and the cultural production of intolerance. In: H. Holmes, & D. Taras (Eds), *Seeing ourselves in Canada: Media, power, and policy* (pp. 59–72). Toronto: Harcourt Brace.

Grayson, E. (1988). *Sport and the law.* London: Butterworths.

Halbert, C. (1997). Tough enough and woman enough: Stereotypes, discrimination, and impression management among women professional boxers. *Journal of Sport and Social Issues, 21*(1), 7–37.

Harries, M., Williams, C., Stanish, W., & Micheli, L. (Eds) (1996). *Oxford textbook of sports medicine.* New York: Oxford University Press.

Hawkins, R. D., & Fuller, C. W. (1998). A preliminary assessment of professional footballers' awareness of injury prevention strategies. *British Journal of Sports Medicine, 32,* 140–143.

Hechter, W. (1976/1977). Criminal law and violence in sports. *Criminal Law Quarterly, 19,* 425–453.

Holmes, D., & Frey, J. (1990). The kind of people who skydive. *Parachutist,* February, 28–32.

Horrow, R. (1980). *Sports violence: The interaction between private lawmaking and the criminal law.* Arlington, VA: Carrollton Press.

Horrow, R. (1982). Violence in professional sport: Is it part of the game? *Journal of Legislation*, *9*(1), 1–15.

Howe, P. D. (2001). An ethnography of pain and injury in professional Rugby Union: The case of Pontypridd RFC. *International Review for the Sociology of Sport*, *36*, 289–303.

Hughes, R., & Coakley, J. (1991). Positive deviance among athletes: The implications of overconformity to the sport ethic. *Sociology of Sport Journal*, *8*(4), 307–325.

Hume, P., & Marshall, S. (1994). Sports injuries in New Zealand: Exploratory analyses. *New Zealand Journal of Sports Medicine*, *22*, 18–22.

Hunt, J. (1996). Diving the wreck: Risk and injury in the sport of scuba diving. *Psychoanalytic Quarterly*, *LXV*, 591–621.

Hyndman, J. (1996). The growing athlete. In: M. Harries, C. Williams, W. Stanish, & L. Micheli (Eds), *Oxford textbook of sports medicine* (pp. 620–633). New York: Oxford University Press.

Johns, D. (1998). Fasting and feasting: Paradoxes of the sport ethic. *Sociology of Sport Journal*, *15*(1), 41–63.

Kirkby, R. (1995). Psychological factors in sport injuries. In: T. Morris, & J. Summers (Eds), *Sport psychology: Theory, applications and issues* (pp. 456–473). New York: Wiley.

Kotarba, J. A. (1983). *Chronic pain: Its social dimensions*. Beverly Hills, CA: Sage.

Larson, M., Pearl, A. J., Jaffet, R., & Rudowsky, A. (1996). Soccer. In: D. J. Caine, C. G. Caine, & K. J. Lindner (Eds), *Epidemiology of sports injuries* (pp. 387–398). Champaign, IL: Human Kinetics.

Lupton, D. (1995). *The imperative of health: Public health and the regulated body*. London: Sage.

Lyng, S. (1990). Edgework: A social psychological analysis of voluntary risk taking. *American Journal of Sociology*, *95*(4), 851–886.

Malcolm, D., & Sheard, K. (2002). "Pain in the assets": The effects of commercialization and professionalization on the management of injury in English Rugby Union. *Sociology of Sport Journal*, *19*, 149–169.

McCutcheon, T., Curtis, J., & White, P. (1997). The socioeconomic distribution of sport injuries: Multivariate analyses using Canadian national data. *Sociology of Sport Journal*, *14*, 57–72.

McNamee, M. (2004). Pain and trust in sport. Paper presented at workshop on 'Pain and Injury in Sport: Social and Ethical Perspectives.' Oslo, February 12–13.

Menard, D. (1996). The ageing athlete. In: M. Harries, C. Williams, W. Stanish, & L. Micheli (Eds), *Oxford textbook of sports medicine* (pp. 596–619). New York: Oxford University Press.

Messner, M. (1990). When bodies are weapons: Masculinity and violence in sport. *International Review for the Sociology of Sport*, *25*(3), 203–219.

Messner, M. (1992). *Power at play: Sports and the problem of masculinity*. Boston, MA: Beacon.

Mills, C. W. (1959). *The sociological imagination*. New York: Oxford University Press.

Morris, D. B. (1991). *The culture of pain*. Los Angeles: University of California Press.

Morse, M. (1983). Sport on television: Replay and display. In: E. A. Kaplan (Ed.), *Regarding television: Critical approaches* (pp. 44–67). Los Angeles: American Film Institute.

Mueller, F., Cantu, R., & Van Camp, S. (1996). *Catastrophic injuries in high school and college sports.* Champaign, IL: Human Kinetics.

Nelson, G. (1996). *Left foot forward: A year in the life of a journeyman footballer.* London: Headline.

Nixon, H. (1992). A social network analysis of influences on athletes to play with pain and injury. *Journal of Sport and Social Issues, 16*(2), 127–135.

Nixon, H. (1993). Accepting the risks of pain and injury in sport: Mediated cultural influences on playing hurt. *Sociology of Sport Journal, 10,* 183–196.

Nixon, H. L. (1994a). Coaches' views of risk, pain, and injury in sport with special reference to gender differences. *Sociology of Sport Journal, 11,* 79–87.

Nixon, H. L. (1994b). Social pressure, social support, and help seeking for pain and injuries in college sports networks. *Journal of Sport and Social Issues, 13,* 340–355.

Nixon, H. L. (1996). The relationship of friendship networks, sports experiences, and gender to expressed pain thresholds. *Sociology of Sport Journal, 13,* 78–87.

Parry, J. (2004). Infliction of pain in sport — Ethical perspectives. Paper presented at workshop on 'Pain and Injury in Sport: Social and Ethical Perspectives.' Oslo, February 12–13.

Pike, E. (2000). *Illness, injury and sporting identity: A case study of women's rowing.* Unpublished Doctoral Dissertation, Loughborough University, UK.

Rail, G. (1992). Physical contact in women's basketball: A phenomenological construction and contextualization. *International Review for the Sociology of Sport, 27*(1), 1–27.

Reasons, C. (1992). *The criminal law and sports violence: Hockey crimes.* Unpublished manuscipt, University of British Columbia, Vancouver.

Roderick, M., Waddington, I., & Parker, G. (2000). Playing hurt: Managing injuries in English professional football. *International Review for the Sociology of Sport, 35*(2), 165–180.

Ryan, J. (1996). *Little girls in pretty boxes: The making and breaking of elite gymnasts and figure skaters.* New York: Doubleday.

Sabo, D. (1986). Pigskin, patriarchy and pain. *Changing Men: Issues in Gender, Sex, and Politics, 16*(Summer), 24–25.

Sabo, D. (1994). The body politics of sports injury: Culture, power, and the pain principle. Paper presented at the National Athletic Trainers Association, Dallas, TX, Nov. 6.

Safai, P. (2001). *Healing the body in the 'culture of risk,' pain, and injury: Negotiations between clinicians and injured athletes in Canada's competitive intercollegiate sport.* Unpublished MA Thesis, University of Toronto.

Shilling, C. (1993). *The body and social theory.* London: Sage.

Smith, E. (1989). *Not just pumping iron: On the psychology of lifting weights.* Springfield, IL: Charles C. Thomas.

Smith, M. (1983). *Violence and sport.* Toronto: Butterworths.

Smith, M. (1987). Violence in Canadian amateur sport: A review of literature. *Report for the Commission for Fair Play.* Ottawa, ON: Government of Canada.

Smith, M. (1991). Violence and injuries in ice hockey. *Clinical Journal of Sports Medicine, 1,* 104–109.

Snyder, E. (1990). Emotion and sport: A case study of collegiate women gymnasts. *Sociology of Sport Journal, 7*(3), 254–270.

Sorensen, C., & Sonne-holm, S. (1980). Social costs of sport injuries. *British Journal of Sports Medicine, 14,* 24–25.

Sparkes, A. C. (1996). The fatal flaw: A narrative of the fragile body-self. *Qualitative Inquiry, 2,* 463–494.

Sparkes, A. C. (1999). Exploring body narratives. *Sport, Education, and Society, 4,* 17–30.

Sports Council (1991). *Injuries in sport and exercise.* London: Sports Council.

Stebbins, R. A. (1987). *Canadian football: The view from the helmet.* London, ON: Centre for Social and Humanistic Studies of the University of Western Ontario.

Sykes, G., & Matza, D. (1989). Techniques of neutralization: A theory of delinquency. In: D. Kelly (Ed.), *Deviant behaviour: A text-reader in the sociology of deviance* (pp. 104–111). New York: St. Martin's Press.

Theberge, N. (1997). "It's part of the game": Physicality and the production of gender in women's hockey. *Gender and Society, 11,* 69–87.

Thomas, C. E., & Rintala, J. (1989). Injury as alienation in sport. *Journal of the Philosophy of Sport, XVI,* 44–58.

Vinger, P. F., & Hoerner, E. F. (1981). *Sports injuries: The unthwarted epidemic.* Littleton, MA: PSG Publishing Company.

Waddington, I. (2000). *Sport, health, and drugs: A critical sociological perspective.* London: Routledge.

Walk, S. (1997). Peers in pain: The experiences of student athlete trainers. *Sociology of Sport Journal, 14,* 22–56.

Watson, R. C., & MacLellan, J. C. (1986). Smiting to spitting: 80 years of ice hockey in the Canadian courts. *Canadian Journal of History of Sport, 17*(2), 10–27.

Young, K. (1990). Treatment of sports violence by the Canadian mass media. *Report to Sport Canada's Applied Sport Research Program,* Government of Canada.

Young, K. (1991). Writers, rimmers, and slotters: Privileging violence in the construction of the sports page. Paper presented at the North American Society for the Sociology of Sport, Milwaukee, Wisconsin, November 6–9.

Young, K. (1993). Violence, risk, and liability in male sports culture. *Sociology of Sport Journal, 10*(4), 373–396.

Young, K. (1997). Women, sport, and physicality: Preliminary findings from a Canadian study. *International Review for the Sociology of Sport, 32*(3), 297–305.

Young, K., & Smith, M. (1988/1989). Mass media treatment of violence in sports and its effects. *Current Psychology: Research and Reviews, 7,* 298–312.

Young, K., & Wamsley, K. (1996). State complicity in sports assault and the gender order in twentieth century Canada: Preliminary observations. *Avante, 2*(2), 51–69.

Young, K., & White, P. (1995). Sport, physical danger, and injury: The experiences of elite women athletes. *Journal of Sport and Social Issues, 19*(1), 45–61.

Young, K., & White, P. (2000). Researching sports injury: Reconstructing dangerous masculinities. In: J. McKay, M. Messner, & D. Sabo (Eds), *Masculinities, gender relations and sport* (pp. 108–127). Los Angeles: Sage.

Young, K., White, P., & McTeer, W. (1994). Body talk: Male athletes reflect on sport, injury, and pain. *Sociology of Sport Journal, 11*(2), 175–195.

Part I

Pain Cultures

Chapter 1

Sport and Risk Culture

Peter Donnelly

> ... why do we embark on that dangerous path when we know that
> a safe path could be followed? (Child 1997: ix).

> There is nothing more rewarding than taking a risk and succeeding
> (Haberl 1997: 1).

> If everything seems under control, you're just not going fast enough
> (Mario Andretti).

The first thing to note about sport and risk is that there are all kinds of ways
to take risks in sports. Risk of injury is perhaps the most common, and it is
related with a more long term risk of ill health — debilitating conditions such as
arthritis, osteoporosis, and other back, joint, neurological or nutritional ailments.
Risk of death is a possibility in some sports, even a probability in others (e.g.
high altitude mountaineering, or free diving). But there are other forms of risk
taking in sports. We might take *economic risks* by betting on sports events, or
by investing so much of our adolescence and early adulthood in an attempt to
become an elite, professional or Olympic athlete that we fail to complete a formal
education or obtain other skills necessary for us to enter the non-sport job market.
And there are also *social risks*, such as reputational risk — champions risk their
reputations each time they go into competition with an underdog, and athletes
who cheat risk being caught; relational risk — becoming so involved in a sport
that it becomes difficult to maintain important relationships in one's life; and even
the risk to one's dignity — imagine appearing on a "sports bloopers" tape, or a

Sporting Bodies, Damaged Selves
Research in the Sociology of Sport, Volume 2, 29–57
Copyright © 2004 by Elsevier Ltd.
All rights of reproduction in any form reserved
ISSN: 1476-2854/doi:10.1016/S1476-2854(04)02001-1

"funniest home videos" broadcast because of something that occurred while you were playing sports. This chapter focuses on the *physical* forms of risk taking — risk of injury, illness, and death. These are the types of risk we usually think of when we study risk taking in sports, and they have certainly garnered the most research.

The second thing to note about sport and risk is that humans, even those of us involved in risky endeavours, have a curiously ambivalent attitude toward risk taking. We admire risk taking, and may even have a sense that it is important that some humans are able to take risks, in the safety services and the military, in order to achieve fame and fortune, or in order to ensure human progress. At the same time we may be horrified by it as a tragic waste of life and limb, an unnecessary medical expense, foolishness that risks the lives of rescuers, and brings trauma and/or hardship to the lives of family and friends. The NASA programme highlights one extreme in the political and moral economy of risk. It brings together risks which are generally acceptable and admired — those taken for material gain, national prestige or security, and public entertainment — although the 1986 Challenger disaster gave pause to those views. Teenage auto accidents resulting from speeding, for example, highlight the tragedy of risk taking and may be seen as the other extreme in the political and moral economy of risk. These views highlight the socially constructed nature of risk, and between these extremes, particularly where sport is concerned, we find ourselves in a dilemma. We frequently admire individuals who appear to put "life and limb" on the line for what, in the greater scheme of things, may be only a symbolic reward (e.g. a record of some kind); but may criticise those same individuals when things do go wrong.

This chapter first considers the definition of "risk culture" in sport, and then attempts to deal with the difficult questions of why people take risks in sports, and why some individuals seem to be more inclined than others to take risks. These questions are addressed briefly from biological and psychological perspectives, and in more detail from a sociological perspective. The chapter concludes with a brief examination of three issues related to the study of risk taking in sports: risk and trust; risk and responsibility; and finally, returning to our ambivalent, or even contradictory attitudes towards risk taking in sports described above, a discussion of the culture of risk vs. the culture of caution.

Defining the Culture of Risk

The phrase "risk culture" or "culture of risk" brings together two of the most complex terms in sociology, and bracketing them together in this way may create even more problems. The use of the term *culture* often depends on context; the term is widely used in the arts and anthropology. For the purposes of this chapter, its sociological use is close to anthropology with reference to the way of life of a population (just as "subculture" refers to the way of life of a group within that population), emphasising customs and traditions, language use, beliefs and behaviours. For example, Donnelly (1980) pointed out that, in the 1970s, two of the distinctive features of the subculture of climbers, often thought of as a high risk subculture, were arrogance and fatalism. Sociology also emphasises the ways in which such characteristics are produced, reproduced, and transformed by those involved.

Giddens (1999) has traced the origins of the concept of *risk* to 16th century Portuguese explorers sailing into uncharted waters. It is a Western concept that stands in contrast to ideas of fate. "Risk isn't the same as hazard or danger. Risk refers to hazards that are actively assessed in relation to future possibilities" (Giddens 1999: 22). Thus, risk taking involves knowing that there is a possibility of failure, but proceeding with the action anyway. Difficulties in using the concept arise not just because of the range of situations (e.g. the physical, economic, and social situations noted in the introduction to this chapter), but also because of our attitudes towards risk. Kasperson (cited in Leiss & Chociolko 1994: 3; see also, Douglas 1992: 44) has pointed out that "the defining of risk is essentially a political act," because once a situation has been defined as risky, it becomes necessary for people and governments to attend to it. Thus, risks are socially constructed, and Douglas has argued that, of the multitude of risks we face, only certain ones are selected for attention. She notes that, "Dangers are selected for public concern according to the strength and direction of social criticism" (Douglas & Wildavsky 1982a: 50, 1982b). Tobacco use and road safety now receive far more attention than the dangers of sport despite, for example, the fact that sport accidents now cause more disability than traffic accidents (MacGregor 2002). But sport has not been beyond social criticism with regard to its dangers (see final section of this chapter on culture of risk and culture of caution).

The particular nature of sport has also assisted in keeping it on the fringes of social criticism. First, sport organizations often function as quasi-legal bodies, continually attempting to maintain their right to deal internally with situations (e.g. fighting, illegal drug use, and deliberate attempts to injure opponents) that would normally attract the attention of the law. Their failure in recent years to deal adequately with a number of well-publicised incidents (e.g. illegal drug use in cycle racing; the McSorley-Brashear incident in ice hockey; deaths in boxing)[1]

---

[1] In 1998, the Tour de France was the source of a major drug scandal, and professional cycle racing has seen a number of deaths resulting from the use of amphetamines and EPO. In 2000, a violent incident

has placed that right more in question. Second, athletes continually point out that they voluntarily and willingly participated in the incidents that led to their injuries, although a number of recent athlete lawsuits against sport organisations and physicians suggests that such participation is not always so voluntary (see Sociological Explanations in next section). Athletes also tend to deny the dangers associated with their involvement in sports, especially when they invoke an "it won't happen to me" attitude. It is necessary for them to suppress any sense of vulnerability in order to continue to participate at a committed level, especially when they see team mates and friends succumbing to serious injuries. This attitude calls into question whether such athletes, if they are denying the dangers, are actually involved in risk taking. However, although awareness of vulnerability may be suppressed, especially during the heat of competition, athletes seem willing to accept the accolades they receive for involvement in risky activities, and awareness of the dangers is usually present at the back of an athlete's mind. Third, there is also an active public denial of danger in the so-called high risk sports — "it's not really dangerous if you know what you are doing" (see Donnelly 1981). There are two intersecting reasons for such denial — pro-commercial, and anti-regulation. If a sport has a reputation as dangerous, it is difficult to attract large numbers of participants to purchase safety equipment, instruction/lessons, and adventure tourism packages in activities ranging from scuba diving to mountaineering. And, if a sport has a reputation for danger, it is more likely to attract the attention of government regulators whose intervention would change the nature of the activity (cf. the early attempts by hang gliders in the United States to avoid Federal Aviation Authority regulations).[2]

Bringing the two terms together to examine risk culture, or the culture of risk places sport in a relatively well-established area of sociological analysis. Since Oscar Lewis (1961, 1965) first coined the term "culture of poverty" to refer to the way of life produced and reproduced among poor people, sociologists have referred to the culture of violence, culture of fear, culture of caring, etc. The "culture of risk" appears to have been used first with reference to the behaviour of some young gay men who were still engaging in "unsafe sex" despite widespread knowledge of its dangers (Douglas & Calvez 1990). It was first applied to sport by Nixon (1992) with reference to the apparent normalisation of injury in some U.S.

---

in a professional ice hockey game in Canada resulted in police charges being brought against Marty McSorley (Atkinson in press). Professional boxing has been an object of medical and legal concern for some 30 years, and each public appearance of Muhammed Ali reinforces that concern; however, the concern peaks each time a boxer dies as a result of brain injuries received in the ring (Donnelly 1988–1989).

[2] Of course, a dangerous reputation will also attract some participants.

university sports, and has since been applied more broadly to sport culture. The rates of injury in many sports are quite astonishing (see Chapters 16 and 17), but do not seem to have attracted the type of social criticism necessary to bring them to the forefront of public attention. If a similar rate of injury, and even death, existed in other areas of social life (e.g. in schools, factories, or the fast-food industry) it would warrant major legal and policy attention. Imagine a fast food industry where there are regular accidents such as burns from the hot fat fryer, or falls on grease-covered kitchen floors; where there is a whole sub-specialty of medicine ("fast food medicine") which included designated clinics, and therapists and specialists in the treatment of such injuries; and where particularly dangerous restaurants have a clinician attached to the workplace. While this may seem absurd with regard to fast food, it is normal practice in sport.

Is it accurate, therefore, to refer to sport as a "culture of risk?" There is a certain vagueness about the use of such terminology. While injury, and even death, may have become a way of life that is produced and reproduced in sport, it is also contested and challenged, and it is also possible to participate in (almost) all sports in relative safety. Porro's (2000) comment that it may be more accurate to refer to "high risk practices in sports" rather than to "high risk sports" is an important qualification. Therefore, given the apparently accepted and normalised rate of injuries and untimely deaths that occur in sports, it is probably a useful shorthand to refer to sports as a "culture of risk" if these qualifications are borne in mind.

Since risk taking involves an active decision taken by an individual, it is necessary — in order to understand the culture of risk — to understand both that individual decision, and the social context in which it is taken, or, as Drasdo puts it, "the internal risk taking sensation,[3] and the external risk taking situation" (Drasdo 1981: 54). The following section deals with precisely these issues of behaviour/experience and context.

Taking Risks and Risk Takers

In order to understand the culture of risk, or high risk practices in sport, it is necessary first to examine the type of people who take risks and/or the circumstances under which people take risks. The questions of why people take

---

[3] As noted in the following section, while genetics and psychology have taken some steps toward identifying which individuals may be more likely to take risks, there is almost no academic research which attempts to understand "the internal risk taking sensation." Donnelly (2000) took some preliminary attempts in this direction by looking at the experiential level, in addition to the macro-social level and the level of social formations in relation to risk taking.

risks, and why some people seem to be more likely to take risks than others, have intrigued scientists for almost 100 years — since Sigmund Freud began to draw our attention to issues of human behaviour and human psyche, and posited that some people have a "death wish" (Freud 1920/1990, 1929/1989). While psychologists seem to have paid most attention to risk taking behaviour, biologists and sociologists have also struggled to explain this behaviour. This section begins with the reductionist explanations[4] — focusing on the individual and the characteristics of individuals who take risks — and proceeds to the sociological — focusing more on the social contexts in which people might take risks.

Biological Explanations

From the earliest days of Pavlov's "orienting reflex" there have been attempts to discover a neurophysiological basis for individual differences in risk and novelty (stimulus) seeking behaviour. In the 1960s and 1970s, various researchers were revisiting Pavlov's "strength of the nervous system," or searching for perceptual differences between stimulus seekers and others (e.g. Petrie 1967; Sales *et al.* 1974). In the 1980s, researchers started to take a more direct biochemical approach in an attempt to understand the predisposition to seek environments that are novel, complex and uncertain. At a 1987 conference ("Self-Regulation and Risk-Taking Behavior") organised by the National Institute of Mental Health in the United States, researchers began to explore the apparently counter-evolutionary proposition that human biology could be implicated in risk taking behaviour that might lead to death or serious injury (Weiss 1987: C10). What psychologist Marvin Zuckerman (1979) terms "sensation seekers" were found to have low levels of monoamine oxidase (MAO, an enzyme that breaks down neurotransmitters) and dopamine beta hydroxylase (DBH, which mediates the conversion of dopamine to noradrenaline; low levels are associated with manic states), and higher levels of testosterone. These findings led Zuckerman to propose a genetic basis for sensation seeking: "What we inherit are different enzymes that regulate our nervous systems. High sensation-seeking is probably not due to high levels of neurotransmitters, but to a lack of certain regulatory controls" (cited by Weiss 1987: C10).

By the 1990s, sensation seekers were beginning to be referred to as "Type-T" (thrill-seeking) personalities, and geneticists in Israel and the United States announced that they had discovered the gene for risk taking. In the United States, Moyzis *et al.* (University of California 2002; see also, Ding *et al.* 2002) declared

---

[4] The area of risk taking has produced a striking convergence of reductionist researchers in evolutionary biology, genetics, and psychology.

that a variant of gene DRD4 (which is associated with one of the brain's dopamine receptors) caused Type-T behaviour. As is often the case, biologists discovering a gene or gene variant are encouraged, often by the media,[5] to overstate their findings and to speculate well beyond their discovery into areas of science in which they have no expertise. For example, Moyzis noted that: "It *may* be that people who are compelled to seek constant stimulation are looking for ways to boost their dopamine levels. . . . People who have this form of the gene *may* also have a quicker physical reaction time — so they *might* have a natural attraction to speed" (cited by Abraham 2002: F6, emphases added).

Both Moyzis, and Frank Farley, a past President of the American Psychological Association who first used the term, "Type-T personality," note the positive aspects of having this gene variant/personality type. Farley points out that society needs Type-Ts — "They tend to be highly creative, outside-the-box thinkers, leaders in the arts, sports, business, science and politics . . . [w]ithout [them] we would not have the modern world. They're at the forefront of human progress" (cited by, Abraham 2002: F6). Moyzis agrees, noting that children with attention deficit disorder and hyperactivity (approximately 50% of whom appear to have variant DRD4) "could be the big entrepreneurs of the future" (cited by, Abraham 2002: F6). Inevitably, there are contradictions. Risk-taking explorers, carrying the gene, *may* have had "an innate survival advantage," despite the counter-evolutionary concerns. And the population distribution of the gene variant is even more paradoxical — 5% in North and East Asian populations; about 20% in Europeans and North Americans of European heritage; and native Americans carry variant DRD4 ranging from 32% in the North to almost 70% in the South (Chen *et al.* 1999). Native South Americans might wonder why they do not rule the world!

Since the limitations of the biological explanations are quite similar to those of the psychological explanations, they are presented following the next section. However, those biologists, geneticists and psychologists who are critical of pure biological determinism or other reductionist interpretations of human behaviour suggest that there is a complex interaction between genes and environment, and it is only in that interaction that we may find the behavioural expression of genes (e.g. Gould 1983; Lewontin 1991; Rose 1984).

Psychological Explanations

When the issue of risk-taking has been raised with respect to high risk sports, it has most often been approached in psychological, and therefore individualistic terms.

---

[5] In this case in response to actor Jason Priestley's (2002) auto racing accident.

Psychological approaches, which clearly overlap with biological explanations, have also invariably assumed that risk taking is male behaviour, and have involved either/or types of explanations: "The whole personality, confronting risk as a whole, is expected to be biased either toward risk-taking or toward risk-avoiding" (Douglas & Wildavsky 1982b). Typical analyses include the following:

- *classical Freudian* — Fuller (1977) explores the sexual symbolism of sports and, in the case of a high risk sport, mountaineering, proposes that climbers are motivated by unresolved infantile anxiety:

    The mountain peak may stand firstly for the father's penis, the apparently unassailable, erect, gigantic object which must be mastered. But its slopes, foothills and crevices may also symbolize the mother's body — that which is to be won by conquering the peak. The act of climbing itself commonly symbolizes erection, or sexual potency in dreams . . . anxiety may be externalized through climbing, and mastered in a way that is both pleasurable and rewarding. . . . In the infantile castration complex, the external threat deriving from the father is only an assumed one. . . . In sports like climbing, the mastery of the anxiety created by an assumed, but unreal, infantile threat is achieved only by putting the self in a situation of real risk (pp. 37–38).

- *pathological behaviour* — clinical psychologists and psychiatrists have invariably treated risk taking as pathological behaviour. Ogilvie has summarised their interpretations as: counter-phobic reactions; fear displacement; dangerous behaviour resulting from unconscious feelings of inadequacy; psychopathic personality; attempts to prove superiority or masculinity; and the classical death wish (1973: 62–63). The death wish, or suicide drive has also become one of the most popular, non-clinical explanations of extremely high risk behaviour.
- *personality profiles* — personality studies of athletes involved in high risk sports, especially when the same test is used, have produced relatively consistent profiles. Participants tend to score high on characteristics such as leadership, independence, emotional detachment, and emotional control. As noted, by the 1990s Farley was referring to this as the "Type-T" personality.
- *akrasia* — refers to loss of control, and is assumed to be associated with the failure — "modular cognitive separation" — of the brain's presumed capacity to make logical decisions. Items of information are separated such that individuals are not able to relate cause and effect, leading to incorrect perceptions of actual risk in sports or other risky behaviours such as smoking.

- *stimulus/thrill seeking* — this has been one of the most popular motivational approaches to the study of risk taking. The approach proposes the existence of a motivational need, the strength of which varies by individual. The motive has been measured by means of questionnaires, the results of which appear to substantiate differences between individuals in stimulus/thrill seeking behaviour.

Let us accept that there are individual differences in thrill seeking/risk taking behaviour, and that such differences may be explained by *biology* and/or *psychology*. These explanations may well be correct, but their reductionism leads to a number of serious limitations. First, they provide no insights into the enormous variety of ways that people may choose to express their genetic and/or psychological predisposition — from criminal to megalomanic behaviour, from hedonistic to altruistic behaviour. Nor do they suggest whether the tendency might be proactive or reactive — do you sit on top of a rocket waiting for it to blast-off, or do you jump in a fast flowing river to rescue a drowning child? Second, they do not take into account the observation that everyone — whether they have the gene/personality type or not — may take physical risks in certain circumstances such as, for example, when a loved one may be in danger, or under circumstances of peer pressure. Related to this is the assumption that risk taking/thrill seeking is a stable disposition that does not vary with, for example, age or the particular circumstances in which one finds oneself. Third, both explanations raise a 'chicken and egg' question — was the gene expressed or the personality disposition achieved as a result of participation in risk taking behaviour, or was the risk taking behaviour a result of having the gene/personality? Fourth, in addition to making masculinist assumptions, the psychological and psychiatric approaches too often assume that risk taking is, at best, irrational behaviour (patently untrue) and, at worst, pathological behaviour. And the personality and stimulus seeking approaches tend to be descriptive and tautological rather than explanatory (you score high on a trait/scale because you take risks; you take risks because you score high on a trait/scale).

Sociological Explanations

While biology and psychology tend to focus on individuals and individual differences, sociology is more likely to focus on the circumstances and conditions under which people are likely to take risks — the social context of risk. First, however, there are two biological characteristics, age and sex, which, in their social manifestations of maturity and gender, help to bridge the divide between biological, psychological and sociological explanations. Younger people seem to be far more likely to take risks than older people, and men seem to be far more likely to take risks than women.[6]

Age

Of the three age groups that are most prone to accidents, 16–24 year olds (the others are the first year of life and the over 60s) are the most likely to die in road accidents, especially in North America (see, for example, Investor Services 2000; Transport Canada 2000), and during participation in high risk sports. Risk taking may be a part of establishing an identity and asserting independence during adolescence, but there is also a sense that risk taking is a part of adolescent culture for both males and females (the forms may be different). Newly won independence and youth have been assumed to combine to create a sense of invulnerability, a feeling that one is "bulletproof." However, two studies (Beyth-Marom *et al.* 1993; Quadrel *et al.* 1993) found no differences in perceived sense of invulnerability between adolescents and adults. The results are not surprising, and lend support to the need to study the social context of risk taking. Not only is there more apparent risk taking between the ages of 16 and 24, but it is easier to take risks during those years than at any other time. Some researchers (e.g. Donnelly 1980) have even suggested that there may be a deliberate acting out of risk at this age before settling down to the "serious business" of work, marriage and parenting.

Gender

Observed differences between males and females in risk-taking behaviour have made it far too easy to propose biology or socialisation as the cause. However, there are reasons to suspect that lack of opportunity might be a more adequate explanation, and one that again returns to social context. While women have been less involved in the safety and social control occupations (e.g. firefighting, military, police), there is no evidence that women have avoided these occupations when the opportunity has been available (e.g. during wartime, or during a time of increasing gender equity). Adolescent females appear to take risks involving substance abuse as often as males, and probably take far more sexual risks than males. And, while

---

[6] Jesse Bernard noted that, "if young people, especially young men, could somehow or other be quarantined or laid away on ice from ages 18 to 25, most violence, even traditional crime, could be eliminated" (1968: 21–22).

there are fewer women than men involved in high risk and high injury sports, the number of women participants is increasing significantly as opportunities are made, or become available. Kevin Young and his colleagues (Young 1997; Young *et al.* 1994; Young & White 1995) have focused on male and female athletes' attitudes toward risk, injury and danger and found very little difference, at least in the populations sampled.

Two additional social characteristics, culture and social class, throw a little more light on the social context of risk-taking.

Culture

There have been popular theories suggesting that certain nationalities or cultural groups are more inclined to take risks than others.[7] Such theories rarely stand up to serious analysis until social context is considered. For example, Thompson (1980) addresses an anthropological puzzle associated with trade involving the risky crossing of the Himalayas between the high plains of Tibet and the lowlands of India: who acts as the intermediary? Either the Hindus of India could move up, or the Buddhists of Tibet could move down, or both could engage in actual travel. In almost every case, it was the Buddhists who undertook the dangerous travel. Thompson argues that risk taking and risk avoidance is associated with conditions of poverty — the collapse into poverty takes place under conditions of risk avoidance while the rise out of poverty takes place under conditions of risk acceptance.[8] However, he also notes that this is a cyclical relationship, although what triggers the cycles in which poor people (or Buddhists here) begin to take risks, and wealthy people (or Hindus here) cease to take risks needs to be determined. The evident growth of risk aversion in wealthy Western societies (see last section) may support Thompson's thesis; but it is also evident that most of the participants in what are normally recognised as high risk sports in the West are of European heritage, relatively wealthy people from advanced industrial societies who have the opportunity to participate.

---

[7] Given Chen's (1999) cross cultural findings, this is another potential biological/sociological characteristic to account for differences in risk taking behaviour. However, his suggestions about gene expression are not borne out by even simple observation (are native South Americans over three times more likely to take risks than Euro North Americans?). There is no sociological or anthropological research to support the differential expression of risk taking behaviour among these populations.

[8] This view recalls the conflicting popular theories that people take risks because they are poor, or that people are poor because they are not prepared to take risks. It also recalls the self-serving neo-liberal view that poor people will work harder if you pay them less, and rich people will work harder if you pay them more!

Social Class

Studies addressing the place of risk-taking in Western working class culture suggest that male status in patriarchal working class cultures has been associated with occupations involving characteristics such as strength, dirt, and risk (e.g. Dunk 1991; Hoggart 1957; Young 1993). To be involved in a dangerous job, or to be invited to do a dangerous job, may have a significant positive impact on an individual's community status. Donnelly (1982) has noted that, in the sport of rock climbing, there was a significant increase in the level of acceptable risk that occurred as a consequence of democratisation of the sport between the 1930s and 1950s to include working class (male) participants. This suggests that, in a class culture or other social context in which risk-taking has come to be approved, one is likely to find more risk taking than might be predicted by genetic or personality predispositions.

Sociological attempts to explore risk taking has fallen into three types — risk assessment/risk management approaches; risk society theory; and response theories.

Risk Assessment/Risk Management

The *risk assessment/risk management* approaches are closely allied to psychological approaches in their assumption that taking risks is irrational, and that risks can, and should, be assessed and managed. It is rooted in economistic cost-benefit analyses and positivist notions that risk may be measured objectively. Our tendency to attribute "real knowledge" to the natural sciences has resulted in a separation between external causality and individual perceptions of risk:

> According to this approach, risk is a straightforward consequence of the dangers inherent in the physical situation, while attitudes toward risk depend on individual personalities. When particular risks are objectively ascertainable, it follows that the gap between the expert and the lay public ought to be closed in only one direction — toward the opinion of experts . . . the lay public must be taught the facts; the scientific message must be clearly labeled (Douglas & Wildavsky 1982a: 49).

The fact that experts so often disagree is perhaps evidence that this approach is seriously lacking in sociological imagination. In addition, risk assessment measures are frequently reported in a way that exaggerates the risk, and may lead to other risks. For example, the announcement in the 1970s that a certain type of oral contraceptive doubled the risk of thromboembolism usually failed to mention that the risk went from 1:14,000 to 2:14,000. The publicity caused an increase in unwanted pregnancies and abortions (Gigerenzer 2002). However, risk assessment and risk management principles form a significant part of sport administration.[9]

Risk Society Theory

The *risk society* approach emerged as the inadequacies of the risk assessment/risk management approach began to become evident after a series of major environmental disasters (e.g. Chernobyl, Love Canal, Walkerton, Bhopal).[10] Beck (1992, 1999), Giddens (1990, 1991), and to some extent Luhmann (1993), in their theories of reflexive modernity, have developed the risk society approach. They note that, as a consequence of the uncertainties of modern life, all individuals have become reflexive risk managers with the primary aim of minimising danger:

> [T]hinking in terms of risk assessment is a more or less ever present exercise . . . because of the shifting and developing nature of modern knowledge, the 'filter-back' effects on lay thought will be ambiguous and complicated. The risk climate of modernity is thus unsettling for everyone; no one escapes (Giddens 1991: 124).

This approach is only beginning to be explored with regard to risk and sport (e.g. Digel 1992; Safai 2002) and, of course, raises all kinds of contradictions for attempts to understand voluntary risk taking (see concluding section on risk vs. caution).

---

[9] Cost-benefit analyses in sport were recently newsworthy (Shoalts 2002) when the Canadian Medical Protective Association (which insures all Canadian physicians against malpractice) announced that it would no longer insure clinicians involved with professional athletes because the lawsuits now involved significant dollar amounts in line with professional athletes' salaries (see Babych decision at end of this section).

[10] See Young (1993) for summaries of several of these disasters. Walkerton was a recent Ontario (Canada) case that involved that involved widespread sickness and a number of deaths when a virulent strain of *E. coli* entered the water supply.

Response Theories

What I term *response theories* are the most direct sociological attempts to explain voluntary risk taking behaviour, and therefore most concerned with risk taking in sport and physical activity. Lyng's (1990) fieldwork with skydivers led to a groundbreaking article in the *American Journal of Sociology*. His work follows a number of attempts to link Marx and Mead, macro- and the micro-sociologies, in an attempt to explain the type of voluntary risk taking that he terms "edgework." At the macro level he points to the alienation felt, even by white collar workers, in the deskilled and bureaucratised workplaces of postindustrial capitalism. Such workplaces are characterised by an absence of spontaneity, by institutional routines, and by the absence of control on the part of the workers. At the micro level, Lyng (following Mead) points to a consequent "hyperextension of the individual's experience of the 'me' and an associated compression of opportunities to experience the 'I' " (Miller 1991: 1531). Lyng notes that the greater (although illusory) sense of control experienced by individuals involved in sports such as skydiving is a psychological need in such conditions of alienation.

Despite Lyng's attempts to distance himself from it, there are some strong similarities here to Mitchell's (1983) earlier work on mountaineering. Commenting on the number of scientists, technicians and engineers in his sample, Mitchell suggested that the alienating working conditions of such individuals — defined as routine and generally non-creative for highly educated individuals who had expected more stimulating work environments — results in a feeling of "relative deprivation" because emotional expectations are not met by career conditions. Therefore, "flow" is sought in activities such as mountaineering.

Katz's (1988) groundbreaking work on *The Seductions of Crime*, in which he attempts to portray crime from the perspective of the criminal, also takes a response approach. He argues that, in the United States, the particular social structure results in the "experience of humiliation" by the underclass. Katz proposes that engaging in risk taking, in the form of "the moral, sensual, and emotional attractions of crime," is a means of resolving the "experience of humiliation." O'Malley & Mugford (1994) complete the circle of this review in their essay attempting to link Katz and Lyng — "Crime, Excitement and Modernity." While adding a number of historical examples and sociological processes to the issue, they retain the essence of both Katz and Lyng's (and Mitchell's) view that voluntary risk taking is a *response* to the social context in which individuals find themselves. There are a number of serious limitations to *response theories*, and I conclude this section on sociological approaches by outlining the limitations, and proposing some alternatives employing ethnography and a critical social constructionist perspective.

There are three basic problems with the accounts of voluntary risk taking addressed by *response theories*:

- since we are all experiencing the conditions of late modernity in advanced societies, why are there relatively few individuals responding to those conditions through risk-taking — whether it be in sports or crime?
- why does so much evidence point to young males taking risks, rather than other population segments? As noted in the previous discussion of age and gender, while the barriers to female risk taking seem to be decreasing, no one has produced a non-speculative account for the youth-risk relationship.
- perhaps the most damning concern lies in the idea that risk taking is a response to circumstances — a reaction, a compensation, a transcendence. Implicit in this view is a value-laden assumption that no one would take a voluntary risk if he or she were not driven to it by circumstances, if they had fulfilling and satisfying lives. In this, we are not far removed from the psychological views of risk taking as irrational or, at least in this case, as a rational response to irrational circumstances. In fact, Lyng and Mitchell come close to characterising voluntary risk taking as a response to lack of job satisfaction.

Years of ethnographic research with people involved in high risk sports does not give me any confidence in this explanation. For example, many of the individuals I studied[11] became involved even before they entered the labour market. Even more significantly, most had fulfilling and interesting lives even before they became involved in the sports.

This is not to dismiss *response theories* completely, but there is an alternative explanation which would apply to many of the participants in my research. Once these individuals became involved in a risk sport, developed skills, and incorporated involvement into their identities and lifestyles, their previous lives and the lives that they often had to return to on Monday mornings may have begun to look mundane in comparison. By restructuring their identities in this way, they may have implied that their lives were unfulfilled, that the "I" was not being fully expressed, but it only seemed so in retrospective comparison.[12] The *response theories* interpretation

---

[11] In addition to my personal involvement in high risk practices in sports (cf. Donnelly 2002), I began studying participants and social structures in "high risk sports" over 20 years ago (Donnelly 1980). Since that time I have maintained links with the mountaineering community, and conducted numerous interviews with participants in sports such as sky diving, scuba diving, hang gliding and surfing, as part of an ongoing interest in issues of risk taking in sport.

[12] The issue of retirement from high risk sport involvement adds support to this reinterpretation, but the argument is beyond the scope of this paper (see Donnelly 1980).

also points to the potential dangers of naive ethnography. It is possible that Lyng and Mitchell spoke to the wrong people, asked the wrong questions, and may have been brushed off as outsiders rather than untrustworthy insiders by hard core participants. Often, forms of talk or a lack of reflexivity among participants may produce a mistaken interpretation among researchers. For example, relatively formal conversations among high risk sport participants may be full of references to safety and control; informal and private conversations, gossip and stories are often full of references to themselves or others at times when circumstances have been extremely unsafe and evidently out of control. Long term contact with individuals who accept the researcher as worthy of respect (in the arrogant world of high risk sports) not only leads to richer data, but also a greater ability to interpret those data.

If some individuals have a psychological or biological propensity to take risks,[13] then it is important for sociologists to understand the social context in which risks are likely to be taken. Risk taking frequently occurs in social settings in which risk is valued, and in which the participants consent to engage in such behaviours (although in some sports there may be an element of coercion that stands in relation to consent). It would probably be a mistake to assume that all of the individuals in those social setting had a similar psychological or biological propensity to take risks. Such social formations might be thought of as "risk subcultures," and these are settings in which *character*, *identity*, and *comradeship* are major motifs.

Since it became part of the *raison d'être* of organised sports in 19th century British public schools, boys and men in particular have been relating to each other in sport (and other areas of life) around the notion of *character*. The four elements of character identified by Goffman (1967), and refined in a sport context by Birrell (1981) — courage, gameness, integrity and composure — are all implicitly related to risk:

- the connection with courage is obvious — knowing the danger you face it anyway. This is why reckless ("crazy") individuals are not often highly regarded in risk sport subcultures — they do not give any impression that they are aware of the danger, and they may endanger others.
- gameness involves returning from a traumatic injury, coming back for more "punishment" despite the odds, playing with injuries, getting up off the canvas

---

[13] Again it should be pointed out that it may not just be individuals with an evident propensity who take risks. There are numerous cases of young women who have taken up, for example, skydiving or rock climbing because their boy friend was involved; or of young men who have become involved in risk taking activities because of peer pressure. They did not initiate, or seek out the involvement, and they may only participate until they feel that they no longer have to — but they did participate.

to fight some more, even when it appears to be over — these are all aspects of risk.

- composure or coolness refers to one's demeanour in the face of danger — not panicking, always being reliable in a dangerous situation.
- integrity involves honesty — not exaggerating, not making false claims (see section on risk and trust).

These elements of character have been socially constructed as highly valued. They encourage risk taking, and they encourage some of the profound problems in modern sport — violence, objectification of the body, high injury rates, etc. — because the dominant structures of sport socialise young people into these values, which are then played out by those with 'the right stuff' in more or less conformist ways. In fact, Hughes and Coakley (1991) specifically refer to many of these behaviours as "overconformity to the sport ethic."

Identity, which becomes fully developed or constructed (Donnelly & Young 1988) during the age period most associated with risk taking, often involves conformity to peer groups, and trying out different identities. Having one's identity accepted (confirmed) by a peer group (*comradeship*) may involve taking physical risks in order to avoid a social/reputational risk — a risk that may be perceived to have even more severe consequences at this time of one's life. The latter has been identified by social scientists who study war as the major motivation for action. In the heat of battle, young soldiers do not fight for their country, or their officers, or for an ideology. They fight for their particular unit in an attempt to ensure the survival of their comrades — they fight for each other. In the parallels between sport and war, this is often a motivation for risky behaviour in sports (e.g. "taking one for the team").

The socially constructed nature of risk is evident in the following scenario:

A group of individuals are on an outdoor wilderness course. They could be a squad on military basic training, trainee managers on a team building exercise, or a patrol at an Outward Bound type of school. The next exercise is an introduction to rappelling/abseiling. While all the individuals are nervous, two in particular are very unhappy about sliding over the edge of a cliff on the rope — despite the instructor's assurances that a safety rope ensures that they are not in danger. There is an element of competition involved for the group (e.g. a race against other groups to be first to return to base, or a point scoring system), and there are requirements that groups learn to function as cooperative and supportive units. The group and the instructor try bribery, reason, group solidarity concerns (e.g. appeals regarding the success or failure of the group), threats, and every other way they can think of to try to encourage these individuals to complete the task. One eventually concedes to the demands and completes the task; the other becomes more and more stubborn, and refuses outright to step over the edge.

Character, identity and comradeship come together in an interesting way in this scenario. The one who completed the task is recognised for her courage and strength of character in overcoming her fears, her identity is confirmed, and she maintains her relationship with the group. The one who refused may lose respect for his presumed weakness of character, his identity is not confirmed, and his relationship with the group becomes difficult, having "let the side down." What is interesting in this scenario, however, is the fact that the first individual receives validation not only for overcoming her fears, but also for conforming to the demands of others. The second individual receives no validation for his courage and strength of character in standing up to what he perceived as the unreasonable demands of others (it was an exercise, it had nothing to do with his job requirements). The second individual could not have been unaware that he was taking a major social risk in defying peer pressure and the demands of an authority figure, and yet such courage is rarely validated. This tends to make a mockery of campaigns to "Just say no!"

Given that risk taking may now be seen to include matters of social context and interpretation, the reason that athletes sometimes appear to take unreasonable risks, even when the potential negative consequences appear to far outweigh the potential benefits, becomes a little more clear. In some cases, the law is now being asked to interpret and rectify the consequences of such actions as professional athletes being pressured into playing while injured. For example, Dave Babych's recent successful lawsuit against the Philadelphia Flyers ice hockey team physician is a case in point. In April 1998, Babych broke a bone in his foot. Because a play-off series was imminent, Babych was pressured to play by the coach, given pain killing injections by the team physician, and had to ice his foot to reduce the swelling enough to fit into his skate. "I told [the coach] I can't go, and didn't want to hurt the team or hurt myself" (all quotes from Associated Press/Kerr 2002: S3). The coach replied, "Well, you have to go. We'll take that chance . . ." The only people who appear to have taken a chance were Babych, who believes that his career was shortened by his decision, and the team physician who was found to have "deviated from the accepted standards in treating the injury." When Babych notes that "there's pressure coming from all round to play," he is indicating that his identity as a hockey player was challenged, his relationship with coaches and teammates was on the line, and his character was questioned. However, his decision to sue the team was also a risk; and he now believes that he has been blacklisted from working for any NHL teams. Babych was 37 years old when he decided/was coerced into playing with a broken bone. One can only imagine the pressure on younger players, or those on the development route to becoming professional players.

From the preceding analyses, is it possible to claim that sport is a "culture of risk?" Clearly, sports constitute a culture in which taking risks is encouraged, sometimes coerced, and rewarded both materially, and emotionally within particular social formations (teams, subcultures) which value character, a shared identity, and comradeship. Sport has produced a culture in which, in Canada, Jacques Plante was initially ridiculed for being the first professional ice hockey goaltender to wear a protective face mask; in which Jackie Stewart was initially ridiculed by his auto racing peers for advocating greater safety at Formula 1 auto racing tracks; and in which, over 20 years later in the same sport, driver Jacques Villeneuve can state, in a critique of new concerns about track safety: "Racing is dangerous . . . nobody obliges you to drive a race car. If you get to the point when you are scared, then stop" (Canadian Press 1997: C16). While I agree with Porro (2000) that it may be more accurate to refer to high risk practices in sports, rather than to high risk sports, it seems that there is a "subculture of risk" associated with certain sports (from football to skydiving). In addition, there are shared elements of risk in all aspect of sport culture, from repetitive strain injuries in bowling, to the non-therapeutic use of beta blockers in target sports. Thus, although the "culture of risk" is a useful descriptor to characterise a set of practices in which physical risk taking is frequently encouraged, it may give the false impression that sport is all about physical risks. The tension between the culture of risk and the culture of caution outlined in the last section perhaps indicates that the term needs to be used with care.

Three Issues in Need of Resolution

I conclude by raising three issues that deserve a more thorough consideration with regard to physical risk taking behaviour in sports: risk and trust; risk and responsibility; and the tension between the culture of risk and the culture of caution.

Risk and Trust

In many ways risk and trust represent the opposite sides of the same coin. We enter risk taking situations trusting that we will emerge safely. Trust involves "the vesting of confidence in persons . . . made on the basis of a 'leap of faith' which brackets ignorance or lack of information" (Giddens 1991: 244); and may be defined as "confidence in the reliability of a person or system" (Giddens 1990: 34). In the past, trust was frequently embedded in social relations. One trusted in one's own abilities and perceptions, and in interactions with others (cf. Donnelly 1994; Donnelly & Young 1988). Giddens has described the development of "disembedding mechanisms," a result of modernity that removes "social activity from localised contexts, reorganising social relations across large time-space distances" (1990: 53). Such disembedding mechanisms placed trust in the sphere of institutional arrangements such as contracts, surveillance systems, forensic accounting, and other expert systems. Granovetter (1985) has argued that trust is still embedded in social relations, but that "while social relations may . . . be a necessary condition for trust and trustworthy behavior, they are not a sufficient condition to guarantee these" (p. 491).

In sport, it is necessary for athletes to trust in expert systems — sport scientists, sports medicine, doping control, manufacturers and testers of safety equipment such as helmets, etc. We may take risks because we trust our equipment, because we trust that medical expertise will be available when a risk has had a negative consequence,[14] or because we trust that rescue will be available to us as mountaineers, adventure racers, or in ocean sailing races. In order to participate effectively in many sports we also need to trust that others will play their part appropriately (e.g. professional wrestling), play by the rules (e.g. that they will not "sucker-punch" you after the bell in a boxing match), and be competent participants who possess the skills that they claim in order to ensure safety. For example, road racing cyclists must trust that others in the race are able to ride in a straight line in a group at speed (see Chapter 9). Climbers must be able to trust that a rope partner will be competent and reliable if things go wrong (see Donnelly 1994; Donnelly & Young 1988). The negotiated relationship between risk and trust is an important part of the social dynamics of sport, and needs more research attention.

Risk and Responsibility

Just as risk and trust stand in relation to each other, risk and responsibility form an interesting counterpoint. On the one hand is Jean Paul Sartre's existentialist position – *on est seul* — individuals taking risks will often declare that they are responsible for and to themselves, that they do not expect others to be responsible

---

[14] Given the economistic principles of risk assessment, it may have been more economically rational to develop the treatment of sport injuries — an ongoing expense — than the prevention of sport injuries (cf. Donnelly 1999).

for them (e.g. to come to their rescue, etc.), and that it is their choice whether they wear a helmet, use a seatbelt, or climb solo. On the other hand is John Donne's declaration that "no man is an island" — we are responsible for each other, and when we are injured or killed it affects others in various ways. This raises interesting social (and legal) questions. In sport, is it possible to take a risk responsibly? Who is, or should be responsible when an individual is seriously injured in sport, or needs rescue from a dangerous situation? Who will take care of the surviving family members of athletes killed because of risk taking, or the caregivers for athletes with serious disabilities as a result of risk taking? These questions have been hotly debated in the mountaineering community (e.g. Powter *et al.* 1997), as has the question of attempting to rescue or care for dying mountaineers on the world's highest mountains (e.g. O'Dowd 2000; Simpson 1997).[15]

There are many positive aspects to risk taking: character development, self-testing, the pleasure of taking risks and being in (relative) control in risky situations, the experiential aspect that makes individuals feel more fully human.[16] But it is also difficult to reconcile taking risks with responsibility. Two related examples also show that there is a gendered aspect to responsibility. In 1995, after the well known British mountaineer, Alison Hargreaves, was killed on K2 in the Himalayas, leaving a husband and two children, her death was severely criticised in the British media (especially tabloid newspapers and women's magazines). She was vilified for her irresponsibility in engaging in a high risk activity as a mother of young children.[17] The next year, during the 1996 "Everest disaster," the New Zealand guide and mountaineer, Rob Hall, died on Mount Everest. In the final hours before he died he held several radio/satellite telephone conversations with his pregnant wife in New Zealand. These heartbreaking conversations, during which they agreed on a name for their unborn child, were heard by all those on the mountain who had a radio; and they were described by John Krakauer and Hall's wife, Jan Arnold, in a television documentary on the "disaster" (ABC Television 1998). At no point was Hall publicly criticised for engaging in a high risk activity when he was about to become a father, and I have never heard criticism of a deceased male mountaineer

---

[15] Simpson (1997) has been particularly critical of the declining moral climate of mountaineering, and the failure of mountaineers to uphold the elements of nurturance and self sacrifice that once characterised the sport.

[16] Drasdo (1981) suggests that risk is "the accelerator of human progress," a view endorsed by Moyzis (2002) and Chen *et al.* (1999) who link the DRD4 gene with historical human migrations. If those who lead such migrations are "adventurers," they would meet with Zweig's (1974) approval: "Man risking his life in perilous encounters constitutes the original definition of what is worth talking about."

[17] Few of the reports mentioned that she was the "breadwinner" for her family, that her adventures paid the bills for the children and their stay-at-home father (Rose & Douglas 2000).

(or any other high risk sport participant) who also happened to be a father with family responsibilities.

Children suffer from adult risk taking in sport — they may lose a father (or mother), or have a parent who has an impairment (e.g. chronic knee problems) which prevents them from playing sports or other games with their children. Spouses (usually wives) also suffer from their partner's risk taking; as do the parents of risk takers. They may be charged with the ongoing care of an impaired person, they cannot enjoy the life that they expected together, or they may suffer the grief of losing a child or a partner. Rescuers, on mountains and oceans or in caves, may be injured as a result of another's risk taking, but that is less of an issue when there are volunteer rescue systems comprised of participants who have developed an expertise in rescue work; or where sport association insurance schemes pay for expert rescue. These are favoured in comparison to the obligation to rescue imposed on park rangers and police and fire services where there may be less expertise. Communities, and societies as a whole may lose the potential contributions of particular individuals who die or become impaired as a result of risk taking. And, at a time of scarcity in the availability of medical resources, risk taking athletes take up a disproportionate share of health care resources. At some events (e.g. Formula 1 auto races, NFL football games), fully equipped medical teams are available exclusively for the competitors.

Whether it is possible in sport to take a risk responsibly is a complex philosophical question. However, the sociological literature on sport injuries is increasing, and a more complete analysis of risk and risk taking would enhance our understanding of the extraordinary rate of injuries that is tolerated in many sports.

Culture of Risk vs. Culture of Caution

Despite everything that has been written previously, there is widespread evidence that we are actually living in a risk aversive culture — a culture of caution. As Hume recently noted:

> The risk-averse, cautious society in which we live is shaped by powerful cultural forces . . . [a] free-floating disposition to panic was discernible long before the terror of 11 September [2001]. That is why, even when there is no hard evidence of any significant risk, and all of the known facts and statistics are explained, many people simply refuse to accept that anything is safe today (Hume 2002: 48).

Thus, despite declining crime rates in North America, people still feel insecure about crime; and despite greater public health and disease control than at any previous time in history, there is more concern about ill health. Concern about our health and welfare is only exceeded, perhaps, by concern about child abduction at a time when the probability of abduction is probably lower than at any time in the last 100 years.

We often claim that play and sports are where children learn to take risks, have adventures, and generally prepare in a relatively safe way for the world that they will enter as adults. However, a growing culture of caution particularly affects children in sport and physical activity, with increased supervision and surveillance, legislation in the face of concerns about injuries, sexual abuse, and other safety concerns. At one level this involves growing surveillance — hidden cameras in children's nurseries to monitor the babysitter or nanny, or parental presence in parks and playgrounds, and at all games and practices to monitor coaches' behaviours and children's safety. At another level, it may involve excessive concerns about safety and lawsuits. The Children's Society and the Children's Play Council in the U.K. recently surveyed children to see what types of behaviour were being controlled in schools and playgrounds. Their findings (www.the-childrens-society.org.uk) were startling. For example:

- yo-yos were banned from school playgrounds because they might cause injury;
- "tag" and running games were banned in case children fell over;
- in one school handstands were banned because a student had injured her elbow doing a handstand;
- one school banned the use of a climbing frame in case children fell.

Playgrounds have been closed because the equipment does not meet new safety standards and insurance cannot be bought. And primary school physical education has been brought to new levels of inactivity, in an already reduced role in the curriculum, by non-specialist teachers who are concerned about injury in their classes.

The tension between a culture of risk and a culture of caution is beginning to become evident in a backlash against the above concerns. In Canada, Teitel signaled it by noting that:

> we're so concerned about our children's emotional safety, their 'feeling good about themselves,' that on at least a certain middle-class level, we've gutted play by taking the risk out of it. We've created a vogue for games without winners, games closely supervised to make sure that there is no gloating or bullying — a moratorium on competition in general (Teitel 1999: 59).

This was followed in the U.S. by Labash's (2001) widely publicised indictment of the "new phys ed" with its concerns about safety and inclusion; and from an academic perspective in a new (2002) report by David Ball for the Play Safety Forum in the U.K. ("Playgrounds: Risks, Benefits and Choices" — www.the-childrens-society.org.uk). The report calls for a balance between safety and some controlled risk and excitement: "Play provision is first and foremost for children and if it is not exciting and attractive to them, then it will fail, no matter how 'safe' it is."

The solution is not to return (regress) to exclusive and dangerous activities, to the "old phys ed." It will take some creative thinking to combine parents' legitimate concerns about safety and security with opportunities for children to take risks, and create excitement. Perhaps we need to return to an old view that sometimes children hurt themselves during play, and it is often nobody's fault, in order to produce a balance between the culture of risk and the culture of caution. Similar concerns are beginning to be apparent in the world of adult risk, where the commodification of adventure tourism and adventure racing seems to be more about "selling safety" than experiencing risk (Safai 2002).

Conclusion

Injuries, and sometimes debilitating illnesses and deaths, are so much a feature of high performance sport, particularly when high risk practices are valued and rewarded, that sport is beginning to be referred to as a "culture of risk." However, this culture of risk is also characterised by a great deal of ambiguity in attitudes towards risk and the negative consequences of risk taking. This chapter examined biological and psychological research on individual propensity to take risks, and found them both descriptive and limited. Even individuals who do not score high on risk taking questionnaires, or carry the DRD4 gene, are seen to take risks in certain circumstances; risk taking behaviour seems to vary by age (which might be unlikely if it was psychologically or genetically driven); and biology and psychology are unable to determine the exact form that risk taking behaviour might take. The focus on individuals carries over into sociological *response theories*, and none of the theories have taken into account the actual experiences of risk taking in sport.

I have suggested that biology and psychology are somewhat less important than understanding the circumstances/contexts under which individuals are likely to take risks, and that risk taking is most likely to occur in social formations that value risk taking, and where risk taking has become normalised. In such social formations, an individual's character and identity are on the line, available for all to see. Individuals will take risks in such settings, perhaps because of their psychological make up or genetic programming, but also because they value the comradeship available because of such behaviour. Neither the explanation nor the behaviour is without problems, and the chapter concludes by examining three related elements (trust, responsibility, and caution), thereby returning to the contradictions associated with risk taking behaviour and our responses to it.

Risk assessment, the culture of caution, and commodification of the culture of risk, have combined to create an interesting cultural moment for the culture of risk in sport. Perhaps the key element here, from a materialist perspective, is that risk assessment has created a huge market for safety and security measures (risk avoidance). In fact, the more the public is panicked by creative, and often contradictory statistical reports, the greater the market for safety and security services (from insurance to gated communities) and equipment.[18] The principle seems to be as follows: identify a risk; provide a notion of its significance by the creative use of statistics; and then sell the cure (pharmaceuticals, policing, equipment, technology, etc.). Such an industry should have had a difficult time dealing with voluntary risk taking in sport and physical activity, but the industry now seems also to be pervading that world. In order to take a risk *responsibly!* (i.e. to show the appropriate level of *caution*) it is necessary to purchase, and *trust* the appropriate equipment (e.g. knee brace, helmet) or service (e.g. lessons from a "certified" instructor) to participate.

In 1972, Harold Drasdo provided a striking experiential critique of the "seven essentials" for mountain hiking:

- always carry waterproof clothing — no more getting wet on the mountain;
- carry spare sweater, gloves, etc. — no more cold on the mountain;
- take a good torch [flashlight] — no more night;
- take watch, map and compass — no more doubt;
- plenty of spare food — no more appetite;
- never go in groups of less than three — no more solitude;
- leave details of your pre-planned route — no more spontaneity;
- study the weather forecast carefully — no more scope for judgment.

Drasdo must be amazed at the way the market has produced even more experiential limits 30 years later. For example:

- wear wicking clothing — no more sweat;
- carry a GPS device — no more need to develop map reading skills;
- carry a cell/satellite phone — no more fear that you won't be rescued.

---

[18] And the greater the opportunity for politically repressive measures.

From space blankets to energy bars, from high tech fabrics to no-blister boots, the mountain hiking experience has been transformed, as have many other sport experiences. The tension between risk and safety is continually being negotiated, and some individuals have taken to retro forms of their sports in an attempt to re-create "authentic" risk experiences — retro surfing (using old-style and heavy Malibu boards); retro skiing (telemark skiing on downhill slopes) and retro mountaineering (using traditional equipment and clothing on old routes) — although no one has yet attempted to "do a Mallory" by ascending Everest in a tweed jacket. In general, sport is a little different from other aspects of modern society — it continues to celebrate risk while it is also troubled by it! Meanwhile, the sport medicine industry thrives on the risk taking behaviour of athletes.

References

ABC Television (USA) (1998). *Mt. Everest: The movie.* ABC News, Saturday Night, March.

Abraham, C. (2002). The genome made me do it. *Globe & Mail,* 17 August, F6.

Associated Press/Kerr, G. (2002). Babych wins $1.37-million judgment. *Globe & Mail,* 1 November, S3.

Atkinson, M. (in press). It's still part of the game: Dangerous masculinity, crime, and victimization in professional ice hockey. In: L. Fuller (Ed.), *Sexual sports rhetoric and violence: Teaming up gender with the language of sport.* New York: Haworth Press.

Beck, U. (1992). *Risk society: Towards a new modernity.* London: Sage.

Beck, U. (1999). *World risk society.* Cambridge: Polity Press.

Bernard, J. (1968). The eudaemonists. In: S. Klausner (Ed.), *Why man takes chances: Studies in stress-seeking* (pp. 6–47). New York: Anchor Books.

Beyth-Marom, R., Austin, L., Fischoff, B., Palmgren, C., & Quadrel, M. (1993). Perceived consequences of risky behaviors: Adults and adolescents. *Development Psychology, 29,* 549–563.

Birrell, S. (1981). Sport as ritual: Interpretation from Durkheim to Goffman. *Social Forces, 60,* 354–376.

Canadian Press (1997). Scared drivers should quit, Villeneuve says. *Globe & Mail,* 11 April, C16.

Chen, C., Burton, M., Greenberger, E., & Dmitrieva, J. (1999). Population migration and the variation of dopamine D4 (DRD4) allele frequencies around the globe. *Evolution and Human Behavior, 20,* 309–324.

Child, G. (1997). Foreword. In: J. Haberl (Ed.), *Risking adventure* (pp. ix–x). Vancouver: Raincoast Books.

Digel, H. (1992). Sports in a risk society. *International Review for the Sociology of Sport, 27,* 257–272.

Ding, Y.-C., *et al.* (2002). Evidence of positive selection acting at the human dopamine receptor D4 gene locus. *Proceedings of the National Academy of Sciences, 99*(8 January), 309–314.

Donnelly, P. (1980). *The subculture and public image of climbers.* Unpublished doctoral thesis, University of Massachusetts, Amherst.

Donnelly, P. (1981). Four fallacies, I: Climbing is not really dangerous. *Mountain,* *80*(July/August), 38–40.

Donnelly, P. (1982). Social climbing: A case study of the changing class structure of rock climbing and mountaineering in Britain. In: A. O. Dunleavy, A. W. Miracle, & C. R. Rees (Eds), *Studies in the sociology of sport* (pp. 13–28). Fort Worth: Texas Christian University Press.

Donnelly, P. (1988–1989). On boxing: Notes on the past, present and future of a sport in transition. *Current Psychology: Research and Reviews, 7,* 331–346.

Donnelly, P. (1994). Take my word for it: Trust in the context of birding and mountaineering. *Qualitative Sociology, 17,* 215–241.

Donnelly, P. (1999). Gulliver's travels: A sport sociologist among the labcoats. *Journal of Sport and Social Issues, 23,* 455–458.

Donnelly, P. (2000, November). *Sticking my neck out!: Taking risks in the sociology of sport.* Presidential address presented at the North American Society for the Sociology of Sport annual meeting, Colorado Springs, CO.

Donnelly, P., & Young, K. (1988). The construction and confirmation of identity in sport subcultures. *Sociology of Sport Journal, 5,* 223–240.

Douglas, M. (1992). Risk and danger. In: M. Douglas (Ed.), *Risk and blame: Essays in cultural theory* (pp. 38–54). London: Routledge.

Douglas, M., & Calvez, M. (1990). The self as risk taker: A cultural theory of contagion in relation to AIDS. *Sociological Review, 38,* 445–464.

Douglas, M., & Wildavsky, A. (1982a). How can we know the risks we face?: Why risk selection is a social process. *Risk Analysis, 2,* 49–51.

Douglas, M., & Wildavsky, A. (1982b). *Risk and culture: An essay on the selection of technical and environmental dangers.* Berkeley: University of California Press.

Drasdo, H. (1972). *Education and the Mountain Centres.* Llanrwst: Tyddyn Gabriel.

Drasdo, H. (1981). The nature and reason of risk taking. *Climber & Rambler, 20* (April), 52–54, 56.

Dunk, T. W. (1991). *It's a working man's town: Male working-class culture.* Montréal & Kingston: McGill-Queen's University Press.

Freud, S. (1920/1990). *Beyond the pleasure principle.* New York: Norton.

Freud, S. (1929/1989). *Civilization and its discontents.* New York: Norton.

Fuller, P. (1977). *The champions: Secret motives in games and sports.* New York: Urizen.

Giddens, A. (1990). *The consequences of modernity.* Stanford, CA: Stanford University Press.

Giddens, A. (1991). *Modernity and self-identity: Self and society in the late modern age.* Stanford, CA: Stanford University Press.

Giddens, A. (1999). *Runaway world.* London: Profile Books.

Gigerenzer, G. (2002). *Reckoning with risk: Learning to live with uncertainty.* London: Allen Lane.

Goffman, E. (1967). *Interaction ritual: Essays on face-to-face behavior.* New York: Anchor Books.

Gould, S. J. (1983). *The mismeasure of man.* New York: Norton.

Granovetter, M. (1985). Economic action and social structure: The problem of embeddedness. *American Journal of Sociology, 91,* 481–510.

Haberl, J. (1997). *Risking adventure.* Vancouver: Raincoast Books.

Hoggart, R. (1957). *The uses of literacy.* Harmondsworth, UK: Penguin.

Hughes, R., & Coakley, J. (1991). Positive deviance among athletes: The implications of overconformity to the sport ethic. *Sociology of Sport Journal, 8,* 307–325.

Hume, M. (2002). You've nothing to fear but fear itself. *New Statesman,* 22 July, p. 48.

Investor Services (2000). *Estimating global road fatalities* (www.factbook.net).

Katz, J. (1988). *The seductions of crime.* New York: Basic Books.

Labash, M. (2001). What's wrong with dodgeball: The new phys ed and the wussification of America. *The Weekly Standard,* 25 June, 17–25.

Leiss, W., & Chociolko, C. (1994). *Risk and responsibility.* Montréal & Kingston: McGill-Queen's University Press.

Lewis, O. (1961). *Children of Sanchez.* New York: Random House.

Lewis, O. (1965). *La vida.* New York: Random House.

Lewontin, R. (1991). *Biology as ideology: The doctrine of DNA.* Concord, ON: Anansi.

Luhmann, N. (1993). *Risk: A sociological theory.* New York: Aldine de Gruyter.

Lyng, S. (1990). Edgework: A social psychological analysis of voluntary risk taking. *American Journal of Sociology, 95,* 851–886.

MacGregor, D. (2002). Sugar bear in the hot zone: Understanding and interpreting the political basis of traffic safety. In: J. P. Rothe (Ed.), *Driving lessons: Exploring systems that make traffic safer* (pp. 125–142). Edmonton: University of Alberta Press.

Miller, E. (1991). Assessing the risk of inattention to class, race/ethnicity, and gender: Comment on Lyng. *American Journal of Sociology, 96,* 1530–1534.

Mitchell, R. (1983). *Mountain experience: The psychology and sociology of adventure.* Chicago: University of Chicago Press.

Nixon, H. (1992). A social network analysis of influences on athletes to play with pain and injuries. *Journal of Sport and Social Issues, 16,* 127–135.

O'Dowd, C. (2000). Don't leave me here to die. *Guardian,* 15 February, pp. 4–5.

Ogilvie, B. (1973). The stimulus addicts. *The Physician and Sportsmedicine* (November), 61–65.

O'Malley, P., & Mugford, S. (1994). Crime, excitement and modernity. In: G. Barak (Ed.), *Criminology: Readings from a dynamic perspective* (pp. 189–211). Westport, CT: Praeger.

Petrie, A. (1967). *Individuality in pain and suffering.* Chicago: University of Chicago Press.

Porro, N. (2000, March). *Response to Donnelly's 'victory at all costs!: Taking risks in 20th century war and sport.'* Keynote address presented at the Japanese Society for the Sociology of Sport annual conference, Tokyo, Japan.

Powter, G. *et al.* (1997). Whose risk is it?: In the always risky and sometimes dangerous world of outdoor pursuits, where does responsibility end and liability begin? *Explore, 87* (August/September), 51–58.

Quadrel, M., Fischoff, B., & Davis, W. (1993). Adolescent (in)vulnerability. *American Psychologist, 48*, 102–116.

Rose, D., & Douglas, E. (2000). *Regions of the heart: The triumph and tragedy of Alison Hargreaves*. London: Penguin.

Rose, S. (1984). *Not in our genes: Biology, ideology and human nature*. London: Penguin.

Safai, P. (2002, November). Risk, risked and risky identities: Articulating risk-taking in sport with Beck's *Risk Society*. Paper presented at the North American Society for the Sociology of Sport annual conference, Indianapolis, IN.

Sales, S. M., Guydosh, R. M., & Iacona, W. (1974). Relationship between 'strength of the nervous system' and need for stimulation. *Journal of Personality and Social Psychology, 29*, 16–22.

Shoalts, D. (2002). Doctors worry about lost coverage. *Globe & Mail*, 22 October, S1.

Simpson, J. (1997). *Dark shadows falling*. Seattle: Mountaineers.

Thompson, M. (1980). The aesthetics of risk. In: R. Schwing, & A. Albers (Eds), *Societal risk assessment: How safe is safe enough?* (pp. 273–285). New York: Plenum Press.

Transport Canada (2000). *The state of road safety in Canada in 1998* (www.tc.gc.ca/roadsafety).

University of California, Irvine (2002). *Press release: Attention-deficit hyperactivity disorder related to advantageous gene: More genetic links found*. 8 January (www.ucihealth.com).

Weiss, R. (1987). Risk-taking behavior 'epidemic'. *Calgary Herald*, 9 October, p. C10.

Young, K. (1993). Violence, risk and liability in male sports culture. *Sociology of Sport Journal, 10*, 373–396.

Young, K. (1997). Women, sport, and physicality: Preliminary findings from a Canadian study. *International Review for the Sociology of Sport, 32*, 297–305.

Young, K., & White, P. (1995). Sport, physical danger and injury: The experiences of elite women athletes. *Journal of Sport and Social Issues, 19*, 45–61.

Young, K., White, P., & McTeer, W. (1994). Body talk: Male athletes reflect on sport, injury, and pain. *Sociology of Sport Journal, 11*, 175–194.

Zuckerman, M. (1979). *Sensation seeking: Beyond the optimal level of arousal*. Hillsadale, NJ: Erlbaum Associates.

Zweig, P. (1974). *The adventurer*. New York: Basic Books.

Chapter 2

The Politics of Sports Injury: Hierarchy, Power, and the Pain Principle

Donald Sabo

> One of the effects of civilization (not to say one of the ingredients in it) is that the spectacle, and even the very idea, of pain, is kept more and more out of the sight of those classes who enjoy in their fullness the benefits of civilization.
>
> J. S. Mill, Civilization (1963)
>
> Power is cautious. It covers itself. It bases itself in another's pain and prevents all recognition that there is 'another' by looped circles that ensure its own solipsism.
>
> Elaine Scarry, The Body in Pain (1985)

Sports injuries have been primarily understood in the context of the biomedical model in which injury and pain are regarded as essentially physiological phenomena. Physicians, athletic trainers, physical therapists, and exercise physiologists generally think about sports injury within clinical frames of reference. The locus of their ministrations is the athlete body. They mend the broken floating rib, the torn cartilage, the sprained ankle. Pain is diagnosed and treated mainly as a side-effect of physical injury, an orthopedic event, a biomechanical mishap, a muscular aberration, or an "isolated biomedical symptom of a discrete body" (Glucklich 2001: 210). But critics of the biomedical model say it ignores human meaning in the interpretation of pain. As David Morris (1991) puts it,

Sporting Bodies, Damaged Selves
Research in the Sociology of Sport, Volume 2, 59–79
© 2004 Published by Elsevier Ltd.
ISSN: 1476-2854/doi:10.1016/S1476-2854(04)02002-3

"...pain is never simply a matter of nerves and neurotransmitters but always requires a personal and cultural encounter with meaning" (p. 267).

Psychologists have been interested in the psychosocial aspects of sports injury, including emotional responses such as denial, fear, anxiety, anger, and depression. Athletic trainers focus on the emotional aspects of rehabilitation and recovery from sports injury. It is assumed that an injured body is attached to an individual psychology — the sprained ankle is attached to the strained psyche. The emotional impacts of sports injury include grief reaction, identity loss, denying feelings, fear and anxiety, loss of short-term goals, and lack of confidence. Injuries are accompanied by social-psychological processes that can shape rehabilitation and recovery. An athlete's coping skills and approach to pain management can also be influenced by his or her social support system. The reactions of parents and peers can lessen the impacts of social isolation that often result from injury, thereby promoting physical and emotional recovery. The behaviours of physicians, coaches, and trainers are also important in framing the athlete's interpretations of the injury as well as promoting effective rehabilitation.

Sociologists focus on social and cultural aspects of sports injury, links between sports violence and injury, and how gender socialisation influences athletes' perceptions of injury (Nixon 1994). The functionalist approach says that many sports entail aggression which, in turn, elevates risk for injury. Norms emerge within sport subcultures that justify aggression and rationalise pain and injury. Critical sport sociologists, in contrast, contextualise violence and injury within relations of power and exploitation (Young 2000). For example, Young and White (2000) discuss sports injury in relation to the social construction of hegemonic masculinity (Connell 1987). Male athletes learn to take physical risks and accept injury and pain partly through their identification with traditional masculinity (Young et al. 1994). Conformity to traditional masculinity, in turn, promises to reap rewards within the larger hierarchy of masculinities that comprise the gender order, such as social recognition and upward mobility. However, many male athletes are exploited and damaged by their struggles to establish masculine adequacy and social advancement within the larger gender hierarchy.

This chapter draws on critical feminist perspectives in order to argue that current thinking about sports injury and pain is infiltrated by cultural beliefs that reflect and reproduce forms of social hierarchy in sport and society. My analysis is situated in what McKay and Rowe (1987) called the "critical paradigm" of sport and media studies, in which strands of structuralism, political economy, and cultural studies find theoretical confluence in an effort to explicate relations of domination in patriarchal capitalist societies. Critical sociologists recognise that we live in webs of hierarchical relationships which, in turn, position individuals and groups in different ways. While some groups are relatively advantaged by the flux of power relations and economic conditions, others are relatively disadvantaged. In North American societies, for example, whites have had it better economically than blacks, just as the upper- and middle-classes enjoyed greater political influence than the lower- and under-classes. Once established, relations of social inequality generate ideas and beliefs that, in turn, tend to legitimate and reproduce the inequities (Bourdieu 2001).

Feminist theories are also deployed in order to call attention to gender as a key linking concept that furthers analysis of a broad configuration of structural, ideological, institutional, semiotic, and psychological processes that surround sports injury and pain (Burstyn 1999; Messner & Sabo 1990; Sabo & Jansen 1998). Feminist scholars emphasise the patriarchal origins and legacies of social hierarchies that are generally dominated by men, where women are relatively powerless in various institutional contexts, and boys grow up and take their place in niches within intermale dominance hierarchies (Hartman 1981; Lerner 1986).

The thesis developed here contends that patriarchy profoundly influences many contemporary customs, religious beliefs, political institutions, family relations, sexuality, medicine, and our understanding of sports, sports injury, pain, and the body itself. My argument builds on a concept developed in the mid-1980's called the "pain principle," which refers to a constellation of patriarchal beliefs and customs that has influenced much of our understanding of sports injury and pain (Sabo 1986).

My interest in pain and injury in sport began when I was a former NCAA Division I defensive football player. I saw a fair share of injuries, giving them and getting them. These athletic exploits resulted in many years of chronic back pain that eventually required a double-level, lower-lumbar fusion. Freed from the grip of pain, I began to systematically analyse how I had encountered so much pain. I realised that many others had been hurt by some of the games people play in our culture. I have since combed anthropological, historical, and sociological writings and research on pain, as well as relevant writing in medicine, epidemiology, gender studies, sports psychology, and sports sociology. I conducted interviews with thirty former athletes (both females and males) who now live with chronic pain which, in their judgement, resulted from over-training or a severe sports injury (Sabo 1994). This chapter draws on these experiences, research findings, and interdisciplinary reading.

The Paradox of Pain and Injury in Sport

Injury is everywhere in sport. Its ubiquity is evident in the lives and bodies of athletes who regularly experience bruises, torn ligaments, broken bones, aches, lacerations, and muscle tears. "Injury reports" appear in daily newspapers and in the jabber of television and radio commentators. *Sports Illustrated* markets its subscription campaign by giving new readers videotaped highlights of football players smashing one another's bodies. Sports medicine has become a burgeoning billion-dollar industry, and professional turf wars are waging among orthopedists, exercise physiologists, athletic trainers, and physical therapists that will decide who will treat the hundreds-of-thousands of sports injuries each year.

Despite the omnipresence of injury in sport, there are curious silences surrounding the pain that injuries produce. First, athletes rarely discuss their pain. Their suffering is hidden behind concentrated gazes, competitive determination, upbeat interview facades, and post-game grins. As a former professional hockey player described the collective blindness of athletes to injuries: "We just take it as an injury. You know the guy is hurt, and that's an injury. It really can't be helped. It happens. You really don't think anything about it." Second, locker room subcultures tend to erase pain from consciousness. Slogans glorify pain only to slickly slide it into non-existence. The phrase "No pain, no gain" beckons athletes to "push yourself to the limit," "sacrifice your body," and "pay the price for victory." Such slogans encourage athletes to disregard pain, or in the words of my interviewees, to "get beyond the pain," to "work through the pain," or to "perform in spite of pain." Coaches often ignore, manage, or minimise the suffering of athletes. Former baseball manager "Sparky" Anderson once remarked about an injured player, "pain don't hurt" (quoted by Mayo 1989: G2).

Third, fans and media also cloak the pain in sport by heroising injured athletes. Fallen competitors who rise from the turf or court are enlivened by applause and cheers. Media commentators extol the courage and dedication of injured athletes who overcome pain in order to play the game. Images of heroic athletes, once produced and disseminated in the culture at large, take on a life of their own. Such heroic images not only belie the pain of individuals, but also the socio-cultural and exploitative processes that precipitate victimisation itself.

And finally, while researchers and medical practitioners profit from the study and treatment of sports injury, they have been generally silent about athlete pain. Few epidemiological studies have calculated the health risks associated with contact sports. Researchers have determined the relative risks for cirrhosis of the liver, hypertension, heart disease, suicide, and homicide by age, race/ethnicity, socioeconomic status, and lifestyle factors such as smoking and alcohol consumption. This means that public health advocates and individual consumers can judge whether or not they should monitor their blood pressure, quit smoking, cut back on alcohol consumption, or see a therapist. Parents and educators can rely on research evidence to advise young people about how to lead healthier life styles. In contrast, there is a lack of research to help inform parents or athletes about long-term risks incurred by contact sports participation for arthritis, chronic back problems, knee pain, or hip replacement surgery. Where are the longitudinal studies of links between youth sports participation and adult health outcomes? Little is known about the relative risk that young gymnasts, divers, swimmers, rugby players, football players, long distance runners, triple-jumpers, or boxers encounter with regard to the experience chronic pain in adulthood. These questions cannot be answered because medical researchers have not done the homework and, I suggest, the paucity of analytical research *is itself* an expression of a wider cultural denial of athletic pain.

Around 1990 I met with two researchers from a university School of Social and Preventive Medicine to propose a retrospective, case-control study of the "long-range orthopedic impacts and pain symptoms among former participants in intercollegiate contact sports." One researcher was enthused about the idea of doing such a groundbreaking study, but the other squashed the project. The latter explained, "We already know what the outcomes will be. Of course they'll be elevated risk levels for the former athletes. And this study would be bad for sport. It'll make sport look bad." In effect, this perception endorsed the status quo of sport while abandoning scientific (and humane) concern for the well-being of athletes. It seems that sport, like war, has obvious casualties. But to focus on the casualties rather than the beneficiaries of an institutional process undermines the credibility of the institution itself. To ignore the casualties, in contrast, bolsters the legitimacy of institutional practices.

In our culture, therefore, we observe a curious paradox. We discuss injury but fail to listen to the pain. We valorise sports injuries but deny their physical and emotional consequences. We capitalise on sports injury without truly empathising with the injured. We diagnose bodies without souls, knees without psyches, and we continue to treat individual symptoms without regard of the institutional realities that produce the symptoms in the first place. We accept sport practices that put thousands of athletes at risk for short-range injury and long-range suffering. In effect, we create small armies of wounded athletes and former-athletes who limp and grimace through their daily routines, but we do not try to understand what the war is all about.

Why are we in denial? What is it about sport in American and other cultures that breeds the collective silences around the emotional and physical pain of athletes? Or, to tap J. S. Mill's quote above, who "enjoys in their fullness the benefits" of the cultural production and denial of pain in sport? Below I argue that the cultural paradox between visible injury and invisible pain in sport derives, in part, from the existence of the "pain principle."

The Pain Principle

The pain principle is a pervasive narrative or cluster of meanings that became insinuated in western Judao-Christian cultural traditions (Sabo 1986). The pain principle is defined as a patriarchal cultural belief that pain is inevitable and that the endurance of pain enhances one's character and moral worth. Pain is regarded as more important than pleasure, and sacrifice is assumed to be required in order to establish self-worth, social acceptance, and status gains.

I speculate that the pain principle emerged coterminously with the development of male-dominated social organisations. Indeed, it served as a kind of ideological crucible within patriarchal societies that allowed male elites to justify their advantaged status and rationalise the oppression of women, lesser-status males, and children. A variety of scholars have woven a conceptual framework for understanding links between pain, culture and power relations. Thomas Szasz (1975) observed that in modern American and Western European culture, pain has been viewed as either good or bad. "Bad" pain is unpleasurable and, therefore, should be removed. "Good" pain indicates to the self and others "that we are good or trying to be good" (p. 249). Pain and suffering are "readily substituted for realistic effort and accomplishment" (p. 249). At work or play, pain and suffering are thus transformed and ennobled.

Ariel Glucklich's (2001) descriptive overview of pain and suffering in religious literatures and practices around the world shows how culture can shift and mould the meaning of pain. He writes, "the task of sacred pain is to transform destructive or disintegrative suffering into a positive religious-psychological mechanism for reintegration within a more deeply valued level of reality than individual existence" (p. 6).

The theoretical recognition that power relations constitute and are constituted by the infliction of pain and its symbolic meanings is developed in Elaine Scarry's (1985) analysis of the structures of war and torture. She contends, "the main purpose and outcome of war is injuring" (1985: 65). Despite the massive injuring in war, however, the perpetuation of war requires that the injuring and pain are "eclipsed from view" (p. 64). Although pain is an individual experience, it is also a linguistic component within the power relations that constitute war itself. Scarry's analysis is supplemented by Kate Millett's (1994) work on the torture of political prisoners, which examines the ties between the infliction of pain, gender identity, and power relations.

Finally, Riane Eisler (1988) studied archeological and mythological evidence in order to track the emergence of patriarchal societies in prehistory. Patriarchal societies adopted a "dominator model" of social organisation, where brutality, warfare, and oppression were common. Dominator societies conquered and displaced those societies organised in accordance with a "partnership model," where men and women enjoyed parity of status and violence was the exception not the rule. In her later work, she argues that dominator societies sacralised and institutionalised pain rather than pleasure, thereby extending and solidifying patriarchal power (Eisler 1995). Eisler sees many forces of cultural transformation in our own time as "an attempt to shift to a system where pleasure — not in the sense of a short-term escape or distraction, but in the sense of healthy, long-term fulfillment — can instead be institutionalized, and even sacralized" (1995: 11).

These scholarly works show that, contrary to many religious and philosophical contentions, pain and suffering are not *universal* aspects of the human condition, but rather, the extent and character of pain vary greatly across persons, groups, cultures, and historical time. Human suffering is socially, culturally, and historically variant. For example, labourers in North America are more likely to experience injury and disability than middle-class managers and corporate executive officers (Young & White 2000); morbidity and mortality are more prevalent among the poor than the rich. In short, pain and suffering are significantly related to social inequality. The pain principle, I suggest, not only disguises the existence of various hierarchies of pleasure and suffering, but it also legitimates and reproduces various forms of male-dominated hierarchies within the current gender order. The biblical story of Abraham helps illustrate this theoretical claim.

In Genesis, verse 22, God said to Abraham, "Take your son, your only son Isaac, whom you love, and go to the region of Moriah. Sacrifice him there as a burnt offering on one of the mountains I will tell you about." The next morning Abraham gathered supplies, saddled his mule, and set off for the mountains with Isaac and two of his servants. They traveled for three days until reaching an appropriate site whereupon Abraham "took the wood for the burnt offering and placed it on his son Isaac, and he himself carried the fire and the knife." Isaac probably feeling a bit ill at ease wonders aloud, "Father? . . . The fire and wood are here . . . but where is the lamb for the burnt offering?" His father assures him that, "God himself will provide the lamb for the burnt offering, my son." Abraham and Isaac build the altar together, arrange the fire wood, and then the dutiful father proceeds to tie up his son, place him on the wood pier, and raise his knife to slay the boy. At the last second, the angel of the Lord calls out from heaven,

> Abraham, Abraham . . . Do not lay a hand on the boy. Do not do anything to him. Now I know that you fear God, because you have not withheld from me your son, your only son. . . . I swear by myself, declares the Lord, that because you have done this and have not withheld your son, your only son, I will surely bless you and make your descendants as numerous as the stars in the sky and

as the sand on the seashore. Your descendants will take possession of the cities of their enemies, and through your offspring all nations on earth will be blessed, because you have obeyed me (Genesis 22).

The testing of Abraham lays bare the two central structural processes within patriarchal societies; that is, sex inequality (inequality between males and females) and intermale dominance hierarchies (inequality among males). First, when commanded by God to murder and burn his son, Abraham does not apparently consult with his wife Sarah, Isaac's mother. Abraham is the elite leader of his people and household, and both Sarah and Isaac are appendages of his patriarchal authority. Likewise, the other husbands and fathers in Abraham's tribe had authority over their wives, children and servants. Second, the story reveals the male status hierarchy within biblical times with God the father residing on top, followed by male angels, Abraham the ranking male on earth, Isaac, and manservants. Whereas Abraham is shown to be in complicity with God's will, so too do Isaac and the two manservants obey the father and master respectively. Abraham's religious motivation masks the fact that he was willing to hurt and kill his son in order to maintain his authority and position. Here the maintenance of the intermale dominance hierarchy depended on the threat of violence and male conformity at several levels. Finally, if Abraham actually cared for his son, it is worth noting that he suppressed his emotions in order to obey God and wreak havoc on those he loved. In the end, the promise of blind obedience paid off for Abraham — his son lived, and he was "blessed" with many descendants, riches, and military victories. The lessons for men are clear: regard women as subservient, obey male authority and prosper, inflict pain and violence if necessary, endure suffering if required.

These Old Testament intersections between patriarchy, gender identity formation, and the infliction of pain are also evident in the anthropological literature on male initiation rites (Benedict 1959; Herdt 1982; Godelier 1986; Moore 1986). Masculinity rites in male-dominated societies contain several common elements. First, older males typically define the cultural situation for younger males. Second, men in authority enact various methods to induce conformity to social rules and appropriate modes of male behaviour. Third, male initiation typically unfolds in sex-segregated settings, and boys are isolated from girls and the taint of femininity. Finally, male initiation rites are filled with the infliction of pain. When boys successfully endure ritualised pain, it guarantees status within the male hierarchy and, furthermore, sets boys apart from and above girls and women.

Many of these elements of primitive initiation rites are also evident in contemporary sport rituals in North American society. For example, Sabo and

Panepinto (1990) studied coach-player relationships in the sport of football. Older male coaches supervise young boys in sex-segregated environments. Cultural lore emphasises manliness, sex differences, and the pursuit of gender-appropriate ideals and goals. Coaches usually insist on conformity to the rules and requirements of the intermale dominance hierarchy. Finally, boys are expected to make sacrifices and to endure the physical and emotional pain associated with training, injury, and loss. In summary, the pain principle is present in sport culture and the life experiences of athletes.

It is impossible to measure or even estimate the extent to which the patriarchal moorings of the pain principle influence contemporary thinking and cultural practices surrounding human suffering and exploitation or, more specifically, the suffering of athletes. Postmodernism has been described as a condition in which overarching, metanarratives lose their cultural pre-eminence (Lash 1990). Yet postmodernists also recognise that these vast explanatory systems may, in turn, encompass many smaller narratives. While it is true that ancient patriarchal beliefs and religious customs pertaining to pain no longer hold as much cultural sway today, there is also a remarkable persistence of male dominance and patriarchal cultural beliefs across world cultures. For example, religious justifications for patriarchal authority are less common in developed nations than in emerging or developing nations. Women's roles in the family and post-industrial workplace have changed during the 19th and 20th centuries, and patriarchal privileges and customs have been challenged by women's liberation movements and progressive forces. However, male-dominated social hierarchies remain largely in tact — even in post-industrial economies. Christian fundamentalism spreads in the west while Islamic fundamentalism grows in the east. In May 2002, the middle-aged American male president, George W. Bush, sat down with the elderly male pope in the Vatican and expressed their respect for life, coded language for a mutual antipathy for women's reproductive rights, the latter a basic tenet of women's rights as outlined by Second Wave feminisms. War, a prototypically patriarchal institution (Connell 2000), is still a feature of 21st century international relations. Worldwide expenditures on the sexual trafficking of women, girls, and boys are comparable to money spent on international drug trade (Herzog 2000). In sport, while women's participation and media presence in developed nations have swelled during the last fifty years, men still control the International Olympic Committee, the Olympic Games, national sport governing bodies, professional sports, sports medicine, sport media, coaching, and athletic administration (Hargreaves 2000).

Contrary to postmodernist claims, therefore, reports of the demise of patriarchy are premature. Patriarchal culture may no longer be unitary, but it is remarkably pervasive. Although male hegemony is being challenged, resisted and eroded, it is still active, resonant, and powerful in countless institutional contexts. So, too, the pain principle continues to influence our lives — outside and inside sport.

Sport, Patriarchy, and the Pain Principle

The pain principle weaves through sport and the bodies and identities of athletes in many ways. Most men and women athletes I have interviewed "grew up" in sport subcultures and embraced tenets of the pain principle. Generally, as their athletic career unfolded, the amount of discipline and punishment encroaching on their daily life, body, and consciousness steadily escalated. When asked about their earliest involvements with sport, they reported "just having fun," "playing," "running," "skating," or "being free just to be physical." They basked in bodily movement and sensation. As training progressed and competitive expertise increased, however, the physical skills required to "play" became progressively specialised, regimented, and habitualised in order to meet the institutional demands of the coach, the team, the organisation, the institution, and ultimately, the hierarchy. Play became work. The athlete body became constituted in ways that maximised the power and autonomy of authorities (e.g. coaches, athletic administrators, owners) and minimised the felt freedom, sensuality, and autonomy of the athlete.

The athletes gradually learned to stifle awareness of their bodies and to limit emotional expression. Learning to suppress emotion and deny pain was often done to please the coach. Coaches value the denial of pain because it facilitates athlete conformity and coach control. Coaches also teach athletes how to interpret the physical sensations and emotions that attend sports injury and pain. In the film *The Program*, a drama about "bigtime" college football, the head coach (played by James Cahn) asks a freshman tailback who has just been hit hard by a monster linebacker, "Are you injured or are you hurt?" The befuddled player asks, "What does that mean?" The coach responds, "Well, if you're hurt, you can still play. If you injured, you can't." The young rookie musters his resolve, sucks it up, and returns to practice.

Learning to Embrace Pain

Varying degrees of injury and pain inevitably accompany athletic training and competition. Athletes not only learn to accept injuries and acute or chronic pain as part of sport, their perceptions of pain and injury also become grafted to their identities and bodies. As a sport career progresses, athlete identity suffuses with the overall identity of the child or adolescent. "Joe" or "Mary" are no longer simply the "eighth-grade boy" and "sophomore university coed" respectively; they become Joe "the soccer player who made the traveling team," and Mary "the distance runner who trains hard and has a decent chance to compete in the Olympic Games someday." So, too, do the tolerance and acceptance of physical and emotional pain become embedded in the constructs of being a "good" or "successful" athlete, the projection of personal identity into the future, and an individual's acceptance by friends, parents, school officials, and coaches. The subjective experience of being in pain or playing with pain, therefore, becomes associated with positive social and psychological outcomes; e.g. pain signifies potential stardom or personal determination. As individuals sharpen the capacity to interpret and signify injury and pain in socially meaningful ways, they get better at tolerating and denying pain. And as the athlete's personal transformation unfolds, as the embrace of pain tightens, he or she becomes more fully integrated into the hierarchical relations that comprise the sport.

Intricate contradictions operate here. When an athlete is said to "have what it takes," it means that he or she has the individual skills and ascetic will to personally succeed. But it also means that he or she will meet the needs of the organisation and those who control it. In short, athlete subservience to pain, whether it takes the cultural form of stoicism or glorification, derives from and reinforces the hierarchical relations within sport and wider society. The following examples from interviews show how the capacity to embrace pain develops across an athletic career.

A former professional ice hockey player who "had to hit in order to survive" recalled getting used to cuts, aches and small injuries as a boy and, later during his junior hockey days (age 16–19), the number and severity of injuries increased. He observed, "When you're young and dumb, it's easier to get through the pain." He listed an array of injuries sustained as a professional player.

> Separated shoulders were bad. I had a lot of those. I broke my ankle, I broke my big toe, I broke my small toe. I tore ligaments in my leg . . . this leg here. I tore ligaments in this knee. I injured the knee cap on this knee here — never did find out what it was, but it was there a long time. I pulled groins. Rib cartilage has been torn numerous times . . . a lot, a lot. My pelvis was thrown out of whack and it had to be put back in. My hips, by the end of the season, from hip-checking, what I did best, everything on the right side was black-and-blue, about half way up my rib cage and halfway down my leg, and everything on this side was one continuous bruise. That wouldn't go away until training camp, and then you started all over again the next year. I had an operation on my shoulder here.

My elbow was dislocated, this thumb was broken, my wrist was broken. I had my first serious concussion playing junior hockey. As a pro, I started wearing a helmet, but I took that off because you were a chicken shit if you wore a helmet. Then the final injury was I fractured my neck. That was the end of my career.

While his early days in hockey were "fun" and "physically exhilarating," he played out his career addicted to pain pills and Valium. He learned early that players who talked too much about their pain and injuries were "whiners" and "complainers."

"Lisa" is a former downhill skier who endured years of knee pain and several surgeries before being forced out of the sport. She has been on skis since the age of two, progressing from being the little girl who went out to the slopes with her parents to a high-powered adolescent competitor with Olympic potential and aspirations. She learned to accept muscular pain, body aches, and minor injuries as "a normal part of training." Though "the training was difficult, as all ski training is," she regarded the pain as necessary and normal. The coach "pushed her physical limits" and put her on diets. She indicated, "When you're a kid everybody in authority, whether they're teachers or coaches, you're not suspicious of them. By their very nature, if they ask you to do something you kind of don't like, you groan and moan and think why is he making me do this, but you do it." For Lisa, chronic bruises became emblematic of self-worth and technical expertise. She explained:

> You get bruised from the gates, by going through the gates . . . You go around the gates so closely and where they spring back up, you can get hit and you can get bruised. I looked like I was being beaten with something, because I had bruises all on my back and my shoulders and my chest and stuff . . . At times I looked like an abused child . . . But these (bruises) were nothing, you know, nothing that I considered an injury.

Lisa did not perceive the bruises as injury and the pain as problematic. Indeed her teammates and coach defined them as a by-product of training and competition and, even favourably, as an indicator of good technique. She recalled how her teammates would show one another their bruises: "Yeah, look at this bruise," and they'd say, "well at least you're keeping close to the gates." Lisa's story shows how the shared denial of injury and positive interpretation of painful bruising fostered cohesion among team members under the coach's supervision. When athletes tell one another war stories or exhibit their scars and braces, they reiterate the pain principle in an effort to telegraph status and inclusion.

Getting Hooked on Getting Hurt

The interviews with former athletes revealed that they do not accept injury and valorise pain because pain feels good. The pain principle is about sacrifice, not masochism. Athletes know that injuries hurt. But they also stay involved with sport long after the pain sets in because, in their minds and identities, both sport and the pain it brings signify something important to them.

John, a former rugby player, for example, reported that he originally played for his father's approval and, later, as he got better at the sport, for recognition from his peers. The external recognition he received from rugby filled the fissures of his developing identity with a kind of epoxy that kept his self-concept whole through the thick and thin of life. Tammy, a 26 year-old former intercollegiate swimmer who "blew out" her shoulders and can no longer raise her arms above her neckline, reported that she competed in order to "maintain a healthy self-image" and "become an independent woman." She explained that swimming "helped keep my body toned" and "enabled me to feel good about myself." She grew up in a traditional family where she consciously identified with her professional father and not her mother who was a traditional housewife. When overtraining and improper coaching translated into chronic shoulder pain, her parents asked her, "Why do you insist on working out when it hurts you so?" Tammy perceived her pain as a physical marker of her growing independence.

Getting hooked on getting hurt is not merely a psychological process. Individual athletes adopt cultural meanings that valorise suffering and edify the experience of injury. Suffering gets linked to tradition and honour or the promise of good things to come. Praise and popularity assuage physical hurt, somehow making injury worth enduring. Moreover, as Foucault (1977) might observe, the structural blueprints and cultural messages surrounding pain in sport are not simply internalised by consciousness, they are mediated through, coded within, and incorporated by the body. It takes discipline to suffer athleticism. As athlete identity is constructed across a lifetime, the body and physical movement are shaped, regulated, and organised in ways that are consonant with and ultimately subjugated by cultural definitions of "injury," "pain," and "athlete."

Meritocratic Pain

As the athletes I interviewed matured into young adults, the pain principle became a strategic formula for upward mobility in their minds. A female distance runner endured pain and suffering to get a university athletic scholarship. A male professional hockey player "played aggressively and took risks" to "keep the owners happy and the money coming in" and to be "somebody who people looked up to." A male "golden gloves" boxer battled chronic headaches "to escape the street and stay out of prison." In each case, the endurance of pain represented individual merit and social success.

"Meritocratic pain" occurs when individuals believe that the endurance of pain will help them achieve upward mobility. The meanings attached to meritocratic pain originate outside the individual athlete as cultural beliefs; that is, suffer now and get ahead later, everybody pays a price for success, you have to pay your dues. In process and effect, meritocratic pain is a form of hierarchical maintenance that expresses and fuels itself through psychological and somatic process. The practice of pain management (emotionally and physically) becomes increasingly internalised, habitualised, and physically incorporated. The experience of pain is subjectively transformed into the promise of moral superiority and upward mobility. And for those athletes who perform ably within the sport hierarchy, the strategy and sacrifice often *actually do* pay off; e.g. high school athletes receive scholarships to university, psychological health is buoyed up by social recognition, travel opportunities accrue, cardiovascular endurance is maintained, or eventually money arrives. Most individuals, however, are processed out of sport early in their careers. Often sacrifices are made in vain, and many athletes end up dealing with chronic pain long after the limelight has faded. Sport hierarchies are highly stratified and, just like other institutional structures within corporate capitalist economies, many are beckoned to scale the heights but few reach the top.

Although their goals differed greatly, almost all the athletes I interviewed perceived their pain at least partly as a life strategy in order to "fit into," "get ahead in," or "climb" a sport hierarchy. Their meritocratic pain was conflated by complex subjective longings which, in turn, fed and reflected multiple systems of domination. For many male athletes, the ascetic practices related directly to intermale rivalry, while female athletes viewed athletic success (and the pain it took to get it) as a benchmark of their struggle for mobility against *both* men and women. A closeted gay male baseball player endured physical injury and a verbally abusive coach in order to "make (a) bid for the semi-pros with the rest of the guys." Race or class fueled other athletes' exchange of suffering for status gains. A former African-American Olympian had used her track-and-field ability to escape southern racism and rural poverty. In her final career years, pain became "normal, a constant." She explained, "I learned to ignore the conscious experience of pain and injury. If my body mechanics could still function, they'd just shoot me up with a pain-killer before a race, and I'd run." Burstyn (1999) argues that violence in sport "functions to maintain a whole superstructure of complex inequalities — between genders, classes, races, abilities, languages, and so forth — structured in the characteristic modes of corporate capitalism" (p. 190). The same superstructure surrounds and animates the infliction, toleration, and uses of pain in sport.

Gender Similarities and Differences

Sport has been a key historical site for the construction of hegemonic masculinity (McKay *et al.* 2000). As sport developed in western civilization, there were significant intersections between athleticism, masculinity, and war (Malszecki 1996), each exhibiting cultural strands of the pain principle. Both athletes and warriors embodied traditionally masculine traits such as emotional inexpressivity, the capacity to objectify the body, violence proneness, and manly denial of physical pain. Sex segregation and stratification mainly kept girls outside of the ranks of athletes and warriors, hemmed in by culturally defined femininities. During the 20th century, however, girls and women entered sport in increasing numbers, and gender theorists and feminists now ask two key questions: Will women's increasing participation and visibility in sport make it more humane, less violent, more body-affirming, and less likely to affirm hegemonic masculinity? Or will women athletes be assimilated into male-dominated sports organisations, thereby adopting similar body-negating cultural practices and masculine traits as men? (Put more succinctly: Will women change sport or will sport change women?)

My interviews revealed similarities between the ways that male and female athletes learned to accept injuries, compete in pain, and comply with the demands of coaches. Both sexes pushed their bodies, downplayed the pain, and often forced themselves to practise when injured. However, the men's narratives about pain and injury typically did not include self-aware references to "macho" values, men's roles, or masculinity. Rather they reported acting out the script of the "athlete" who trains, gets strong, competes unrelentingly, expects to get injured, fights off the pain of injury, keeps his feelings to himself, and is loyal to the team and the coach. Pain and injury simply came with the territory of being an athlete, competing against other males, enjoying male camaraderie, and vying for status. Actions spoke louder than words.

In contrast, women's commentaries on sport injury and pain displayed a consciousness of gender that the men's commentaries did not. Several women athletes voiced skepticism about masculine approaches to sport and risk for injury. They distinguished themselves from male athletes even though, ironically, in many ways, they followed similar behavioural pathways to injury and chronic pain. As one female basketball player who was eventually hobbled by knee and ankle injuries stated, for example, "I always went out to play and the pain was always there, but I didn't see it as a macho thing. You simply had to play." A female swimmer observed that her coach "had us doing like men's workouts. The women were supposed to be just as good as the men. He thought the women would be just as good as the men. When they weren't, he'd scream at us, just like the men." While she resisted the perceptions that her chronic pain was a badge of masculine achievement or honour, she also did the same workouts as the men. Finally, a female tri-athlete who "could take low-grade pain forever" expressed her criticism of more manly approaches to pain and injury with this anecdote:

> He was a world champion and he won the Ironman the last couple of years. At the end of one Ironman, he ended up in the hospital with internal bleeding and took eight pints of blood. He has this ability to go into kind of a trance and run beyond his ability, and he is on such overdrive at that point, still functional, still running pretty hard, and still able to go at that level of pain. If he had backed off, he would have done better. He can push himself and is very similar to the movie *They Shoot Horses Don't They*. There are people who have the mind and ability to push physically until they kill themselves. Not me. I don't ever want to get there.

Some women athletes consciously adopted masculine rationales for dealing with their injury and pain. They are reminiscent of how Leslie Heywood's (1998) critical memoir of her formative years as a distance runner depicts a woman's identification with hegemonic masculinity in sport. Highly competitive, she aspired to dominate the field, to run against and beat the women and men. She aspired to be like male athletes, preferring what she perceived as masculine styles and cultural practices to what the girls were doing. Extreme training practices resulted in the development of chronic pain that she endured for years until becoming so crippled that she left the sport. In Third Wave feminist terms, she saw herself as a "male-identified woman" (Heywood & Drake 1997) who played out the masculine script only to become victimised like so many male athletes who preceded her.

There are contradictions at play here in both individual and social contexts. Male athletes commonly integrated traits associated with hegemonic masculinity (e.g. denial of pain, competitiveness, dominance striving, emotional inexpressivity) into their experiences with injury, but they did not recognise that these meanings are gendered in any way. Put simply, male athletes did not link their suffering to any critique of masculinity. Women athletes *were* aware that gendered meanings surrounded sports involvement and injury, and they were often skeptical of masculine scripts that glorified pain and underplayed suffering. Despite their insights, female athletes still complied with many of the same body-negating sport practices that the men did.

The interviews also revealed that male athletes were not as likely as female athletes to talk about injury and pain. Most male athletes were silent in the midst of their pain. A former World Football League "defensive end" with "bad knees" was typical. He saw everyday pain as "part of the game and you're going to bounce back from it. There's nothing you can do." While he assumed that the other players "knew" what he was going through, he never talked to them about his or their physical and emotional suffering. He added, "Once in a while I'd mention it to my fiancée." Several women athletes, in contrast, did talk to teammates about their injuries and pain, while most kept their suffering secret from coaches. One former female goalie for a junior hockey team (who ended up with a knee that "felt like a bowl full of oatmeal") said her coaches were "educated" and that she felt comfortable talking about her injuries.

Conclusion

The pain principle beckons athletes to sacrifice their bodies in order to attain merit and victory through various athletic rituals and body practices. At the individual level, the meanings associated with pain become grafted to identities, habitualised by physiology. The pain principle also hides athlete pain behind socially structured silences which, in turn, constitute dominant group interests and hierarchically organised power relations in sport. Many athletes "play along" and "suffer through" protracted injuries because to cry out in pain, to resist bodily risk and harm, would challenge the hierarchical status quo. Speaking out would jeopardise one's immediate status and long-range opportunities. As women enter sport in increasing numbers, they seem to be buying into the pain principle *behaviourally* but, in contrast to men athletes, many are disavowing its cultural associations with masculinity.

When young people enter sport and kick their first soccer ball, shoot their first basket, or run their first foot race, they take their first steps into a hierarchy. They soon learn that hierarchy breeds inequity, and inequity breeds pain. To remain stable, the hierarchy must either justify the pain or explain it away (Sabo 1986). Athletes, for better and worse, become increasingly caught up by and in complicity with multiple systems of domination. Some profit from athletic participation in the form of educational mobility, popularity gains, health benefits, bolstered confidence, and community prestige (Melnick *et al.* 2002; Miller *et al.* 1998; Sabo *et al.* 2002). Others are cut from teams, get their confidence shattered, suffer serious injury, or end up with chronic pain.

There is sad irony in an athlete's compliance to pain. The athlete is a powerful symbol of healthful vitality in our culture, and yet, the bodies of many athletes end up broken, battered, and in varying states of chronic pain (Messner 1992). The culture valorises the athlete who surmounts injury, endures pain, and returns to the field of hierarchical endeavour. Often, the greater the heights of athletic achievement, the greater the extent of objectification of the body and ascetic denial of pain. Paradoxically, as the body is "built up" in order to "move up" the competitive hierarchy, the body is increasingly "worn down." Many athletes become embroiled in a larger set of exploitative power relations inside and outside sport that lead to physical entropy. Within the context of the competitive hierarchies that comprise early 21st century capitalist patriarchy, athletes can be compared with success-striving, upwardly mobile middle managers who drive themselves into exhaustion and, after millions of little concessions to the pain principle over a period of years, get depressed or develop stress-related illness. Many athletes are like factory workers who accept unsafe working conditions or acquiesce to daily exposure to potentially harmful chemicals in order to make a living.

Recent discussions in critical sport studies recognise the paradoxes between positive and negative health outcomes in athletics (Sabo *et al.* 2004). Eitzen (1999) argues that sport is both healthy and unhealthy. Hargreaves (2000) notes that athletic participation can instill pride in women's bodies or facilitate pathogenic weight loss behaviour. Whereas athletic participation reduces risk for tobacco use and illicit drug use among USA high school students, the risk for alcohol use increases (Melnick *et al.* 2002; Miller *et al.* 1998; Sabo *et al.* 2002). Some youth sports experiences foster violence while others quell its expression (Gatz *et al.* 2002).

The pain principle resonates in the minds and hearts of many athletes, making risk for injury the norm. Male-dominated social hierarchies are still firmly entrenched in sport, and injury risk is built into its organisational dynamics. Individual survival and mobility require taking physical risks and, to one extent or another, learning to take pain in the bargain. In the process, some athletes are elevated and others are debilitated, some are empowered while others are subjugated. Competition in sport yields differential results, as it does in other hierarchical relations. Some people get rich from the ownership and management of fast food restaurants, while many people who eat fast food become obese, develop diabetes and hypertension, and die prematurely. Some investors cashed in on the rise and fall of Enron, while most were shattered by its collapse. Black and Latino men in the United States are imprisoned in record numbers, while corrections officers get their houses painted and buy new automobiles, and politicians use the fear of crime to get elected and solidify their power base (Sabo *et al.* 2001). In all social hierarchies, sacrifice and pain are distributed unequally and, in their quest for inclusion and advancement, individuals take their chances and, in effect, make their bargains with the devils of inequality. In sport, alternatives to male-dominated hierarchies mainly exist in the utopian visions of intellectuals and reformers but, in reality, they are few and far between. The vast majority of athletes — both females and males — end up dreaming their dreams and taking their competitive risks beneath the historical and cultural shadow of patriarchy.

Finally, biomedical and psychological approaches to understanding sports injury locate the source of the pain and responsibility for coping with the pain *inside* the individual. However, I have tried to show that each athlete's pain is also an expression of an outer world of people, events, inequalities, and cultural practices. The origins of our pain are *outside*, not inside, our skins. My hopes for reform are minimal. One feasible strategy is to make athlete pain visible and palpable, and to gradually replace the discourse of pain in sport with one that affirms physical and emotional health. Ennoble fitness not sacrifice, ensure safety not risk, seek pleasure and vitality and not pain, and construct partnerships not hierarchies.

References

Benedict, R. (1959). *Patterns of culture*. Boston: Houghton Mifflin.

Bourdieu, P. (2001). *Masculine domination*. Stanford, CA: Stanford University Press.

Burstyn, E. (1999). *The rites of men: Manhood, politics, and the culture of sport*. Toronto: University of Toronto Press.

Connell, R. W. (1987). *Gender and power: Society, the person, and sexual politics*. Stanford, CA: Stanford University Press.

Connell, R. W. (2000). *The men and the boys*. Berkeley, CA: University of California Press.

Eisler, R. (1988). *The chalice and the blade: Our history, our future*. New York: HarperCollins.

Eisler, R. (1995). *Sacred pleasure: Sex, myth, and the politics of the body*. San Francisco: Harper.

Eitzen, D. S. (1999). *Fair and foul: Beyond the myths and paradoxes of sport*. Boulder, CO: Rowman & Littlefield.

Foucault, M. (1977). *Discipline and punish: The birth of the prison* (A. Sheridan, Trans.). New York: Pantheon Books.

Gatz, M., Messner, M. A., & Ball-Rokeach, S. J. (Eds) (2002). *Paradoxes of youth and sport*. Albany, NY: State University of New York Press.

Glucklich, A. (2001). *Sacred pain: Hurting the body for the sake of the soul*. New York: Oxford University Press.

Godelier, M. (1986). *The making of great men: Male domination and power among the New Guinea Baruya*. Cambridge, England: Cambridge University Press.

Hargreaves, J. (2000). *Heroines of sport: The politics of difference and identity*. London: Routledge.

Hartman, H. (1981). The unhappy marriage of Marxism and feminism. In: L. Sargent (Ed.), *Women and revolution: A discussion of the unhappy marriage of marxism and feminism* (pp. 1–41). Boston: South End Press.

Herdt, G. (1982). Fetish and fantasy in Sambia initiation. In: G. H. Herdt (Ed.), *Rituals of manhood: Male initiation in papua new guinea* (pp. 44–98). Berkeley, CA: University of California Press.

Herzog, P. (2000). *Commentary on global aspects of women's health.* A presentation for the World Congress on Medicine and Health, Medicine Meets Millennium, July 30, Hannover, Germany.

Heywood, L. (1998). *Pretty good for a girl: A sports memoir.* New York: Free Press.

Heywood, L., & Drake, R. (Eds) (1997). *Third wave agenda: Being feminist, doing feminism.* Minneapolis: University of Minnesota Press.

Lash, S. (1990). *Sociology of postmodernism.* London: Routledge.

Lerner, G. (1986). *Creation of patriarchy.* New York: Oxford University Press.

Malszecki, G. (1996). *He shoots, he scores: Metaphors of war in sport and the political linguistics of virility.* Dissertation Abstracts, DAI-A-56/10, p. 4151 (April).

Mayo, D. (1989). Tigers' Sparky sly and successful. *Kalamazoo Gazette*, 2 April, G2.

McKay, J., Messner, M. A., & Sabo, D. (Eds) (2000). *Masculinities, gender relations, and sport.* Thousand Oaks, CA: Sage.

Melnick, M., Miller, M., Sabo, D., Farrell, M., & Barnes, G. (2002). Tobacco use among high school athletes and non-athletes: Results of the 1997 Youth Risk Behavior Survey. *Adolescence*, *36*(144), 727–747.

Messner, M. A. (1992). *Power at play: Sports and the problem of masculinity.* Boston: Beacon Press.

Messner, M. A., & Sabo, D. (Eds) (1990). *Sport, men and the gender order: Critical feminist perspectives.* Champaign, IL: Human Kinetics Books.

Mill, J. S. (1963–1991). *Collected works: John Stuart Mill.* Toronto: University of Toronto Press.

Miller, K., Sabo, D., Farrell, M., Barnes, G., & Melnick, M. (1998). Athletic participation and sexual behavior in adolescents: The different worlds of boys and girls. *Journal of Health and Social Behavior*, *39*, 108–123.

Millett, K. (1994). *The politics of cruelty: An essay on the literature of political imprisonment.* New York: W. W. Norton.

Moore, H. L. (1986). *Space, text and gender: An anthropological study of the Marakwet of Kenya.* Cambridge, England: Cambridge University Press.

Morris, D. B. (1991). *The culture of pain.* Berkeley, CA: University of California Press.

Nixon, H. (1994). Social pressure, social support, and help seeking for pain and injuries in college sports networks. *Journal of Sport & Social Issues*, *13*, 340–355.

Sabo, D. (1986). Pigskin, patriarchy and pain. *Changing Men: Issues in Gender, Sex and Politics*, *16*, 24–25.

Sabo, D. (1994). The body politics of sports injury: Culture, power, and the pain principle. Paper presented at the National Athletic Trainers Association Annual Meeting, Dallas, TX (June 11).

Sabo, D., & Jansen, S. C. (1998). Prometheus unbound: Constructions of masculinity in sports media. In: L. Wenner (Ed.), *MediaSport: Cultural sensibilities and sport in the media age* (pp. 221–232). Boston: Routledge & Kegan Paul.

Sabo, D., Kupers, T. A., & London, W. (2001). *Prison masculinities*. Philadelphia, PA: Temple University Press.

Sabo, D., Melnick, M., Miller, K., Farrell, M., & Barnes, G. (2002). Athletic participation and the health risks of adolescent males: A national study. *International Journal of Men's Health, 1*(2), 173–195.

Sabo, D., Miller, K., Melnick, M., & Heywood, L. (2004). *Her life depends on it: Sport, physical activity, and the health and well-being of American girls*. East Meadow, NY: Women's Sports Foundation.

Sabo, D., & Panepinto, J. (1990). Football ritual and the social reproduction of masculinity. In: M. A. Messner, & D. Sabo (Eds). *Sport, men and the gender order: Critical feminist perspectives* (pp. 115–126). Champaign, IL: Human Kinetics Books.

Scarry, E. (1985). *The body in pain: The making and unmaking of the world*. New York: Oxford University Press.

Szasz, T. S. (1975). *Pain and pleasure: A study of bodily feelings*. New York: Basic Books, originally published in 1957.

Young, K. (2000). Sports-related pain an injury: A research agenda and prognosis. Paper presented at the 21st Annual Conference of the North American Society for the Sociology of Sport, Colorado Springs, CO, November 8–11.

Young, K., & White, P. (2000). Researching sports injury: Reconstructing dangerous masculinities. In: J. McKay, M. A. Messner, & D. Sabo (Eds), *Masculinities, gender relations, and sport* (pp. 108–126). Thousand Oaks, CA: Sage.

Young, K., White, P., & McTeer, W. (1994). Body talk: Male athletes reflect on sport, injury, and pain. *Sociology of Sport Journal, 11*, 175–194.

Chapter 3

Cultural, Structural and Status Dimensions of Pain and Injury Experiences in Sport

Howard L. Nixon II

Introduction: Dimensions of Pain and Injury Experiences and the Sociological Perspective

Pain and injury are not experienced solely in physical or physiological terms, and athletes who ostensibly have the same injury do not necessarily experience pain or other reactions in the same way or to the same degree. Pain and injury also have cultural and social dimensions. Without this broader and deeper understanding, injury prevention and intervention approaches are less likely to be effective. Cultural context, social structure and social status factors are important filters that shape how athletes perceive, experience and respond to pain and injuries in sport.

Waddington (2000) recently pointed to the growing literature on physical activity and health. He noted that nearly all of this literature reflected a physiological perspective and that it tended to concentrate on how physical activity related to conditions such as cardiovascular health and weight control. Waddington shifted the perspective on exercise, sport and health to sociological concerns. My chapter on pain and injury in this volume has a parallel focus. It reviews work largely published over the past decade focusing on sociological perspectives of risk, pain and injury in sport, and it concentrates on the ideas and findings of my own work in this area. In view of the limited body of sociological literature about

Sporting Bodies, Damaged Selves
Research in the Sociology of Sport, Volume 2, 81–97
Copyright © 2004 by Elsevier Ltd.
All rights of reproduction in any form reserved
ISSN: 1476-2854/doi:10.1016/S1476-2854(04)02003-5

risk, pain and injury in sport, this chapter should be seen more as suggestive than definitive.

My research was inspired by a series of studies, including: Kotarba's (1983) analysis of social dimensions of chronic pain; Ewald & Jiobu's (1985) work on positive deviance and pain tolerance among runners and body builders (see also Hughes & Coakley 1991); Sabo's (1986) linking of masculinity to a "pain principle"; Curry & Strauss's (1988) study of the normalisation of sports injury in college wrestling (see also Curry 1993, 1994); Duquin's (1991) examination of "the meaning, myth and reality of self-inflicted pain in sport" and McTeer & White's (1991) investigation of masculinity and injured bodies in sport (see also Messner 1992). Also in this vein, I had explored self-destructive tendencies among "obsessed" middle-aged male runners and anorexic adolescent females as gender-related problems of identity and role adjustment (Nixon 1989).

Taken together, these various studies provided important conceptual leads and some empirical substance for the development of a body of literature showing how and why cultural and social factors influence pain and injury experiences in sport. Despite this work, however, one could argue that sociologists of sport had generally neglected pain and injuries, perhaps assuming it was so central to the experience of athletes that it needed little exploration or explanation. What drove my own work was a desire to understand more fully why athletes were willing to endure injuries and pain over and over again and, more specifically, how cultural and social factors influenced pain and injury decisions and experiences. In this context, the concept of risk taking became a key concept. It was always my aim to encourage my colleagues in the sociology of sport to make the study of risk, pain and injuries a major focus of their own research, so that cultural and social dimensions of pain and injury in sport would be better understood and interventions to limit the severity and long-term effects of pain and injuries would be more successful.

The review of my own work in this chapter is meant to provide a blueprint of various cultural and social dimensions of pain and injury experiences that can be investigated to learn more about how and why athletes play hurt and endure painful surgeries and rehabilitation repeatedly so that they can play again. My work provides no definitive conclusions, but it offers suggestive leads for a number of lines of sociological research into pain and injury in sport, which I hope will propel this research into a more central place in the field of sport sociology. This volume edited by Kevin Young is the most comprehensive collection of sociological studies of sports-related injury and promises to make a major contribution to efforts to advance the sociological study of pain and injury in sport.

Mediated Cultural Influences on Playing Hurt

The social factors and relations that influence pain and injury in sport must be understood in a cultural context. Thus, I began my research by trying to understand how cultural messages about risk, pain, injury and comebacks in sport were conveyed by a popular American sports magazine (Nixon 1993a). A content analysis of 44 relevant *Sports Illustrated* magazine articles from 1969 to 1991, with nearly 90% between 1980 and 1991, provided data about these cultural messages. The articles focused exclusively on male athletes, due to the very limited coverage of female athletes by the magazine during the period studied. The sources of the messages were active and retired athletes, journalists, doctors, trainers, coaches, management officials, owners, and others, such as a judge in a negligence suit and legal counsel for the National Football League Players' Association. I was especially interested in what these types of people had to say about the grey or ambiguous area between disabling and nondisabling injuries; that is, the injuries with which athletes could "play hurt."

The content analysis produced six major thematic categories for understanding why athletes accepted the risks of pain and injuries. The categories, listed in order of frequency of occurrence of items, are (Nixon 1993a: 186–187):

(1) *Structural role constraints*, which refer to perceived expectations, demands and obligations associated with role performance, included perceptions of being disposable, having a precarious career, being stigmatised for being disabled, being expected to push the body to perform and having a responsibility to perform for the team.

(2) *Structural inducements and support*, which refer to rewards and encouragement that make the athlete's role appealing, included perceived opportunities for immediate financial rewards and future financial security, status recognition, being part of a team and hearing the cheers of the crowd.

(3) *Cultural values*, which refer to shared general beliefs about what is important, included statements about the importance of good character, the tolerance of pain and demonstrating masculinity.

(4) *Institutional rationalisation*, which refers to managerial or organisational reasons for accepting risks and pain of injuries and disability, included perceptions of the need to see pain and injuries as necessary or inevitable in sport, to minimise or ignore injuries and pain, to rely on (team) medical personnel and to subordinate personal interests and sacrifice one's body for the good of the team.

(5) *Socialisation of athletes*, which refers to the learning process through which athletes internalise ideas about the self, roles and acceptable beliefs and feelings, included expressions about character, having to prove oneself as an athlete and man, being competitive, an uncritical love of sport, having pride in one's ability, fitness and invincibility and trusting medical personnel.

(6) *Accepting the risk and pain*, which refers to explicit and implicit expressions of the acceptance of the risks and pain of sports injuries, included statements about minimising or ignoring pain and injuries and learning to play hurt, accepting personal blame for getting hurt and pushing the body and accepting the risks of doing so.

"Sportsnets" and the Culture of Risk, Pain and Injury in Sport

I have argued that these cultural themes constitute a relatively coherent "culture of risk" (Nixon 1992, 1993a). The combined effect of this culture of risk is a powerful message that athletes must accept, minimise or ignore the risks of pain and injuries and be willing to play hurt if they are to succeed, or even compete, in sport. In a broader societal context, the decision to play hurt and risk more serious injuries and chronic pain and disability would seem irrational. In the context the culture of risk in sport, however, which the content analysis described, we can understand why the decision to play hurt might seem rational.

As a seriously competitive physical activity, sport can only exist if athletes are willing to accept the risks of pain and injury, since pain and injury actually are inevitable to some extent in all sports over time, at least at the most competitive levels. Indeed, Frey (1991) has linked risk to the social meaning of sport. Thus, successful socialisation or institutional rationalisation of pain and injury is necessary for sport to exist. This means that the culture of risk must be effectively communicated to athletes. I have argued that the cultural messages justifying risk, pain and injury are communicated within individual sports through social networks, called "sportsnets" (Nixon 1992). Social networks are sets of relations among persons, positions, roles or social units (Berkowitz 1982), and sportsnets are webs of social interaction directly or indirectly linking members of a social network in an individual sport or sports-related environment. We begin to appreciate the influence of sportsnets when we think of them as "athletic subcultures" in which members share a common set of cultural beliefs, including the culture of risk.

Athletes are socialised from young ages by a variety of influences, including the mass mediated messages about the culture of risk found in popular publications such as *Sports Illustrated for Kids* and then the "adult version" of *Sports Illustrated*. When they learn sports roles as athletes and become part of one or more sportsnets, they are confronted with a culture of risk that is further reinforced by an institutional rationalisation process in the more organised realms of sport. I have theorised that within sportsnets, a "risk transfer" process occurs to reduce uncertainty among those who control the sportsnet (Nixon 1992). That is, administrators and coaches minimise their own financial, commercial, status-related or career-related risk (of failure or losing) by getting athletes to be willing to sacrifice their bodies "for the good of the team." Unable to define the boundaries of acceptable risk themselves, athletes assume substantial physical risks as "part of the game" and absolve management of its responsibility to assure the safety of athletes. This institutional rationalisation process tends to insulate sportsnets and its authority figures from challenges to the essence of their sports as inherently risky or dangerous activities.

I do not want to claim that all or most sports authorities intentionally expose athletes in their sport to serious risks or that they resist all efforts to make their sports safer. In fact, it is not in the interest of sports authorities to have all their athletes, and especially their stars, injured. Furthermore, I will present evidence showing that coaches believe that they are protecting the welfare of their athletes. It nevertheless is true that it is impossible to avoid pain and injuries in sport, especially as it becomes more intense and serious. Thus, as previously argued, the culture of risk must be internalised to some extent by athletes for serious sport to occur.

The more athletes confine their social relations to members of their sportsnets, the more likely they are to be influenced by these other sportsnet members. Thus, athletes' efforts to deal with pain and injuries are likely to reflect prominent beliefs from the culture of risk held by coaches, medical practitioners or teammates to whom they turn within their sportsnet. When they turn to others with a vested interest in competitive success in their sport, these others may convey an unintentionally or intentionally biased and illusory or mistaken impression of the control athletes have over their own bodies. This kind of support tends to reinforce the culture of risk while it misleads athletes trying to decide what to do about their pain and injuries and whether to play hurt. Athletes with subversive thoughts about the wisdom of playing hurt are challenged by committed sportsnet members who reiterate prominent themes from the culture of risk. The structural location of most athletes within sportsnets, with little authority or power, makes them potentially very vulnerable to coaches, trainers and team doctors who are more committed to team success than the welfare of athletes (Nixon 1992). When athletes turn to these other sportsnet members for social support to cope with their pain and injuries, the "support" they receive is likely to be biased by the culture of risk and people with a vested interest in their own sports success (Nixon 1993b).

Some empirical support for this conception of the vulnerability of athletes within sportsnets was provided by Kotarba (1983). He found in his study of chronic pain among professional athletes that social networks of fellow athletes enabled them to communicate information about how to disguise pain and return to action as quickly as possible. These interaction networks of athletes depended on trust and secrecy to conceal the actual extent of pain and injuries, since such information could be used against athletes to threaten their active playing status. Trust was especially important in relations between athletes and trainers, who had knowledge important to team doctors, coaches and team management personnel as well as the athletes themselves. Kotarba found that trainers generally were highly committed to ethical standards protecting athletes from painful and serious physical conditions that could portend further damage or disablement.

Huizenga (1994), on the other hand, reported often feeling indirectly or directly pressured by team management, coaches and even his medical superior to returning players to action on the football field under risky or questionable circumstances. He was a team doctor for the Oakland Raiders of the National Football League for nearly ten years and a past president of the National Football League Physician's Association. Huizenga observed an environment in which players used drugs to mask their injuries and steroids to enhance their play and played despite severe pain and injuries that could have threatened their careers or caused chronic pain and disability.

Stebbins's (1987) investigation of Canadian football players indicates that the pressure to take physical risks and play hurt may be intense despite players' skepticism about the motives of coaches and team medical personnel. He suggested that the players he studied sensed their manipulation or exploitation by club authorities and focused on self-preservation instead of team sacrifice concerning pain and injuries. Yet, for a variety of reasons, they still typically decided to play hurt. According to Messner (1990, 1992), who interviewed male former athletes, one of the compelling reasons for men to play hurt despite reservations or concerns is a deeply internalised stereotypical sense of masculinity and the need to prove it on the playing field. Furthermore, one could argue that generalised male socialisation as well as socialisation into sport for males engenders a perceived need to demonstrate toughness, which is translated into risk taking in sport (see Nixon 1996a, 1997). We will see that this interpretation is somewhat complicated by data about female athletes.

From a humanistic standpoint, what athletes do about their pain and injuries is ultimately the most important question in this line of research. From a sociological perspective, we are ultimately interested in learning how and why cultural and social structural conditions and social status factors shape what athletes do about their pain and injuries. Major purposes of my research were to discover the pervasiveness of the culture of risk in sportsnets below the most commercialised and professionalised levels of sport and to learn how beliefs about risk, pain and injury and social relations, statuses and roles within sportsnets affect what athletes do about their pain and injuries.

Belief in the Culture of Risk

Even in a volume about pain and injury in sport, it is important to remember that the realities of pain and injury are at odds with popular beliefs about the fitness and health benefits of sport that Edwards (1973) found to be part of the "dominant American sports creed." Edwards proposed that the creed, espoused by prominent authorities in sport over much of the previous century, was an ideology that helped legitimise sport as a social institution. We would argue that the culture of risk reconciles the realities and popular beliefs about sport, pain and injury by minimising or normalising them or in some cases, glorifying these realities as heroic or manly. Hughes and Coakley (1991) suggested that accepting the need to play hurt was part of a "sport ethic" that defined what it meant to be serious about sport. They hypothesised that athletes were especially likely to overconform to this sport ethic — or engage in "positive deviance" — when they had low self-esteem, identities defined mainly in terms of sport and relied on sport for social mobility and status.

How much do athletes accept the culture of risk? I constructed a questionnaire that included items about risk, pain and injury from my prior content analysis (Nixon 1993a) and surveyed athletes and coaches at a medium-sized NCAA Division I institution, which was probably representative of a large cross-section of comprehensive universities in the U.S. at the time. Nearly 200 male and female varsity athletes in 18 different sports responded (see Nixon 1993c, 1994a, 1996a, b, 2000; Nixon & Frey 1996). Approximately 80% of these athletes reported experiencing significant injuries, nearly all of these athletes said they played hurt and nearly 45% of the previously injured athletes indicated that they had lingering effects of their injuries. About half of these athletes who said they had significant injuries said that they felt some influence from significant others to play hurt. A majority or near-majority of the male *and* female athletes agreed with the following questionnaire items:

Being an athlete means that you have to be willing to accept risks (91% males and females).
Athletes need to push themselves to their physical limits (88% males, 77% females).

It is very difficult for athletes to quit, even after serious injuries (92% females, 88% males).

Every athlete should expect to have to play with an injury or pain sometime (86% males, 76% females).

Injured athletes should trust team doctors and trainers (84% females, 83% males).

Playing with injuries and pain demonstrates character and courage (77% males, 58% females).

Only athletes understand what it is like to play with injuries and pain (74% females, 73% males).

Athletes should try to recover quickly from injuries (73% males, 65% females).

Athletes who say they can't play because they are hurt usually are telling the truth (78% females, 72% males).

Athletes trying a comeback have something to prove (72% males, 58% females).

Athletes who endure pain and play hurt deserve our respect (70% males, 65% females).

No pain, no gain (75% females, 69% males).

Athletes who care about their team will try to play with injuries and pain (69% males, 57% females).

Fans lose interest in athletes who are injured and out of action (64% males, 51% females).

Serious athletes have to play with injuries and pain (64% males, 55% females).

Any athlete can be replaced (61% males, 46% females).

You can't worry about injuries and pain if you are going to be an athlete (60% males, 47% females).

Athletes will do everything possible to play despite injuries and pain (80% females, 60% males).

While 46% of male athletes agreed that "In sport, winning is everything and losing is nothing," only 24% of female athletes agreed with this statement. Most of the athletes rejected the idea that coaches did not care about their physical welfare. Slightly more than 40% of the males and 26% of the females agreed that coaches only care about their players who are healthy and able to play. In addition, less than 30% of males and females agreed that team trainers and doctors cared more about the needs of the team than about the needs and feelings of the athletes they are treating; that athletes should ignore pain and injured teammates; that athletes should "tough it out" with an injury or pain today and not worry about the effects tomorrow; that athletes should never complain and that athletes who get injured can only blame themselves.

Along with the item regarding caring about their health and ability to play, there were several other coach-related items. As with the other items, there are some interesting apparent contradictions. For all except the last item, the majority of males and females agreed with the following statements:

Coaches and other athletic officials do everything possible to protect athletes from injuries (77% females, 74% males).
Coaches make athletes feel guilty if they don't want to play hurt or with pain (71% males, 61% females).
Coaches are impressed with athletes who play with pain and injuries (71% males, 51% females).
Coaches say they don't want athletes to play with serious injuries but they actually push them to play if they are needed (65% males, 68% females).
Athletes who complain about pain and injuries ought to be worried about losing their position on the team (50% males, 41% females).

There are numerous ways to interpret these results. The most general conclusion is that although there were some contradictions, most of the surveyed athletes expressed strong or reserved agreement with this interpretation of the "culture of risk" in American sport. About two-thirds of the items expressed or implied a willingness to play hurt. We will examine more closely in a future section the gender differences in these results, but it should be reiterated here that these items were constructed from a content analysis based on statements about male sports. For about half of the items, there was less than a 10 percentage point difference between male and female agreement, and in a few cases, females more strongly subscribed to the culture of risk. Before considering gender differences and other status dimensions of these results, we will examine results from a parallel study of 26 of the 32 coaches at the institution of the surveyed athletes (Nixon 1994b).

How much do coaches accept the culture of risk? Coaches were asked to respond to the same 31 items about the culture of risk to which their athletes responded. The statement with which coaches expressed the widest and strongest agreement concerns athletes needing to push themselves to their physical limits, with over 92% agreeing and 54% agreeing strongly without reservations. Despite this strong expression of support for the culture of risk, the picture of coaches' beliefs about risk, pain and injury is not easily interpreted. For 10 of the 31 items, a majority of the coaches agreed with reservations, and for 20 of the items, at least one-third of the coaches agreed with reservations. Coaches expressed substantially less agreement (10 percentage point difference or more) than their athletes with the following statements:

No pain, no gain (54% vs. 75% females, 69% males).
In sport, winning is everything and losing is nothing (12% vs. 46% males, 24% females).
Team trainers and doctors care more about the needs of the team . . . (4% vs. 31% males, 15% females).

Among the other items with which they expressed little agreement are items indicating that athletes: ought to ignore pain (8% agreement); that athletes should "tough it out" today and not worry about the effects tomorrow (8%); that athletes who get injured can only blame themselves (8%); that athletes should never complain (23%) and that athletes ignore injured teammates (27%).

What the coaches said about themselves as coaches provides insight into the complex and apparently contradictory process by which coaches rationalise physical risks for athletes. Eighty-five percent agreed that coaches and other athletic officials do everything possible to protect athletes from injuries (54% strongly agreed) *and* that coaches are impressed with athletes who play with injuries and pain (15% strongly agreed). Furthermore, over 46% of the coaches agreed (none strongly) that coaches make athletes feel guilty if they don't want to play hurt or with pain, while 31% agreed that coaches say they don't want athletes to play with serious injuries but they actually push them to play if they are needed (4% strongly agreed) and that athletes who complain about pain and injuries ought to be worried about losing their position on the team (none strongly agreed). Just 8% agreed (4% strongly) that coaches only care about their players who are healthy and able to play. The picture that emerges from the coaches' responses reveals widespread support for the culture of risk but also reservations about a number of the beliefs and a very strong belief that they take care of their athletes and protect them from injuries. That is, coaches recognise that sport involves risk taking for athletes, but they do not seem to want to acknowledge fully or explicitly the connection between their endorsement of the culture of risk and the dangers to which they expose their athletes.

Gender Differences in Coaches' and Athletes' Beliefs in the Culture of Risk

We begin to understand some of the gender differences in athletes' beliefs when we look at the gender differences in what coaches said they believed. There were statistically significant (and substantial) differences between male and female coaches on three items: respect for playing hurt (95% male vs. 50% female agreement); playing hurt impressing coaches (95% male vs. 50%

female agreement); and coaches making athletes feel guilty (60% male vs. 0% female agreement). There were two additional items for which there were statistically significant (and substantial) differences between coaches of male and female teams: athletes making comebacks having something to prove (81% male team vs. 40% female team agreement) and demonstrating character and courage by playing hurt (94% male team vs. 60% female team agreement).

These results help explain some of the differences between male and female athletes' beliefs. Although the gender differences between coaches were much larger, all of the coaching results were paralleled by differences between male and female athletes. The difference between the athletes was substantial, greater than 10%, in all cases except the respect item. Although we cannot say that the coaches rejected or fully accepted the culture of risk, both male and female coaches and coaches of male and female teams, like their athletes, embraced many of the beliefs legitimising and normalising taking physical risks and playing hurt. Either through effective socialisation, institutional rationalisation or simply, acknowledgment of the realities of serious sport, both coaches and athletes seemed to reconcile the contradictions in what I have called the "risk-pain-injury paradox": that is, sport compels athletes to push their bodies to their limit, but it is in the self-interest of athletes not to take excessive risks with their bodies, which are the instruments of their engagement in sport (Nixon 1994b). Both coaches and athletes overwhelmingly accepted the idea that being an athlete means that you have to be willing to accept risks and most accepted, at least with reservations, that athletes should expect to play hurt sometime. Although the influence of coaches on their athletes seems obvious, we need to explore the dynamics of this influence process more extensively. We will gain some insight into it later in this chapter by examining results about relations between athletes and coaches in regard to help-seeking and avoidance behavior concerning pain and injuries.

It is striking how much males and females agreed about the culture of risk which, after all, is a set of beliefs rooted in stereotypically masculine notions about risk, pain and injury. In the same vein, Young & White (1995) found that elite female athletes in Western Canada seemed to be as unreflective about the implications of playing with injuries as we would expect their male counterparts to be. In my research, there were some large gender differences in beliefs, but they were relatively few and generally related to identity and esteem issues, such as character, courage, respect, proving oneself and impressing authorities. Although sport was important for the female athletes I studied, it still may not have been as centrally tied to their sense of self as it was for their male counterparts.

It is noteworthy that female athletes were significantly more likely than male athletes (80% vs. 60%) to agree that athletes will do everything possible to play despite injuries and pain. It is not clear, however, whether they were observing what they saw in the male-dominated realm of media sports, because they were less likely than their male counterparts to say things such as athletes ought to push themselves to the limit or be expected to play hurt. Overall, then, my research suggests a degree of moderation of the culture of risk in female sportsnets, but still widespread and often deep acceptance of a set of beliefs that minimise, normalise, rationalise or glorify the risks of playing with damaged bodies in sport.

Social Influences on Responses to Pain and Injury in Sport

As I wrote earlier, the most important question about pain and injury in sport from a humanistic perspective is how athletes respond, since serious "re-injuries" could have long-term debilitating consequences. That is, we must ultimately be interested from this perspective in how athletes interpret and react to the condition of their bodies in the context of the culture of risk. We have seen that gender has some effect on what coaches and athletes believe about risk, pain and injury. Now we will examine what my research revealed about gender differences in how athletes behaved in relation to pain and perceived injuries.

Based on results from attitude scales about expressed toughness and perceived pressure from coaches and fans to play hurt, I found that male athletes were more likely than their female counterparts to express a general attitude of toughness and to feel pressed to play hurt (Nixon 1996a). Male athletes were also more likely to have injuries requiring surgery and to have significant periods of inaction — that is, disabilities — due to sports injuries. Despite gender differences in expressions of attitudes of toughness, male and female athletes did not express different levels of tolerance of pain (Nixon 1996b). In addition, perhaps due in part to similar expressed pain thresholds, no gender differences were found in help-seeking or attempts to avoid or hide pain and injuries from teammates when teammates pressed them to play hurt (1994a). More specifically, there were no statistically significant effects of gender on nine different help-seeking and avoidance items, concerning talking to coaches, teammates or trainers or physical therapists about their own or others' sports injuries; turning to coaches, teammates or trainers or physical therapists for help or encouragement with sports injuries; or avoiding or hiding pain or injuries from coaches, teammates or trainers or physical therapists. Related to these results is the additional finding that there were also no gender differences in encouragement or pressure (or discouragement) felt from coaches, teammates or trainers to play hurt.

Other social factors, including sports status and social relations within sportsnets, were related to athletes' pain and injury experiences and how they reacted to them (Nixon 1994a, 1996a). For example, line-up regulars were more likely to have lingering effects of sports injuries and to have more injuries, and holders of athletic scholarships had more surgeries for athletic injuries. These results validate the seemingly intuitively obvious idea that playing sports more often and at a higher level is more damaging to the body. Athletes more often talked to athletic trainers or physical therapists and doctors about their pain and injuries when they seemed sympathetic and caring. Athletes were also more likely to seek medical attention when they saw their coaches as sympathetic and caring, but they avoided or hid their pain and injuries from authorities in their sportsnet, such as coaches, trainers and physicians, when these people were perceived as pressing them to play hurt. In this context, it is important to emphasise that over 50% of the athletes I surveyed said they had *not* been discouraged by coaches or teammates from playing hurt. Furthermore, almost two-thirds of the athletes said they had avoided coaches or had tried to avoid or conceal their pain and injuries from trainers and teammates. More than 40% felt pressed by teammates to play hurt, and nearly 50% felt such pressure from coaches.

Getting hurting athletes into the training room or doctor's office is essential to protect their physical welfare and health. In a study of student interns in a university athletic training programme, Walk (1997) revealed the complicated relations surrounding the treatment of student athletes. On the one hand, athletes frequently looked down upon the student trainers and tried to avoid their help, but they also used the student trainers to help them fake injuries, avoid tough workouts and misuse the services of the training room in other ways. At times, student trainers conspired with athletes to help them get around what coaches expected them to do. At other times, the student interns worked with staff trainers to handle resistance to their treatment from athletes and coaches.

Athletes faced a complex array of influences when they decided to enter the training room. The athletes in my study were more likely to avoid trainers when they felt pressure from teammates to play hurt, which means that the encouraging influence of a sympathetic trainer could be offset by team pressure discouraging the athlete from going to the training room. In the complex relations of the sportsnet, it also seems that hurting athletes avoid coaches when trainers are sympathetic, coaches press them to play hurt and the athletes are not white.

The racial aspect of this relationship may reflect some general mistrust of coaches across racial lines. This racial interpretation is reinforced by the additional finding that white athletes were more likely than non-white athletes to turn to coaches for help and encouragement with their pain and injuries. Like many other American universities, head coaches and nearly all assistant coaches at the university in this study were white. This white-dominated sportsnet also explains why non-white athletes were more likely than white athletes to avoid or conceal their injuries from coaches and teammates. Non-white athletes may have had more difficulty disclosing their pain and injuries to others in their sportsnet because they feared that their playing status might be jeopardised or simply because they felt uncomfortable getting close to others of a different race. This aspect of the research is among those requiring more attention.

Another finding is that individual sport athletes were more likely than team sport athletes to talk to teammates about pain and injuries. At the same time, individual sport athletes were less likely to avoid teammates regarding pain and injuries. These findings may be explained by generally less frequent and less intense or personal interaction with teammates among individual sport than team sport athletes. If contacts with teammates are less frequent and personal among individual sport athletes, they may be both more willing to talk about pain and injuries and be less strongly influenced by what their teammates say. If team sport athletes are more closely tied to their teammates, it may be more difficult for them to ignore what their teammates say. Thus, they will not want to talk to teammates if they are afraid what they will say. It must be added, though, that it was found that when individual *and* team sport athletes perceive a sympathetic or caring attitude from teammates about pain and injuries, they will be more likely to turn to them for help or encouragement.

Despite ambivalence, suspicions or other reservations, most of the athletes nevertheless said they turned to coaches and teammates for support when they were hurt, and three-quarters said they turned to trainers or physical therapists for help or encouragement when they were hurt. Relatively few felt pressure from trainers or physical therapists to play hurt; most indicated that coaches, teammates and medical personnel expressed some sympathy or caring about their sports injuries and pain; and more than 60% said they had been discouraged by trainers or physical therapists from playing hurt (Nixon 1994a).

Implications for Managing Physical Risk, Pain and Injuries in Sport

While athletes may feel encouragement or discouragement, or support or pressure, from coaches, teammates and others in their sportsnets, relations with trainers and physical therapists clearly seem most important in determining whether or not athletes actually go to the training room or doctor's office for help with their pain and injuries. Thus, ties to sympathetic and caring trainers seem essential to protect the long-term welfare of athletes. My research showed, however, that when athletes depend more on sympathetic trainers, they are more likely to avoid conversations with their coaches about their pain and injuries. This trust and confidence in trainers can be undermined when trainers press athletes to play hurt. When athletes feel such pressure, they are more likely to turn to coaches for support. This support may be biased or compromised by the implicit or explicit commitment of coaches to the culture of risk, which justifies pressing athletes to push their bodies, even when hurting, to achieve team success.

Athletes want to believe that coaches, other sports officials and medical personnel are committed to protecting their welfare, but they hold many beliefs and act in a variety of ways suggesting that they still feel they are expected to play hurt. Coaches say that they are committed to their athletes' welfare, but their own welfare depends on athletes taking risks with their bodies. Both athletes and coaches, especially at the highest levels, are immersed in sportsnets that emphasise values and beliefs that minimise, normalise, legitimise or glorify risk, pain and injury.

The professional ethics of medical personnel exist outside and even to some extent in opposition to the culture of risk in sport. Getting hurting athletes to see medical personnel is essential for their welfare, and we have seen that athletes will seek medical personnel when they seem sympathetic and caring. On the other hand, Huizenga's (1994) experience shows that medical personnel may find themselves compromising their professional ethics when their positions are embedded within the structure of a powerful sportsnet, such as a professional or high-level intercollegiate sports team. For medical personnel to gain the trust of athletes and feel that they can act responsibly on behalf of athletes, they must be independent of the authority of coaches, management and owners in the sportsnet in which they practice. For athletes to feel comfortable about seeking help from medical personnel, they must believe that their playing status and relations with teammates will not arbitrarily be jeopardised by having their pain and injuries treated.

The biggest obstacles athletes may face in feeling comfortable about not playing hurt could be the culture of risk they learn when they become athletes and the social relations within sportsnets that reinforce this culture. The results concerning individual and team sport athletes are suggestive in this regard. It may be that athletes who are more loosely tied to social relations in their sportsnet but who are still committed to proficiency in their sport may be more insulated from compelling effects of the culture of risk. I did not explicitly examine this idea in my research, but it should be a fruitful line of research if my assumptions about the influence of sportsnets and this culture are valid. Evidence about the permanently disabling long-term effects of athletes' ignoring the risks of their pain and injuries (see Nixon 1997, 2000: 432–433; Waddington 2000) underscores the importance of this kind of research so that we can learn more about what influences athletes to play hurt and what influences them to avoid taking excessive risks with their bodies. My social network approach to this research has been challenged (e.g. see Nixon

1998; Roderick 1998), but it is less important to find the definitive theoretical or analytical approach to this research than it is to find perspectives and data that show how cultural, structural and social factors influence the pain and injury experiences of athletes and enable athletes to cope effectively with pressures to play hurt.

References

Berkowitz, S. D. (1982). *An introduction to structural analysis: The network approach to social research.* Toronto: Butterworths.

Curry, T. J. (1993). A little pain never hurt anyone: Athletic career socialization and the normalization of sports injury. *Symbolic Interaction, 16,* 273–290.

Curry, T. J. (1994). A little pain never hurt anybody: A photo-essay on the normalization of sports injuries. *Sociology of Sport Journal, 11,* 195–208.

Curry, T. J., & Strauss, R. (1988, November). *On the normalization of sport injury: A little pain never hurt anybody.* Paper presented at the North American Society for the Sociology of Sport annual meeting, Cincinnati.

Duquin, M. E. (1991, November). *Choosing pain: The meaning, myth and reality of self-inflicted pain in sport.* Paper presented at the North American Society for the Sociology of Sport annual meeting, Milwaukee.

Edwards, H. (1973). *Sociology of sport.* Homewood, IL: Dorsey Press.

Ewald, K., & Jiobu, R. M. (1985). Explaining positive deviance: Becker's model and the case of runners and bodybuilders. *Sociology of Sport Journal, 2,* 144–156.

Frey, J. H. (1991). Social risk and the meaning of sport. *Sociology of Sport Journal, 8,* 136–145.

Hughes, R., & Coakley, J. (1991). Positive deviance among athletes: The implications of overconformity to the Sport Ethic. *Sociology of Sport Journal, 8,* 307–325.

Huizenga, R. (1994). *"You're okay, it's just a bruise."* New York: St. Martin's Griffin.

Kotarba, J. A. (1983). *Chronic pain: Its social dimensions.* Newbury Park, CA: Sage.

McTeer, W. G., & White, P. G. (1991, November). *Sport, masculinity and the injured body.* Paper Presented at the North American Society for the Sociology of Sport annual meeting, Milwaukee.

Messner, M. (1990). When bodies are weapons: Masculinity and violence in sport. *International Review for the Sociology of Sport, 25,* 203–220.

Messner, M. (1992). *Power at play: Sports and the problem of masculinity.* Boston: Beacon Press.

Nixon, H. L., II (1989). Reconsidering obligatory running and anorexia nervosa as gender-related problems of identity and role adjustment. *Journal of Sport and Social Issues, 13,* 14–24.

Nixon, H. L., II (1992). A social network analysis of influences on athletes to play with pain and injuries. *Journal of Sport & Social Issues, 16,* 127–135.

Nixon, H. L., II (1993a). Accepting the risks of pain and injury in sport: Mediated cultural influences on playing hurt. *Sociology of Sport Journal, 10,* 183–196.

Nixon, H. L., II (1993b). Social network analysis of sport: Emphasizing social structure in sport sociology. *Sociology of Sport Journal, 10*, 315–321.

Nixon, H. L. II. (1993c, August). *Cultural beliefs, status factors, and vulnerability to pain and injuries in sport.* Paper presented at the American Sociological Association annual meeting, Miami, FL.

Nixon, H. L., II (1994a). Social pressure, social support and help seeking for pain and injuries in college sports networks. *Journal of Sport & Social Issues, 18*, 340–355.

Nixon, H. L., II (1994b). Coaches' views of risk, pain and injury in sport, with special reference to gender differences. *Sociology of Sport Journal, 11*, 79–87.

Nixon, H. L., II (1996a). Explaining pain and injury attitudes and experiences in sport in terms of gender, race and sports status factors. *Journal of Sport & Social Issues, 20*, 33–44.

Nixon, H. L., II (1996b). The relationship of friendship networks, sports experiences, and gender to expressed pain thresholds. *Sociology of Sport Journal, 13*, 78–86.

Nixon, H.L II. (1997, October). *The culture of risk, playing hurt and being a man in the NFL.* Invited presentation to the annual meeting of the Treating Clinicians, NFL/NFLPA Program for Substances of Abuse, Essex Junction, VT.

Nixon, H. L., II (1998). Response to Martin Roderick's comment on the work of Howard L. Nixon II. *Sociology of Sport Journal, 15*, 80–85.

Nixon, H. L. II. (2000). Sport and disability. In: J. Coakley, & E. Dunning (Eds), *Handbook of sports studies* (pp. 422–438). London: Sage.

Nixon, H. L. II., & Frey, J. H. (1996). *A sociology of sport.* Belmont, CA: Wadsworth.

Roderick, M. J. (1998). The sociology of risk, pain and injury: A comment on the work of Howard L. Nixon II. *Sociology of Sport Journal, 15*, 64–79.

Sabo, D. (1986). Pigskin, patriarchy, and pain. *Changing Men: Issues in Gender, Sex and Politics, 16*, 24–25.

Stebbins, R. A. (1987). *Canadian football: The view from the helmet.* London, Ontario: Centre for Social and Humanistic Studies of the University of Western Ontario.

Waddington, I. (2000). Sport and health: A sociological perspective. In: J. Coakley, & E. Dunning (Eds), *Handbook of sports studies* (pp. 408–421). London: Sage.

Walk, S. R. (1997). Peers in pain: The experiences of student athletic trainers. *Sociology of Sport Journal, 14*, 22–56.

Young, K., & White, P. (1995). Sport, physical danger, and injury: The experiences of elite women athletes. *Journal of Sport & Social Issues, 19*, 45–61.

Chapter 4

Professional Athletes' Injuries: From Existential to Organisational Analyses

Joseph A. Kotarba

This collection of essays is a tribute to the sophisticated attention social and behavioural scientists have recently been giving to the analysis of sports-related injuries. This interest has been driven by a number of factors, including growing awareness of the centrality of sports to society, the increasing presence and appreciation of women in sports, the sheer expansion of sports across cultures and generations, and so forth (Coakley 2001: 181–186). In this chapter, I will examine sports injuries and health care delivery from two analytically distinct perspectives — the very personal, existential perspective, and a social class-driven, organisational perspective. I want to highlight the paradoxical wonder of modern sports which remains an inherently private, visceral and embodied experience played out in an increasingly wide range of (primitive as well as sophisticated) organisational settings. The two approaches adopted also reflect the evolution of my research and thinking on sports injuries.

I derive the primary methodological and analytical framework for the present analysis from a metaphor that has informed my research on sports injuries and pain for over twenty years; that is, *viewing professional sports as work and occupation.* As Young (1993: 373) has noted, professional athletes work in an occupational arena "that requires routine violence be done both by and to athletes, and ultimately guarantees injury." If we conceptualise professional athletes as workers who get hurt, then we are able to see the service used to treat work-related injuries as occupational health care. Occupational health care refers to the delivery of health

Sporting Bodies, Damaged Selves
Research in the Sociology of Sport, Volume 2, 99–116
Copyright © 2004 by Elsevier Ltd.
All rights of reproduction in any form reserved
ISSN: 1476-2854/doi:10.1016/S1476-2854(04)02004-7

services to workers who occupy the role of patient. The delivery of occupational health care has evolved as the capitalistic economy has become more sophisticated and the relationship between owner and worker has grown enormously complex (Navarro 1981).

In the remainder of this chapter, I will examine the social organisation of health care delivery to professional athletes. I define professional athletes as those individuals who participate in sports for a living. I would be naïve, of course, to assume (let alone argue) that some amateur athletes, such as those who perform as student-athletes at colleges and universities, do not perform for remuneration. A simple Marxian analysis would argue that amateur athletes are productive cogs in the bigger "wheels" of Western capitalistic societies by either suffering as unpaid athletes whose labour brings profit to university administrators, athletes who are preparing themselves for professional careers, or as quasi-professionals who are paid under-the-table by anxious alumni or zealous agents (see Zimbalist 1999). In spite of these economic similarities, I will discuss health care delivery only to those athletes who explicitly play sports for a living. Commonsensically and journalistically, this type of health care appears universally available, increasingly technologically-based, and effective. I will argue that there is great variation in the delivery of this health care that correlates with social class differences among professional athletes. These differences can only be partially accounted for by type of sport, and specific physical activities and stressors. Other factors include the economic value of athletes and the various cultures informing their sports. The delivery of health care to professional athletes has evolved from a personalistic model to a model increasingly diverse in terms of technological sophistication and organisational complexity.

The Existential Experience of Pain

My earliest work on the sociology of athletic injuries and pain was a component of a broader ethnographic study of the emerging practice of acupuncture in the U.S. (Kotarba 1975). Following the historical visit of President Nixon to China in 1972, the American mass media quickly disseminated the promise of this Asian healing modality throughout the U.S. Among all the problems for which proponents claimed acupuncture was a miracle cure (e.g. obesity, chemical dependencies, and hearing loss), it appeared that the vast majority of clientele were drawn to acupuncture's effective management of pain. Although the TV news proclaimed the amazing ability of doctors to perform surgery on conscious patients under acupuncture anesthesia, the spotlight in the U.S. was on *chronic* pain. Chronic pain is "an ongoing experience of embodied discomfort that fails to either heal naturally or to respond to normal forms of medical intervention" (Kotarba 1983a: 13).

The phenomenon of chronic pain is sociologically fascinating because it is *existential* in two distinctively *social* ways. First, chronic pain is social to the degree that it requires concerted effort to make it social; that is, to disclose its existence to others. With the absence of visible physical symptoms, people who suffer from chronic pain appear normal. They can be young and otherwise healthy looking. There are no visible lesions and, in many cases, no behavioural evidence (e.g. a traumatic accident) to point to the likely presence of pain. For example, I am aware that someone has chronic pain, in the form of, say, migraine headaches or low back pain, because that person can convince me of it in interaction. Existentially speaking, chronic pain is first and foremost embodied and only secondarily social and cultural (Kotarba 1977).

Second, chronic pain is existential because people who suffer from it embark on a long, difficult, and only occasionally successful journey to make sense of it. Western culture tells us that we should not hurt without cause, and that modern medicine should either mask the pain or eliminate its cause. For people with chronic pain, neither statement is true. Existential social thought instructs us that we cannot live for long in a state of meaninglessness or absurdity. Therefore, people with chronic pain routinely spend much time and energy trying to locate (medical and/or non-medical) meaning for their suffering that will ideally result in a cure (Kotarba 1983b: 682). This search for meaning is essentially and inevitably *social.*

Thus, chronic pain is embodied and personal, but its management occurs in the presence of others. Existential social thought also tells us that the person with pain, like all of us with pain, exercises *agency*; that is, the power and responsibility to decide how to respond to inevitable problems in everyday life (Douglas 1977). One decides when, how, and to whom to disclose pain. The situational management of chronic pain is well illustrated by its relevance to the most common of everyday life concerns — work — and professional athletes even have their own particular way of talking about this dilemma.

"Play with Pain, Talk Injury"

It is obvious that the pain-afflicted person will decide to disclose — make social — suffering to those who can offer affective, moral, sympathetic, philosophical or medical help. The pain-afflicted person will decide to hide suffering from others when the costs of disclosure appear too high: shame, guilt, stigma, loss of credibility, and — for the purposes of the present argument — loss of a job.

During my early research on athletic injuries and chronic pain,[1] I was struck by a members' expression I heard repeatedly: "play with pain, talk injury." As I noted then:

> This expression . . . neatly summarizes the options a player has in deciding what to do about physical problems. Put simply, *play with pain* refers to the decision to prevent a physical problem from interfering either with one's athletic identity or with one's play. *Talk injury* refers to the decision to disclose a physical problem to potentially helpful (or discrediting) audiences such as coaches, trainers, management, the press, or the public. The variables that influence these decisions include visibility and severity of the injury, age, and the location of the problem in the athletic career continuum. The major factor influencing this decision, however, appears to be the athlete's perception of his or her job security (Kotarba 1983a: 137).

Players with insecure athletic identities are those who feel that the active disclosure of a non-restrictive injury or pain problem threatens job security. An insecure identity can be based upon such factors as ethnicity, rookie status, veteran status, low skill level, poor minor league career, and so forth. If the athlete chooses to not disclose the problem, he or she may deal with the problem outside of the team organisation. Options have traditionally included consulting one's own physician, seeking alternative health care (e.g. acupuncture or chiropractic), or self-care. More recent options include things like nutritional regimens.

Micropolitical and Interactionist Components

The athletic injury and pain scenarios I explored in my earlier research highlighted the micropolitical and interactional components of professional athletic careers that dominated sports until quite recently. Professional athletes were able to largely manage their non-visible injury problems through personal relationship and negotiations with team officials such as the team trainer (Kotarba 1983a). Trust, confidence, and friendship were critical to minimising risk of disclosure to those team officials, such as general managers who could use injury and pain data to make personnel decisions. The situation has become much more complex through the great expansion in the number and types of professional sports, the

---

[1] See Kotarba (1980, 1983a) for descriptions of the methods used to study acupuncture and chronic pain.

globalisation of professional sports, the growing presence of women in professional sports, and the explosion in the economic dimension of professional sports. The strength of a sociological approach to understanding these complex phenomena lies in structural and cultural analysis (see Chapter 3).

Toward a Sociology of Professional Sports Medicine

In a recent paper (Kotarba 2001), I proposed a framework for conceptualising professional sports medicine as a variety of occupational medicine. The numerous styles of occupational health care provided to workers today reflect the variety and complexity of work in our post-industrial society. Specifically, there are two principles — based upon *structural* and *cultural* characteristics of work — which largely determine the configuration of any occupational health program.

Structurally, the quality and complexity of occupational health care is a function of the relative value of the worker to the employer. The recent emergence of wellness-in-the-workplace programmes demonstrates how the most highly valued employees (e.g. executives and managers) receive the highest quality, individualised preventive health care services (e.g. health and country club memberships), in contrast to lower status employees (e.g. line and staff employees) who are offered group services at the work site (e.g. aerobics and smoking cessation classes) (Conrad 1988; Kotarba & Bentley 1988).

The style, tone, and meaning of occupational health care delivery (e.g. practitioner-patient interaction and ongoing relationships) are largely a function of the work culture. For example, the delivery of comprehensive health care to astronauts by NASA flight surgeons is only partially shaped by the requirements and stressors of space flight. The flight surgeon-astronaut relationship is also a function of the more general culture of flying with its attendant values on individuality, adventure, mastery of the environment, and optimal work performance (Kotarba 1983c).

For analytical purposes, I summarise the variety of occupational health care systems according to three types: *elite, managed,* and *primitive.* This three-category model also applies to occupational health care delivered to professional athletes, or sports medicine.

Elite Occupational Health Care

Elite occupational health care is delivered to the most highly valued workers in an organisation. Employers provide the very best in preventive and curative medicine to top executives, managers, and skilled workers for two reasons: to maximise their crucial productivity, and to avoid the tremendous expense of replacing them (Kotarba & Bentley 1988). Structurally, elite health care is the most expensive and medically sophisticated care corporate or governmental money can buy. Culturally, elite health care is framed in the value of *individuality*, since the most highly valued workers are perceived as special. Elite employees receive country club memberships, personal trainers, wellness retreats, and other amenities not often made available to lower status employees.

Elite occupational health care is denoted by *technological sophistication* and *diagnostic creativity*. Technologically, elite workers receive state-of-the-art treatment representing the full range of medical specialties. Diagnostically, elite workers' health problems are analysed and interpreted through an open horizon of healing models. For example, NASA astronauts and their families are provided with comprehensive health care that addresses the astronauts' physical, psychological and even spiritual well-being in a distinctively holistic manner (Kotarba 1983c).

Major league players (i.e. the National Basketball Association, the National Football League, the National Hockey League, and Major League Baseball in the U.S.) receive elite health care. A common practice for NFL teams is to station orthopedic physicians on the sidelines during a game, in addition to the traditional team trainers and physicians. In terms of technological sophistication, the degree to which teams can intervene with and control their highly-priced players' bodies is remarkable in contrast to the sports medicine described above. For example, the nascent Houston Texans NFL team chose "left tackle" Tony Boselli first in the 2002 expansion draft. The five-time "Pro Bowler" did not come cheaply — his annual salary will be U.S. $7.5 million. Before the draft, there was considerable concern with his health, since he has recently undergone major surgery to repair torn cartilage in his right shoulder and arthroscopic surgery on his left shoulder. The Texans' management put Boselli through lengthy and intensive medical tests, but the medical findings were sufficiently positive to result in a major team investment. Nevertheless, professional teams can continuously intervene in cases of players like Boselli beyond the traditional orthopedic surgery and hope for recovery. During Spring practice, Boselli underwent a "minor arthroscopic procedure" to remove scar tissue from his healing left shoulder. The team's general manager announced to the press:

> There was some scar tissue in there, and we wanted to clean it out. We felt it would accelerate his 'rehab' if we cleaned it out. His range of motion increased after the procedure, so the doctor (one of the most famous orthopedic surgeons in Texas) feels good about how everything went (Thompson 2002: C1).

Whether or not the Texans' efforts with Tony Boselli pay off, the fact is that all professional sports in the U.S. exercise similar technological sophistication in caring for their expensive players, perhaps best exemplified by the famous "Tommy John Surgery" that has extended the careers of numerous major league pitchers. Briefly, this term refers colloquially to tendon replacement surgery first performed in 1974 on Los Angeles Dodgers baseball pitcher Tommy John. Dr. Frank Jobe extracted a tendon from John's right arm and used it to replace the torn ligament in his left, pitching arm. Tommy John went on to win 170 additional games. Dr. Jobe and other orthopedic surgeons have since performed well over two hundred of these operations (see http://espn.go.com/trainingroom/s/2000/0315/427112.html).

In terms of diagnostic creativity, the holism practised at NASA with astronauts has its equivalent in professional sports. Teams routinely hire sports psychologists and nutritionists to supplement the work of traditional team physicians and trainers. Perhaps the most glamorous example of diagnostic creativity is the philosophy of Phil Jackson, the former coach of the World Champion Los Angeles Lakers NBA team and former coach of the six-time champion Chicago Bulls. Jackson routinely invokes talk about stress management, centering, meditation, Zen Buddhism, and other "New Age" phenomena to motivate his players and solve team problems (Kaye 2002). It is also worth noting that those professional athletes competing and succeeding in individual sports (e.g. golf, sailing, and tennis) can afford to take the best care of themselves, just as independent businessmen do in the corporate world.

Managed Occupational Health Care

Managed occupational health care is delivered to typical workers in an organisation. Structurally, managed health care must be responsive to economic contingencies, as employers constantly seek ways to control the ever-rising costs of health care for the bulk of their employees. Culturally, managed health care is framed in the value of *rationality*, most commonly in terms of managed care. The modal health care worker in managed health care is the primary care physician who serves as much as bureaucratic gatekeeper for HMO (Health Maintenance Organization) or PPO (Preferred Provider Organization) services — as they are known in the United States — as he or she does as healer. Although managed care can be high quality care, its availability and delivery are bureaucratically-grounded (Ritzer & Walczak 1988).

Managed care is delivered to the middle-class of professional athletes. In the U.S., these athletes perform for "Pro-Pop" sports teams. The term *Pro-Pop sports* refers to professional team sports whose status is lower than that of major league sports in terms of overall popularity, fan attendance, level of remuneration to players, and so forth. Unlike minor league sports, such as the Continental Basketball Association and Minor League Baseball, Pro-Pop sports do not ordinarily serve as training grounds for future major league stars. Instead, Pro-Pop sports teams function to provide arena business when the major league sport is not in season, and to attract families and other budget-conscious entertainment consumers who have been priced out of the major leagues. Pro-Pop sports include, for instance, the Continental Indoor Soccer League, the Arena Football League, and the Women's National Basketball Association.

Pro-Pop athletes receive all their health care from companies that specialise in comprehensive managed care service, such as HealthSouth, Inc. The Pro-Pop team does not ordinarily employ its own team physicians or trainers — these are provided by the contractor. The team, therefore, can save a lot of money. The contractor makes money by providing health care to numerous teams, thus maximising the work of each physical therapist, athletic trainer, massage therapist, exercise physiologist, and physician who work for it. As is the case with traditional HMOs, the managed care company does not promise that the same trainer will always show up before each game. In effect, this is the latest stage in the rationalisation of sports medicine. The impersonality of this relationship replaces the warm and intimate image of the trainer-athlete relationship commonly portrayed in pop culture: a cigar-stomping old guy, accompanied by towel and pail, giving a rub down and fatherly advice to a young boxer/outfielder/defenseman/running back.

Primitive Occupational Health Care

Primitive occupational health care is delivered to the most marginal or least valuable workers. Structurally, primitive occupational health care is low-quality and low-cost health care because the employer has very little invested in the worker. The worker can be easily replaced, given low skill requirements or the abundance of potential alternative workers. Culturally, primitive health care is framed in the value of *benevolence*. Health care is given either as charity or for extra-productivity objectives such as public relations or employer image. No real effort is made to achieve optimal health or productivity. Instead, the goal is at best to "patch up" the worker in an incidental manner — when care is available and when there is an immediate need for care. The modal worker is the allied or ancillary health care practitioner who patches up the worker, but who also conveys the conservative ideological belief that good health (or poor health) is primarily the responsibility of the worker. In the lowest-status professional sports, these workers include athletic trainers, physical therapists, and lay or indigenous healers.

In order to explain this process, I will briefly describe the delivery of health care to rodeo cowboys, local professional wrestlers, and boxers.[2]

The Rodeo Cowboy

In their definitive study of rodeo in the United States, Wooden & Ehringer (1996) describe the way professional rodeo has emerged to become a great national pastime. Rodeo originated in the common work needed to operate cattle ranches in America. Professional rodeo now involves more than U.S. $22 million in annual prize money and nearly 20 million spectators in attendance. Professional rodeo cowboys freely admit that rodeo is as much a lifestyle as it is a professional, potentially lucrative, and dangerous sport. Among professional athletes, cowboys are unusual because they do not get paid to compete. The rodeo contestant must pay an entrance fee that allows him the opportunity to compete for a share of the "purse." If the cowboy's animal must be "turned out" because the cowboy is too ill to compete, or if the cowboy is injured in a preliminary event, or even if there is a foul-up in travel plans, he forfeits the entrance fee.

Professional rodeo cowboys ordinarily do not have sponsors to help cover their expenses. They may have "patch sponsors" (similar to the advertisements posted on race cars), and they may make a few personal appearances at local western boot and hat stores, but they cannot live on these sources of income. For this reason, many rodeo cowboys hold second or off-season jobs to help cover expenses.

From all indications, the injury rate among rodeo cowboys is very high (see Chapter 11). The Justin Sportsmedicine Program, headquartered in Dallas, Texas, has compiled extensive data on the relationship of specific rodeo events to specific injuries. From 1983 to 1998, the percentages of injuries by specialties were: 46% in bull riding; 24% in bareback riding; 17% in saddle bronc riding; and 13% in various timed events. Major types of injuries include: spine injuries (20%); hand, wrist, and elbow injuries (17%); knee injuries (13%); foot, ankle and leg injuries (13%); shoulder injuries (11%); groin or hamstring injuries (10%); head or face injuries (9%); and miscellaneous injuries (7%) (Justin Sportsmedicine Program 1999; see also Nebergall *et al.* 1992).

Since injuries are a common and expected risk in professional rodeo, they have become a common feature of rodeo culture. For example, the most dramatic

---

[2] See Kotarba (2001) for a description of the methods used to study rodeo cowboys and local professional wrestlers.

examples of contestants being "bucked off" the animals or missing the catch in some timed event are replayed for the entire audience on the giant TV screens at the end of each day's competition at the annual Houston Livestock Show and Rodeo. By the volume of their applause, the audience selects the cowboy to receive the "Hard Luck Award," which in recent years has been a round-trip airplane ticket. The applause reaches a crescendo at the sight of life-threatening events, such as a bull stomping on a thrown cowboy's head. Conversely, the audience has been known to boo minor events, such as a saddle bronc rider merely being thrown from a horse.

In her anthropological analysis, Elizabeth Atwood Lawrence (1982: 65) notes that the term "individualism" most forcefully marks the identity of the rodeo cowboy. This identity is a residue of the image of the traditional cowboy who worked on ranches. When we think of the rodeo cowboy as a professional athlete, this identity is dramatic. The rodeo cowboy is an individual participant in his sport. No one is there to "carry" an injured cowboy or substitute for him when he is injured, as is the case in team sports. Rodeo cowboys commonly help each other out on the circuit, sharing a truck or a room at night. There is, however, little your friend or buddy can do for you when you are injured — he is likely to be hurt himself.

The essence of health care for rodeo cowboys is last resort, charity-like services offered more for catastrophic injuries than for routine injury management or prevention. These services address public relations at least as much as healing functions. The Justin Boot Company supports the Justin Cowboy Crisis Fund (JCCF), established in 1989 through a cooperative effort with the Professional Rodeo Cowboy Association (PRCA). The overall purpose of the Fund is to provide need-based financial assistance to persons injured through their participation in the sport of professional rodeo. Since its inception, the JCCF has provided over U.S. $1.4 million in financial help to approximately 180 individuals in need. A board of directors consisting of celebrities from other sports and the music industry administer this fund. An award may be used for rehabilitation expenses or, as one official from Justin put it, "to help an injured cowboy make his truck payment." There are medical insurance policies available. These policies are very expensive for most cowboys, and many cowboys have too many pre-existing conditions to qualify.

The Justin Heeler

The most comprehensive and most widely-recognised form of health care for rodeo cowboys is the Justin Sportsmedicine Program (Justin Sportsmedicine Program 1999). Founded in 1981, the programme takes into account the nomadic nature of rodeo and the rather independent and solitary style of rodeo cowboys.

The programme consists of two elaborately furnished truck/trailer units stocked with state-of-the art equipment and supplies and over-the-counter medications for the on-site care of rodeo injuries. These trailers are staffed by health care workers known as the "Justin Heelers," with backgrounds as university-educated athletic trainers. Each Justin Heeler treats, on average, approximately 70 cowboys during a typical rodeo, while providing education, preventive information, and pre-competition preparation to a great many more over the course of the season. In addition, he coordinates back-up services with local physicians, athletic trainers, and physical therapists. Coordinating activities serves to educate local health workers about rodeo injury care, while insuring their ready availability if serious injuries should occur.

As Justin Heelers, individuals find themselves at the intersection of two cultures. One world is that of sophisticated health care workers who use their training and expertise to get young athletes back into competition as quickly as possible. The second world is that of the nomadic cowboy, traveling around the rodeo circuit and enjoying the excitement and atmosphere of the rodeo world. The Justin Heelers share the personality and persona of their clients. Their work uniform consists of traditional cowboy attire (i.e. pressed Wrangler jeans, crisp western-cut shirt, a pair of Justin boots, large silver belt buckle, seasonally appropriate hat and, above all else, a jacket or vest with the logo of the sponsoring corporation emblazoned on the back). Their hair is always closely cropped and freshly trimmed. They "chew" and "spit" (tobacco).

The Justin Heelers' style of work follows from their very personalistic relationship with the cowboys. One stock handler remarked, "If a cowboy gets bucked off and lands hard, the first face he sees when he opens his eyes is usually Bill's" (Kotarba & Haney 1995: 16). Much of the Justin Heelers' credibility and effectiveness derives from their direct, pragmatic, and holistic style of healing. Many cowboys come to the trailer to receive some good, practical health and career advice. The lasting value of any information or advice offered by the Justin Heeler is that it may be the last health and/or injury intervention the cowboy may receive for an injury.

Clearly, the Justin Sportsmedicine Program offers battlefield-style health care — it is designed to treat acute injuries and get the cowboy back to work as soon as possible. Long-term care is still a problem, and the establishment of viable long-term care for cowboys is only an organisational goal at this time.

The Wrangler Chiropractor

The Wrangler Chiropractic Sports Medicine Program is a second, albeit smaller, system of health care available to professional rodeo cowboys in the U.S. The

Wrangler company sponsors the programme by providing promotional materials and supplies. The programme is staffed locally by chiropractors who volunteer their services. In tune with the culture of their profession, the chiropractors set up adjustment tables in the open areas behind the actual floor of the rodeo where the cowboys queue for their events. Cowboys seek a preventive spinal adjustment *before* their events. The chiropractors do not respond to injured cowboys during or after the actual events. Unlike the Justin Heelers who organise their work in terms of their employment by the Justin Sportsmedicine Program, the chiropractors promote their local private practice quite heavily with business cards and brochures on chiropractic stamped with their name and office information.

The presence of the medically-oriented Justin Heeler and a chiropractor in the same rodeo functions as a microcosm of the larger professional relationship between medicine and chiropractic. Privately, each practitioner acknowledges the potential value of the other's work, but publicly ignores the other's existence and does not ever refer cowboys to him (see also Kotarba 1983a: 96).

Local Professional Wrestling

The world of local professional wrestling is a far cry from its glamorous, international counterpart. There are approximately 100 local wrestling organisations stretching across the U.S. The southern states seem to be the mainstay of local wrestling, with four organisations in the Houston, Texas, area alone. Local professional wrestling is a low-profit venture. Events are typically held in bingo halls, Veterans of Foreign Wars (VFW) clubhouses, or community centers. Crowd sizes typically range from a few dozen to three or four hundred. Tickets are very inexpensive: $9.00 for general admission (rows four to seven) and $10 for reserved seats (rows one to three). It appears that most income is derived from snack stand sales of nachos, sausage-on-a-stick, beer and the like.

Local professional wrestlers' remuneration ranges from nothing to several hundred dollars per match. Most participants maintain day jobs or other sources of income in order to support their major love and thrill in life: beating up each other with open fists or folding chairs. Typical day jobs range from nightclub bouncer and construction worker to loan shark collector and bodyguard. Those wrestlers who do not work can be found taking college courses or working out in the gym. Local professional wrestlers are young men in their twenties whose athletic careers typically include a little high school football, perhaps some high school wrestling, and considerable fighting, playful or otherwise. They love physical contact; they love to hit and be hit.

Managing Wrestling Injuries

The major structural principle organising health care in professional wrestling is that the promoter assumes no responsibility either for injury or the provision of injury care. Local wrestlers sign standardised waivers by which they assume all the responsibility for injuries. The revenues produced by professional wrestling are simply too low and unpredictable to support regular provision of health care. Furthermore, most local wrestlers do not have contracts with promoters, so that any sort of work-related health insurance would be prohibitively expensive.

That does not mean, however, that health care is not available. There are, in fact, four typical sources of care. First, some wrestlers who hold day jobs have medical insurance through work. They can receive care for wrestling injuries if they either claim that the injuries occurred at their day jobs, or if they claim that the injuries occurred during leisure time. Second, those younger wrestlers who are full-time college students or are dependents of their parents can file insurance claims based upon these statuses. Third, injuries that require immediate medical care are taken to local hospital emergency rooms where stitches and X-rays are paid for out-of-pocket. Fourth, the promoter can offer injury care directly through, for example, a friend who is a chiropractor or physical therapist and is willing to work for free.

The major cultural principle organising health care in professional wrestling is that the provision of injury care fits the local wrestling subculture. The wrestlers conceive of themselves as very physical, manly, and tough. They crave the action in the ring and use pain and injuries as signs of both their dedication to and success in the ring. Like professional rodeo cowboys, professional wrestlers seek health care less to verify disability than to get them back into the ring as soon as possible. The pragmatic approach of chiropractic fits in well. Furthermore, the small scope of local professional wrestling requires participants to act out multiple identities at different times. Wrestlers can, for example, serve as managers, corner men, promoters, and security workers. Thus, they get involved with injuries from a number of perspectives relevant to the local wrestling culture.

Interestingly, local wrestling fans are confederates in the staging of wrestling and wrestling injuries. They contribute to the mass illusion of pain and suffering with their "oohs" and "aahs" when a wrestler is punished. Yet, one event illustrates the limits to the fantasy mutually created during a wrestling event. During one recent match held in a small town near Houston, Texas, a manager, who was standing just outside the ring, handed his wrestler what appeared to be a beer bottle (I later discovered that the bottle was made of a soft, sugary, and harmless material). When the wrestler hit his opponent with the bottle, it shattered all over the ring. Several fans at ringside, who are typically the most vocal and obnoxious of all fans, immediately shouted to the referee and pointed out the sharp-edged broken "glass" littering the ring. The referee ignored their cries and, consequently, placed the combatants at great risk of head and facial cuts as they dragged each other across the canvas. Two ring attendants/guards/crowd control agents eventually swept the ring during the following intermission. This event suggests that the fans really do not enjoy or favour real injuries to their heroes in the ring.

The Cut Man in Professional Boxing

Boxing is one of the oldest sports. At its professional level, it is also the classic working-class sport (Wacquant 1992). Boxing is also the most violent of sports. The first and last objective in boxing is to hurt one's opponent, while putting up with pain and even injury oneself. At the highest professional level, boxing is an extremely lucrative business. Individual purses for heavyweight division, championship bouts are now in the eight-figure range, given the added economic impact of pay-per-view television coverage. At the local level, young men from predominantly minority and lower/working-class backgrounds, punch and jab in the hope of achieving the elusive big payday.

Accordingly, local professional boxers receive health care that is appropriate to the structure and culture of their occupation. This care is organised primarily through the training system responsible for getting the boxer in physical and psychological shape to work. There is also, by law, a ring physician present at all sanctioned boxing matches. The focus here is on the critically important health care worker who is responsible for healing the boxer during the actual match — the *cut man* (Kotarba & York 1983).[3]

Cut men come from the same working-class world as most boxers. A cut man is primarily responsible for closing cuts and stopping bleeding during a boxing match. Two different types of individuals can occupy this role. First, one of the regular trainers can perform this role as one of many corner activities. Second, and the focus of this analysis, there are men whose sole activity in the corner during the bout is to close cuts to the skin. They are the true — and often mythical — cut men. The cut man is very important to the boxer's corner because cuts acquired during a bout can end a fight. On the one hand, cuts around and above the eyes can blind a boxer and preclude him from continuing. On the other hand, heavy bleeding, even if it does not impair the boxer's vision, looks bad to ring officials who may use it as an excuse to call a fight off.

There is no formal training *per se* for becoming a cut man. Like most roles in the world of local boxing, one learns how to close cuts through informal apprenticeship

---

[3] See York (1982) for a description of our study of local boxing.

and on-the-job training. There is no one best technology available for closing cuts. The best cut men are notorious for maintaining great secrecy over the composition of their "special salve" or "magic lotion." Thus, the cut man is much like any other indigenous healer whose healing strategy is idiosyncratic (Bakx 1991).

The myth of the cut man extends beyond his magical formulae. Cut men are generally thought to be somewhat independent of the politics of the gym, and willing to help out with any boxer in need of their services. Consequently, the cut man is generally viewed as a humanitarian in an otherwise dog-eat-dog world. An example from our study of local boxing (Kotarba & York 1983: 5–7) illustrates this point:

> A talented local fighter was stopped on cuts by his more heralded out of town opponent. Prior to this fighter's bout his manager dismissed the cut man who had accompanied the fighter throughout his local career. Since the bout was on the undercard of an internationally televised event, the number of "seconds" allowed in the ring was limited. The manager chose himself to be in the corner and share the media limelight. As the fight unfolded the local fighter, despite inflicting severe damage on his favored opponent, was retired due to cuts. Dejected and dazed, the local fighter returned to the dressing room unaccompanied by either his manager or the trainer. The cut man recalled: "Larry came back all alone, still bleeding. That son of a bitch (the manager) hadn't even tried to patch him up. I went over to him and told him to let me look at it. I got him patched up so he wouldn't scar, and talked to him a little bit."

The cut man is the archetype of the primitive occupational healer, working in perhaps the most primitive of professional sports — local boxing. Structurally, the cut man gets paid very little, a "few bucks" at most per match. Quite often, he is remunerated no more than the opportunity to hang around and achieve status in an exciting sports scene. Culturally, the cut man makes his work meaningful by integrating it into a very traditional scene. Boxing is notorious for its rituals and superstitions, so that the claim that one's healing skills are "magic" makes perfect sense to everyone else in the social world of boxing.

Discussion and Conclusion

As we have seen, the quality and quantity of health care delivered to professional athletes vary according to the social class membership of the athlete. The best care goes to those athletes who are most valuable and most difficult to replace, as is also the case in the more general corporate world. We have also seen a trend over the years by which health care for professional athletes at all levels has become more sophisticated and bureaucratic. The trend is most true, however, for team athletes and the elite individual athletes. The working-class athlete is very much a sole proprietor who shoulders overwhelming responsibility for his health and illness. Like the day labourer or contract worker in the more general corporate world, the working-class athlete is not afforded the protection of a collective work environment. Without regular job status, union membership, or occupational legislation/regulation, the working-class athlete not only stops working but also ends a career when injured.

Many observers have noted that effective communication in the health care encounter is critical to healing. As sports medicine for team athletes becomes increasingly sophisticated and bureaucratic, personal communication between athletes and practitioners becomes more problematic. Ironically, the best personal communication I have observed over many years of research on this topic occurs at the working-class level, as we have seen in rodeo and boxing. Health care workers and patients either share or are close in social class membership — or at least closer in social class membership than, say, the medical specialist and a typical patient. From an interactionist perspective, they also share the same social world, including language, values, goals, routine procedures, and feelings (Unruh 1980). This finding corresponds to the high quality personal communication that occurs between chiropractors, holistic healers, and pediatrician and patients and clients in the more general world of health care delivery.

The theory presented here can be expanded and refined by applying it to other athletic worlds. The most obvious are non-American sports worlds. The structure and culture of professional soccer and rugby are much different than those of American sports, for example, leading us to look for different styles of health care delivery. Another athletic world to explore would be that of amateur sports, where the status of athletes as worker becomes quite complex.

In conclusion, what can we say about the contrast between existential and organizational levels of analysis? Athletic injuries and pain are still present in the world of professional sports. Existentially, the athlete still controls much of their disclosure. When the athlete discloses pain, however, it is most likely disclosed to a more formal, more highly trained, yet affectively distant health care worker than was previously the case. In any event, the athlete still has the right as well as the responsibility to ultimately decide when to *play with pain, talk injury.*

References

Bakx, K. (1991). The 'eclipse' of folk medicine in Western society. *Sociology of Health and Illness, 13*(1), 20–38.

Coakley, J. (2001). *Sport in society* (7th ed.). Boston: McGraw-Hill.

Conrad, P. (1988). Worksite health promotion: The social context. *Social Science and Medicine, 26*(5), 485–489.

Douglas, J. D. (1977). Existential sociology. In: J. D. Douglas, & J. M. Johnson (Eds), *Existential sociology* (pp. 3–73). New York: Cambridge University Press.

Justin Sportsmedicine Program (1999, November 24). *Justin sports medicine injury report.* Fort Worth, Texas: Author. Available: http://www.prorodeo.com.

Kaye, E. (2002). *Ain't no tomorrow.* New York: McGraw-Hill.

Kotarba, J. A. (1975). American acupuncturists: The new entrepreneurs of hope. *Urban Life, 4*(2), 149–178.

Kotarba, J. A. (1977). The chronic pain experience. In: J. D. Douglas, & J. M. Johnson (Eds), *Existential sociology* (pp. 257–272). New York: Cambridge University Press.

Kotarba, J. A. (1980). Discovering amorphous social experience: The case of chronic pain. In: W. B. Shaffir, R. A. Stebbins, & A. Turowetz (Eds), *Fieldwork experience* (pp. 57–67). New York: St. Martin's Press.

Kotarba, J. A. (1983a). *The chronic pain experience.* Beverly Hills: Sage.

Kotarba, J. A. (1983b). Perceptions of death, belief systems and the process of coping with chronic pain. *Social Science and Medicine, 17*(10), 681–690.

Kotarba, J. A. (1983c). The social control function of holistic health care: The case of space medicine. *Journal of Health and Social behavior, 24*(3), 275–288.

Kotarba, J. A. (2001). Conceptualizing sports medicine as occupational health care: Illustrations from professional rodeo and wrestling. *Qualitative Health Research, 11*(6), 766–779.

Kotarba, J. A., & Bentley, P. (1988). Workplace wellness participation and the becoming of self. *Social Science and Medicine, 26*(5), 551–558.

Kotarba, J. A., & Haney, C. A. (1995). Taking care of rodeo cowboys. Paper presented at the annual meeting of the Society for the Study of Symbolic Interaction, Los Angeles, CA (August).

Kotarba, J. A., & York, J. (1983). Professional boxing in Houston. Paper presented at the annual meeting of the Southwest Sociological Association, San Antonio, TX (March).

Lawrence, E. A. (1982). *Rodeo: An anthropologist looks at the wild and the tame.* Chicago: University of Chicago Press.

Navarro, V. (1981). Work, ideology, and science: The case of medicine. In: V. Navarro, & D. M. Berman (Eds), *Health and work under capitalism* (pp. 11–32). Farmingdale, NY: Baywood.

Nebergall, R., Bauer, J., & Eiman, R. (1992). Rough riders: How much risk is rodeo? *Physician Sports Medicine, 20*, 85–92.

Ritzer, G., & Walczak, D. (1988). Rationalization and the deprofessionalization of physicians. *Social Forces, 67,* 1–22.

Thompson, C. (2002). Boselli's shoulder cleaned. *Houston Chronicle,* April 30, Section C, p. 1.

Unruh, D. R. (1980). The nature of social worlds. *Pacific Sociological Review, 23,* 271–296.

Wacquant, J. D. (1992). The social logic of boxing in Black Chicago: Toward a sociology of pugilism. *Sociology of Sport Journal, 9*(3), 221–254.

Wooden, W. S., & Ehringer, G. (1996). *Rodeo in America: Wranglers, roughstock & paydirt.* Lawrence, KS: University Press of Kansas.

York, J. (1982). *Professional boxing: A social constructionist perspective.* Masters Thesis, Department of Sociology, University of Houston.

Young, K. (1993). Violence, risk and liability in male sports culture. *Sociology of Sport Journal, 10,* 373–396.

Zimbalist, A. (1999). *Unpaid professionals: Commercialism and conflict in big-time college sports.* Princeton, NJ: Princeton University Press.

Chapter 5

Weight Management as Sport Injury: Deconstructing Disciplinary Power in the Sport Ethic

David P. Johns

One of the many paradoxes that exists in modern sport is to be found in the way that certain behaviours, normally considered deviant or extreme, have become acceptable when practised within the institution of sport. This normalising effect can be attributed to an ethic that seems to influence individuals into adopting expected patterns of behaviour that define what it means to be an athlete in a particular sport in contemporary society. Sporting practices, particularly at the high performance level, require, even demand, unquestioned and unqualified acceptance of certain discursive practices. This conformity has become embodied in what has become known as "the sport ethic" (Hughes & Coakley 1991). In their paper, Hughes and Coakley describe the sport ethic as the willingness of an individual to adopt a cluster of beliefs involving sacrifice, risk, striving for distinction, and accepting no limits in order to be acknowledged as an athlete. Consequently, many of the injuries, conditions and disorders from which athletes suffer are directly related to their desire to conform to such an ethic. While this phenomenon is interesting from a moralistic point of view, it is of greater interest for sociologists to understand the relationships of power that operate to bring about injuries and disorders than to examine the biological or structural disorders themselves. This chapter attempts to analyse the organisational power that exists between athletes and their supervisory or administrative superiors (Gruneau 1993: 85) in order to understand how such power relationships facilitate extreme corporeal practices involving dietary control that often result in unjustified injury and suffering.

Sporting Bodies, Damaged Selves
Research in the Sociology of Sport, Volume 2, 117–133
© 2004 Published by Elsevier Ltd.
ISSN: 1476-2854/doi:10.1016/S1476-2854(04)02005-9

How Power Shapes Action

Sociologists of sport have been remarkably reticent in their discussions about corporeal practices, considering their interest in the social significance of sport and the importance of the body in such a human activity (Theberge 1991). Nevertheless, after a decade of interest in this aspect of the discursive practice of sport, scholars in this field have returned the body to the culture that surrounds sport (Loy *et al.* 1993). This resurgence of interest has kindled an awareness of the body and the part it plays in the social interaction related to sport settings. The rise in interest now devoted to the body has been due to several factors. These are what Frank (1990) has termed modernism, postmodernism and feminism. Of these three developments, the most salient is postmodernism which has succinctly addressed prominent issues that are highly relevant to sport through the concepts developed by Foucault (1977, 1978, 1985, 1986a, b, 1988).

In this chapter, a Foucauldian framework will be engaged in order to explore the way in which disciplinary power is linked to sport. The focus will be at the point where the sport ethic intersects with those discursive practices of high performance athletes that are especially related to severe weight loss practices and the deliberate denial and elimination of one or more food groups from their diet. This framework will permit the body to be situated at the center of the research question and will allow an investigation of questions usually not posed by the more traditional biomedical discourses. In this way, it is possible to explore the connection between knowledge and power as it relates to high performance athletes, not only from a macro level but also at the specific site of action (Fox 1994). This connection can be analysed in the context of a discourse of expertise that legitimises the preparation of athletes and uses power coercively to ensure the production of a compliant and passive participant.

It is interesting to note that Foucault makes no mention of sport in his analysis of social relations. However, his concept of power is useful when analysed as a micropolitical influence that is "implicit in everyday interaction and the normalized practices demanded in various institutional settings" (Gruneau 1993: 101). What Foucault has termed "procedures of power" was developed out of the 17th century view of the need for political power over the body, from birth to death. At that time, the body was understood to be a bipolar entity. The first pole was seen as being anatomical or machine-like, while the second was thought to be biological and political in nature. Foucault described the whole structure as being linked together by an "intermediary cluster of relations" (1978: 139). With such importance ascribed to the appropriate function of the body, surveillance of the population was introduced to regulate the performance of the body, requiring deployment of an entire series of regulatory controls or "disciplines of the body." Thus evolved the notion of power over performances of the body, based on the coercive discourse of expertise.

Foucault's intention was to understand the way in which power became the type of constraint on action (Fraser 1989) that shaped and enabled rather than distorted or inhibited action. Using the example of discourse in sport, such constraint can be construed as the means to provide boundaries beyond which the discourse is no longer relevant. Through prescription, proscription and description (Shogan 1999), the discursive practice of athletes and coaches can define the constitution and acquisition of sport skills within the terms of the sport ethic. By focusing on some of the preparatory practices of the sport, it becomes clear how difficult it is to distinguish between those ethically and morally prescribed boundaries. This is particularly challenging when winning can make a significant difference to the lifestyle of an athlete who has made considerable sacrifices to excel at his or her sport. Exploring the concept of disciplinary power illustrates how groups within sport such as athletes, coaches, administrators and others contend with prescribed practices within the proscriptive constraints that are established for the sport.

Sport Studies and a Foucauldian Perspective

In making the case for use of a Foucauldian analytical framework, Rail and Harvey (1995) have shown how Foucauldian concepts such as technologies of power and technologies of the self can be applied to contemporary sport. Using postmodern terminology, it can be described as a "site that embodies the tensions between regimentation and excess" (Miller 1998: 81). Within the sociology of sport literature there is now an increasing number of examples of the way in which researchers have explored Foucault's conceptualisation of the body to explain how technologies of power and domination operate in different social contexts (Bordo 1993; Cole 1993; Duncan 1994; Spitzack 1990). The following are only a few of the many examples of efforts to provide an explanation of sporting practices from a Foucauldian perspective. For example, Chapman (1997) has examined the subjective experiences of female rowers to understand how weight management, a technology of the self, is governed by normalising assumptions used to ensure that their bodies become the site of domination. Similarly, Johns and Johns (2000) have examined the binary relationships that are formed in settings where athletes in particular are often dominated by coaches and administrators and their presumed expertise. In another study, Duncan (1994) has employed the image of the panopticon, a Foucauldian analogy of prison architecture. In this case, it is used to illustrate how modern athletes are subjected to the surveillance of the public especially when they are exposed to the uninvited gaze of others through the photographic, printed and electronic media.

These studies of competitive sport interrogate, deconstruct and frequently discover paradoxical configurations in the discourse, but unfortunately they do not necessarily mean that solutions will follow because critics "work from positions that locate change and movement in strategies other than the resolution of contradiction" (Cole 1998: 273). Not surprisingly, different perspectives reveal different realities. For example, a cursory glance may suggest that athletes have been empowered by their goal-orientation and the self-chosen means to achieve it. Alternatively, a critical interrogation of the discourse reveals a discursive practice that privileges coaches and officials and, in the process, subordinates the athletes. Thus an "agency of discipline" is created (Miller 1993: 38) that produces "docile bodies that monitor, guard and discipline themselves" (Eskes *et al.* 1998: 319).

Body Images and the Pre-occupation with Weight Loss

There can be no doubt that modern sports provide a public forum for the production of images made apparent through the presentation of the sporting body. These images cover a wide spectrum and extend from the way in which the athletic body conforms to trends and styles set by the fashion and fitness industries (Johns 1998) to broader issues of national identity. The latter is illustrated by the way in which a nation is somehow represented by the child-like bodies of gymnasts (Chisholm 1999). In her examination of U.S. Women's Olympic gymnastics, Chisholm suggests that the multi-ethnic team is seen as the embodiment of Americanisation that mediates the cultural anxieties of the popular U.S. imagination. Such examples serve to emphasise the emergence of the sporting body in a form that has ignited social and cultural interests in the body as a site for a critical discourse.

In spite of considerable research in this area, there is no conclusive evidence to suggest where the modern image of the ideal body originated. However, it is clear that in today's consumer-driven market place, the advertising industry has played a major part in shaping the culture of the young (Klein 2000). Certainly, images of the ideal body have continued to change throughout history, from the Rubenesque female forms depicted in many of the masterpieces of art to the waif-like figures that parade down the "cat walks" in the fashion houses of Paris, London and New York. For women, the normal body shape and size has been redefined. Women's health and beauty magazines, following the lead of men's magazines, are devoting more attention to exercise as a means of creating the ideal body (Eskes *et al.* 1998). Reinforced by the sylph-like images of fashion models and those in the film industry, it is not surprising that for many contemporary women, self-esteem seems to be linked with physical appearance. Achieving the perfect shape has become even more difficult, because in most physically active pursuits, the design of clothing "barely disguise(s) the form underneath, and instead of using garments to reshape themselves, women are relying on diet, exercise and the tools of the plastic surgeon" (Tucker 1990: 95). While it would be unusual for female athletes to subject themselves to plastic surgery, the emphasis on exercise, diet and weight loss is increasingly emphasised more to enhance appearance than to improve performance. The emphasis on the cosmetic body shape as opposed to physiological preparation for performance has only recently been examined in terms of how body shape impacts on sporting outcomes (Chapman 1997; Chisholm 1999; Johns 1998).

In high performance sport, where the visual appearance of the body plays a major part in the eventual outcome, dieting is a form of preparation deemed necessary for the purpose of gaining, losing and maintaining body weight. As such, it is experienced as a technology of power that dominates individuals "bringing them to define themselves in particular ways" (Miller 1993: xiv). This power has, until recently, been more clearly illustrated by female athletes because of the attention that has been drawn to an apparent predisposition to eating disorders (Sundgot-Borgen 1994). In contrast, the male physical form has received less attention from a biomedical perspective than from the sociologists who have focused on its value as a commodity and the related exploitation of the body in that context (Miller 1998; Young 1993). Nevertheless, this differentiation is amplified in various subjective sports where the female body image rather than that of the male is a major factor in the performance outcome. This is particularly evident in sports such as gymnastics, synchronised swimming, figure skating, and diving where athletes are guided by unwritten rules to mold an ideal body shape for performance. The impact of this pre-occupation with body shape and the devastating results of unhealthy eating habits have been thoroughly and dramatically chronicled by Ryan (2000).

Perhaps to the less informed, the male body has not been subjected to the same scrutiny as the female body. However, Martin and Miller have pointed out that not only does "sport allow men to watch and dissect other men's bodies in fetishistic detail" (1999: 20) but, as society moves towards a sexually inclusive audience, the sporting body, male or female, has become "the master signifier of the fashion-magazine industry" (Miller 1998: 105). It is significant that the interest in the male body has not only paralleled the rise in the commodification of sport over the last two decades but is now raising similar questions of overconforming practices leading to injury (White & Young 1997; Young *et al.* 1994) that have until recently focused primarily on women in sport. The sport injury process in male sports has traditionally been considered in biomedical and biomechanical terms but, as White and Young point out, little attention has been paid to "the way in which hegemonic styles of playing and organizing sport interface with gender dynamics" (1997: 3). In response to this observation, this chapter departs from the biomedical perspective in order to examine how the power arrangements in sport influence the injury process by means of the discursive practices of the athletes.

Current Discursive Practices of the Sport Ethic

As these practices are subjected to closer scrutiny by sociologists of sport (Chapman 1997; Johns & Johns 2000), it has become apparent that technologies of power in sport are either associated with the subjectification of the body and the image (gymnastics, figure skating) it represents, or the body as instrument (boxing, weightlifting) and how it is maintained to meet specific sport requirements. Although these technologies are not usually linked to structural injury such as broken bones and torn ligaments, they should be identified as serious psychological disorders that often lead to unnecessary suffering, debilitating injuries (Ryan 2000) and even death (Hawaleshka 1994). A common misconception has been that eating disorders related to weight control were primarily a problem for female athletes involved in subjective sports. However, this is not the case as the problem has also extended to male athletes in many sports where body mass is a critical factor. Sports such as boxing, rowing and wrestling require athletes to conform to the weight class in which they have chosen to compete. If they are unable to meet these stringent requirements, they are not permitted to enter the competition. To ensure that they conform to the weight class, athletes in these sports often use severe weight-loss practices (sauna exposure, fluid restriction, diuretic use) and in doing so expose themselves to the risk of micronutrient deficiency, dehydration, hypohydration and hyponatremia (American College of Sports Medicine 2000: 2137) which, in some cases have resulted in the death of athletes. Three American collegiate wrestlers died in 1997 while attempting to rapidly lose weight before a match (quoted in Kiningham & Gorenflo 2001). In their fatal attempt they used fasting and dehydration which, according to Kiningham and Gorenflo, "can adversely affect cardiovascular function electrical activity, thermal regulation, renal function, and electrolyte balance" (2001: 813).

Classification by weight also is used in ocean racing where the crew of each boat must conform to a predetermined total weight. In the case of the 2001 Volvo "Round-the-World" yacht race, one particular all-women crew appealed to the organisers because they were underweight and wished to add additional crew to make up the deficit, as the women competitors were generally lighter than their male counterparts. The outcome was that the yacht sailed with 13 female crew members whereas the all-male crews sailed with 12.

Athletes who aspire to weigh more are more unusual in most sports than those who desire to shed weight. Clinical psychologists have observed that dancers are pre-occupied with weight loss because a lighter body helps the dancer to conform to a specific image and also enables them to jump higher. Male and female divers use pathogenic weight-loss methods to lose weight in order to improve the visual effect of the body in flight (Murphy 1995). In ski jumping, the ability to lose weight is also considered crucial for better performance because it is now recognised that lighter athletes jump significantly further than heavier athletes. In these disciplines, clinical psychologists have reported disturbed eating behaviours among ski jumpers, divers and dancers because athletes in these sports believe that in order to jump higher, further or to appear more aesthetic during flight, it is imperative to lose weight. Superficially, these disciplines of the self appear to promote sport as a wholesome, natural and liberating experience. However, observers who have examined the validity (Chapman 1997), ethics (Shogan 1999) and paradoxes of the sporting experience (Johns 1998) have indicated that to achieve these acceptably contoured bodies and to meet weight class restrictions requires a "transgression of the body's natural limits" (Franklin 1996: S100).

Discursive Practice or Athletic Excess?

Fox compellingly argues that modern cities provide evidence that the surface of the body is probably the most "discussed, imagined, prescribed and proscribed, disfigured, disguised and disciplined surface in the physical world . . . and in the main street, in the clinics, and in the private rooms experts inscribe the body, be they doctors, sports instructors or lovers" (1994: 25–26). Clearly, athletes signify and inscribe their bodies by marshalling technologies that will produce athletic-looking bodies. This strategy can be deconstructed to expose discursive practices that are associated specifically with athletic performance. For athletes, the body is the focus of the discourse and consequently becomes the most discussed, prescribed and disciplined aspect of the process of subjectification, a process easily identified through the modalities used in sport preparation (Rail & Harvey 1995). Immersed in this process, athletes learn to be intensely aware of the importance of the body. They adopt the appropriate technologies. This technique permits them to effect what Foucault describes as, "a certain number of operations on their own bodies and souls, thoughts, conduct, and way of being, so as to transform them-selves in order to attain a certain state of happiness, purity, wisdom, perfection, or immortality" (1988: 18). It is obvious that in sports such as rowing, boxing and wrestling it is essential that an athlete conforms to the declared weight class. The consequence for non-compliance is to be eliminated before the competition begins, thus dashing any hopes of achieving those states of happiness, immortality or perfection that Foucault describes. As an added incentive for adherence to the prescribed standard, wrestlers are weighed in public, yet another technique to ensure that they comply with the rules. They maintain their diet right up to the point of stepping on the scales and as soon as they have assured the officials that they have conformed to their declared weight class, they are no longer weighed or monitored.

In her research, Franklin has observed that high performance preparations for sport "are enacted along the impossibly thin edge of the acceptable and the unacceptable transgression of the body's natural limits" (1996: S100). These fine lines of transgression are more discernable in some sports than in others. For example, wrestlers, synchronised swimmers and track athletes consider nutrition as a necessary dietary proscribed behaviour essential to athletic preparation. Although stringent dieting is required, they do not generally consider themselves to be transgressing any natural biological parameters as in the case of the three unfortunate wrestlers who died. Proscribed boundaries are more clearly understood than those that are prescribed within the excesses of elite sport (Johns 1998). This is because proscribed constraints are usually set out by the sport governing body and are established on what is considered to be acceptable and normal whereas an athlete's behaviour in high performance sport is grounded in an "uncritical acceptance of rules" (Coakley 2001: 145) that permit, encourage and even demand practices that can only be considered to be beyond proscription. Weight management has become one of the regulatory modalities that frequently can transgress proscriptive constraints. This particular practice may include a combination of behaviours that are performed to regulate the body such as compulsive exercise, excessive weight training, the consumption of ergogenic aids and performance enhancing drugs that may or may not be legal. Ironically, the latter practice has not received the attention that perhaps it deserves considering the apparent prevalence of these behaviours among high performance athletes (Reiterer 2000).

By most normal standards, a description of weight management in sports is extreme and would include a range of aberrant eating habits such as fasting, "crash" dieting, purging, use of diuretics, diet pills and fluid restriction (Murphy 1995). Other techniques used regularly include the avoidance of food consumption or eating in public but, when eating at a team or family meal is unavoidable, self-induced vomiting immediately after the meal occurs to eliminate the food before the body begins the digestion process. The following extracts from an interview I conducted with Sarah, an 18-year old Canadian rhythmic gymnast who battled with weight loss for many years during her competitive career, illustrate the conflict encountered in weight management:

> (Extract 1) They (coaches) told me to eat like the young gymnasts on the junior team, which was completely ridiculous because a twelve or thirteen year old's metabolism is totally different to an eighteen year old. The coaches were always watching you and that forces you to 'pig out' in seclusion. Anyhow, they had me sign contracts and weighed me 4 times a day. In frustration and anger the coach made me drop my tights so that she could examine my butt to see how fat I was. She also made me tell her my weight in front of other gymnasts. You can't imagine how humiliating that is.

> (Extract 2) One instant sticks out in my mind. My teammate was a pretty good gymnast and the coaches felt she was the ideal athlete because she was quiet, did what she was asked and was thin as a rail. I was always being compared with her because I was eating healthily and was not as thin and did not always do what I was told. The thing the coaches didn't know was that she was a full-blown bulimic. In front of the coaches she was restrained and didn't eat a thing but when she was back in her room she stuffed herself with all sorts of junk food and then threw it up in the toilet.

Such accounts indicate the efforts athletes make to manage an appropriate impression because they are the subjects of a clinical gaze that exercise a technology of power that could define them as fat, indifferent, lazy, or rebellious. In contrast, athletes who effectively manage impressions that others have of them apply a technology of the self through inscriptions of docility, compliance and productivity involving "humiliation, extraordinary work and blind obedience" (Ryan 2000: 27) that are reaffirmed in the gaze of the coaches and officials. The effort to transform is aimed at heightened awareness of the ideal body form and regulation of the body in order to meet the criteria of compliance and outcome or what Foucault referred to as the essential qualities of "docility-utility" (1977: 138).

As a so-called spectator sport, women's gymnastics places particular emphasis on the importance of appearance (Johns 1998). The importance of this image of the body has been observed by Chisholm, who writes: "Not coincidentally, judges and television commentators for women's gymnastics assess gracefulness and elegance, and concurrently perfect performances, not only in relation to the execution of elements derived from dance but also in relation to overall appearance" (1999: 133). The achievement of this ideal representation involves more than merely poise, confidence and a winning smile. Gymnasts express concern with their shape and size because "their appearance may affect the judges' ratings of their performance" (Chapman 1997: 207). Regardless of the warnings of sports medicine practitioners, most gymnasts follow a stringent regime of dieting (Sundgot-Borgen 1993) to lose weight so that their appearance indicates low fat ratios and well-defined musculature. These standards, imposed by a sport ethic, define what it is to be an athlete but fail to prescribe how this is to be attained without deleterious effects. This has been recognised by sport psychologists as a serious problem among coaches and athletes: "The greatest danger to an athlete's health exists when pressure is applied to lose weight in the absence of knowledge concerning safe and effective weight-management procedures" (Murphy 1995: 316).

Unfortunately, those in positions of authority such as coaches and judges are free to demand achievement of unwritten "gold" standards. Often these standards are based on knowledge derived from sport science that show it is possible to draw a positive relationship between low percent body fat and high performance success in sports. However, the exact percentages of body fat have not been correlated to specific performances nor have they been generalised to populations of athletes in any one sport. Thus the suitability of the gymnast for the sport is often based on the coach's notion of whether her body shape is acceptable or can be transformed into a particular ideal. Consequently, gymnasts, under the powerful influence of coaches, work long hours without adequate levels of nutrition or fluid intake to ensure that their appearance meets the requirements defined by judges and endorsed by coaches. In particular, female gymnasts are often subjected to manipulation and harassment (as exemplified by public weighings) by coaches because they are young and over-willing to conform to standards that are subjective and arbitrary and that dictate the way in which the individual is to present herself in the competition (Johns 1998).

Similar to that ideal demanded in synchronised swimming and gymnastics, presentation of the ideal body shape is even more important in bodybuilding because the athlete is subjectively judged on the volume and proportion of the musculature of the body (Klein 1993). This sport focuses on ways of increasing the size and improving the shape of muscles through tortuously long hours of resistance training using machines and free weights to accomplish cosmetic goals. In keeping with overconforming behaviours of the sport ethic, athletes in this sport go far beyond what would be considered normal by augmenting their physical workouts with ergogenic aids that result in the accentuation and even distortion of the shape and volume of muscles. To realise this extraordinary achievement requires a great deal more than long and punishing workouts in the weight-room.

Since bodybuilding became highly competitive, it has become common discursive practice to be able to discuss, know about and consume a range of supplements such as chromium, creatine and HMB (beta-hydroxy-beta-methyl-butyrate). Some athletes go even further and are knowledgeable about and even practice with precision the use of drugs such as anabolic steroids and growth hormones (American College of Sports Medicine 1999; Coakley 2001). Finally, to achieve the ideal of body appearance in the hours leading to the competition, bodybuilders severely restrict food and fluid intake (leaving them malnourished and dehydrated) in order to drain the fluids in the superficial tissues covering the muscles to create an image of pure muscle in the complete absence of body fat. Bodybuilding as a sport is the ultimate paradox in which the athlete's body in the quest for excellence is reduced to its lowest and most compromised state in terms of physical performance.

Ways and Means to Accomplish the Impossible

The preceding examples reveal a complex inter-relationship of power and domination in the sport setting (Birrell & Cole 1994; Chapman 1997; Rail & Harvey 1995). These are omnipresent and well dispersed in a web-like structure throughout society. In everyday routines, they act to normalise technologies of the self. This begs the question of how it is possible to sustain the use of such self-disciplined technologies in the unbridled preparation of the self for sporting competition. A Foucauldian response to this dilemma is to focus on the politics of the body through its visibility. In his analysis, the panopticon — a prison tower and an "exemplar of modern surveillance" (Fox 1994: 28) — became a useful metaphor in which those who are guarded cannot see who is guarding them or if they are being guarded at all. By this means, Foucault has shown that society no longer requires structural mechanisms to maintain and reproduce power relations. External control would be replaced by an internal equivalent. Similarly, many aspects of modern society, including sport participation, are controlled by mechanisms that are widely dispersed and difficult to locate (Eskes *et al.* 1998). Surveillance, from the Foucauldian perspective, is more than simply a comprehensive management of everyday life. By means of an invisible but ever-present force, society is held together. It is also constituted as a sense of personal responsibility, one that incorporates personal rights and freedoms. In sport, this force is evident in the way athletes express obligation and commitment particularly when they are engaging in extreme acts referred to by Hughes and Coakley (1991) as "positive deviance" or a zealousness to over-conform.

As we have seen in the examples above, the commitment of athletes to their sport is evident through their adherence to the sport ethic. However, there is considerable variability in the discursive practice of athletes and how far beyond the natural boundaries of the body athletes are prepared to go. While athletes, in so-called "power sports" such as field events, are unable to excel in competition without with the assistance of growth hormones (Reiterer 2000), others seem more able to cope within those boundaries. Middle- and long-distance runners, by natural selection, are endowed with a lean muscle mass and are well suited to the demands of their sport. Normally, they express no concerns with body weight or body shape because the level of anaerobic training required to excel in their sport ensures the effective use of body fat as a source of energy resulting, usually, in 6–15% body fat (American College of Sports Medicine 2000: 2133). Their disciplinary practice is concerned with function rather than form because the performance is based on the objective measure of distance against time. Athletes perform in a public forum that permits the anonymous engagement of the normalising gaze of coaches and other athletes in "a surveillance that makes it possible to qualify, to classify, and to punish" (Foucault 1977: 184–185). Understandably, athletes are very aware of the scrutiny of their peers. These feelings of being watched have been recognised and can be summed up in the following extracts by Greg, a 24-year old Canadian middle-distance runner, and Sarah, the gymnast previously mentioned:

> (Extract 3) I feel a certain pressure to maintain my body so that it looks fit and prepared because people soon notice and make all sorts of remarks that make you feel they are sizing you up.

> (Extract 4) This sport is about appearance and everyone is totally aware of it. Coaches and judges come to the workouts to scan you and stare at you when you are working out. They are not only looking at how you are doing the skills. They are eyeing you off to see how fat you are. And of course we all look at each other to see if we are getting fat or if we gained over the weekend.

These excerpts illustrate the fact that surveillance is based on the athlete's perception of unspoken proscriptions and accepted standards. These are learned by athletes and guide them as members of the group to conform in order to retain their membership. While coaches interpret messages that are inscribed on the bodies of athletes that signify them as worthy members of the sport, athletes feel they must engage in technologies they believe will sustain that membership. Dieting, as a technology of the self, for the purpose of weight management, operates within the power relationship between athlete and coach creating a disciplinary structure in which power effectively shapes the discursive practice through constant surveillance and manipulation.

Modifying the Coach/Athlete Power Relationship

This chapter has considered the ramifications of aberrations in eating patterns in athletes as part of a health-related disorder that has the potential to injure the body and the mind. The sociological explanation for this particular injury seems to be more complex and much less conclusive than those offered from a biomedical perspective. This type of injury is so serious that it is capable of eclipsing a promising sports career in which the disease process, in particular cases, has been fatal. Nevertheless, there is a certain consistency in the willingness of athletes to expose themselves to the inherent risks associated with sport and in the way they engage in a discursive practice that is excessively sacrificial, driven by distinction and accepts no limits. It seems that athletes such as ski jumpers, divers, and gymnasts are faced with the possibility that they will sustain serious injuries. However, they do not regard abnormal eating behaviours to be as serious as a bad fall even when such behaviours render the athlete incapable of performing at the levels that such practices were designed to achieve. The reasons for this are that discursive practices involving eating have become normalised and the outcomes are insidious rather than traumatic. Another distinct difference between the usual injuries sustained by athletes and the disorders associated with eating is that, unlike muscular-skeletal injuries, eating disorders are preventable. Behaviours associated with dietary intake for weight-management purposes do not occur accidentally but are processes through which power arrangements are permitted to foster practices that lead to over-conformity and eventual breakdown of normal health.

It is clear that there is a disciplinary power structure that exists within the boundaries of the sport ethic that can be defined in Foucauldian terms as a binary opposition between the authority and power of the coach and the over-conforming willingness of the athlete. Deconstruction of these distinct but related entities enables us to uncover "the logic of grammar" (Cole 1998: 273) upon which these binary terms depend and upon which the structure of the present argument is based. We have witnessed that more salience and importance is accorded the privileged and presumed expertise of coaches and administrators than to athletes who are sanctioned and resource-dependent. This logic is located in the signifiers and behaviours of athletes, whose practices otherwise would be considered "unconscionable assaults" (Fox 1994: 40) on the individual outside the discourse. However, for reasons peculiar to sport, these practices are created when "technologies of power and technologies of the self" (Miller 1993: xiii) constitute the discourse within its boundaries.

In speaking about educational planners, Cherryholmes has suggested that "[u]nless those who are privileged voluntarily and actively refuse the benefits of their position, oppressive conditions and situations are likely to continue" (1988: 165). Although they may have a profound effect, such voluntary actions are no more likely to happen in sport than they are in educational reform. Nevertheless, a strategy is required to challenge the present arrangement in many sports and the employment of a Foucauldian deconstruction strategy is proposed. This technique calls for the interruption and contradiction of the discourse in order "to multiply the levels of knowing" (Lather 1991: 12–13). Such a strategy of displacement requires the reversal of "the dependent term from its negative position to a place that locates it as the very condition of the positive term." This permits an alternative subjectification in which the reformulation "creates a more fluid and less coercive conceptual organization of terms" (Lather 1991: 13). This, in effect, disrupts the discourse, challenges and demystifies the privileges that have been created by coaches and as such provides a safeguard against the dominant system of beliefs. Adoption of this strategy would provide a healthier perspective for high performance sport. By allowing athletes to "explore the constitution of themselves as subjects of sport" (Shogan 1999: 91) they would be released from the grip of power that embroils them in a sport ethic that demands but never rewards, and overemphasises success without evaluation of personal loss.

The willingness to conform will remain, and as "long as athletes accept without question or qualification the norms of the sport ethic, they will continue to voluntarily try or take anything to remain in sports" (Coakley 2001: 168). Such disciplinary power is not confined to sport institutions but may be found in other settings such as those found in high school physical education where participants are encouraged to indulge in a "risk-focused, body obsessed, calorie counting, sports mad" (Tinning 2001: 8) discourse. An alternative approach, suggested by Tinning, is one that could be equally applied to athletes as well as to high school students. It emphasises the need to physically educate citizens who are "critical consumers of the sports, fitness and leisure industries" (2001: 8). As long as the power relationship of coach to athlete exists in its present form in the disciplinary structure of sport, critical thought leading to liberating action is unlikely to develop. What is needed is the development of a relationship where the opportunity exists "to encourage an active and ongoing questioning by participants of the ways in which sport discipline 'normalises' practices that would otherwise be considered harmful and that produce athletes capable of and willing to engage in these prac- tices" (Shogan 1999: 91). Therefore, a plausible response to inherent problems in high performance sport would be to facilitate the disruption of the discourse and set aside the power arrangements upon which the discourse is founded. Then, it would be vital to allow the relationship between coach and athlete to develop into one of mutual respect in order to re-evaluate the norms of the sport ethic and to set limits that are likely to be adopted, respected and maintained. Without such changes, the strength of the sport ethic will continue to dehumanise the athlete by demanding that they adjust to structures imposed upon them while they remain silent about the exercise of power within those structures.

References

American College of Sports Medicine (1999). *Anabolic steroids: Current comments* (April).

American College of Sports Medicine, American Dietetic Association and Dietitians of Canada Joint Position Paper (2000). Nutrition and athletic performance. *Medicine and Science in Sports and Exercise, 32*(12), 2130–2145.

Birrell, S., & Cole, S. (1994). *Women, sport and culture.* Champaign, IL: Human Kinetics.

Bordo, S. (1993). *Unbearable weight: Feminism, western culture, and the body.* Berkeley, CA: University of California Press.

Chapman, G. E. (1997). Making weight: Lightweight rowing, technologies of power, and technologies of the self. *Sociology of Sport Journal, 14,* 205–223.

Cherryholmes, C. (1988). *Power and criticism: Post-structural investigations in education.* New York: Teacher's College Press.

Chisholm, A. (1999). Defending the nation: National bodies, U.S. Borders, and the 1996 U.S. Olympic Women's gymnastic team. *Journal of Sport & Social Issues, 23*(2), 126–139.

Coakley, J. J. (2001). *Sport in society: Issues and controversies* (7th ed.). New York: Irwin and McGraw-Hill.

Cole, C. (1993). Resisting the canon: Feminist cultural studies, sport, and technologies of the body. *Journal of Sport & Social Issues, 17,* 77–97.

Cole, C. (1998). Addiction, exercise and cyborgs: Technologies of deviant bodies. In: G. Rail (Ed.), *Sport and postmodern times* (pp. 261–275). Albany: State University of New York Press.

Duncan, M. C. (1994). The politics of women's body images and practices: Foucault, the panopticon, and Shape magazine. *Journal of Sport and Social Issues, 18,* 48–65.

Eskes, T. B., Duncan, C. M., & Miller, M. M. (1998). The discourse of empowerment: Foucault, Marcuse and the women's fitness texts. *Journal of Sport and Social Issues, 22*(3), 317–344.

Foucault, M. (1977). *Discipline and punish: The birth of the prison.* New York: Pantheon Books.

Foucault, M. (1978). *The history of sexuality* (Vol. 1). New York: Vintage Books.

Foucault, M. (1985). *The history of sexuality: The use of pleasure* (Vol. 2). New York: Random House.

Foucault, M. (1986a). *The history of sexuality: The care of self* (Vol 3). New York: Random House.

Foucault, M. (1986b). *The care of the self.* New York: Random House.

Foucault, M. (1988). *Technologies of the self: A seminar with Michel Foucault.* Amherst: University of Massachusetts Press.

Fox, N. J. (1994). *Postmodernism, sociology and health*. Toronto: University of Toronto Press.

Frank, A. W. (1990). Bringing bodies back in: A decade review. *Theory, Culture and Society, 7*, 131–162.

Franklin, S. (1996). Postmodern body techniques: Some anthropological considerations in natural and postnatural bodies. *Journal of Sport and Exercise Psychology, 18*, S95–S106.

Fraser, N. (1989). *Unruly practices: Power, discourse, and gender in contemporary social theory*. Minneapolis: University of Minnesota Press.

Gruneau, R. (1993). The critique of sport in modernity: Theorising, power, culture, and the politics of the body. In E. G. Dunning, J. A. Maguire, & R. E. Pearton (Eds.), *The sporting process: A comparative and developmental approach* (pp. 85–109). Champaign, IL: Human Kinetics.

Hawaleshka, D. (1994, July 28). Pressures cited in gymnast's death. *The Globe and Mail* (p. 15).

Hughes, R., & Coakley, J. (1991). Positive deviance among athletes: The implications of overconformity to the sport ethic. *Sociology of Sport Journal, 8*(4), 307–325.

Johns, D. P. (1998). Fasting and feasting: Paradoxes of the sport ethic. *Sociology of Sport Journal, 15*, 41–63.

Johns, D. P., & Johns, J. S. (2000). Surveillance, subjectivism and technologies of power: An anaylsis of the discursive practices of high-performance sport. *International Review for the Sociology of Sport, 35*(2), 219–234.

Kiningham, R. B., & Gorenflo, D. W. (2001). Weight loss methods of high school wrestlers. *Medicine & Science in Sports & Exercise, 33*(5), 810–813.

Klein, A. (1993). *Little big men: Bodybuilding subculture and gender construction*. Albany: State University of New York Press.

Klein, N. (2000). *No logo: Taking aim at the brand bullies*. Toronto: Vintage Books.

Lather, P. (1991). *Getting smart: Feminist research and pedagogy with/in the postmodern*. London: Routlege.

Loy, J. W., Andrews, D. L., & Rinehart, R. E. (1993). The body in culture and sport. *Sport Science Review, 2*(1), 69–91.

Martin, R., & Miller, T. (Eds.). (1999). *Sportcult*. Minneapolis: University of Minnesota Press.

Miller, T. (1993). *The well-tempered self: Citizenship, culture, and the postmodern subject*. Baltimore: Johns Hopkins University Press.

Miller, T. (1998). *Technologies of truth. Cultural citizenship and the popular media*. Minneapolis: University of Minnesota Press.

Murphy, S. (1995). Eating disorders and weight management. In: S. M. Murphy (Ed.), *Sport psychology interventions* (pp. 307–329). Champaign, IL: Human Kinetics.

Rail, G., & Harvey, J. (1995). Body and work: Michel Foucault and the sociology of sport. *Sociology of Sport Journal, 12*, 164–179.

Reiterer, W. (2000). *Positive: An Australian Olympian reveals the inside story of drugs and sport*. Sydney: Pan Macmillan Australia Pty Limited.

Ryan, J. (2000). *Little girls in pretty boxes*. New York: Warner Books.

Shogan, D. (1999). *The making of high-performance athletes: Discipline, diversity, and ethics.* Toronto: University of Toronto Press.

Spitzack, C. (1990). *Confessing exercise: Women and the politics of body reduction.* Albany, NY: State University of New York Press.

Sundgot-Borgen, J. (1993). Prevalence of eating disorders in female elite athletes. *International Journal of Sport Nutrition, 3*, 29–40.

Sundgot-Borgen, J. (1994). Eating disorders in female athletes. *Sports Medicine, 17*(3), 176–188.

Theberge, N. (1991). Recent developments in the theory of the body. *Quest, 43*, 123–134.

Tinning, R. (2001, June). *Physical education and the making of citizens: Considering the pedagogical work of physical education in contemporary times.* José-Marié Cagigal Lecture, Association Internationale Des Ecoles Superieures D'Education Physique International Congress, Taipei, Taiwan.

Tucker, S. (1990). What is the ideal body? *Shape Magazine*, July, 95–11.

White, P., & Young, K. (1997). Masculinity, Sport, and the injury process: A review of Canadian and international evidence. *Avante, 3*, 1–30.

Young, K. (1993). Violence, risk, and liability in male sports culture. *Sociology of Sport Journal, 10*(4), 373–396.

Young, K., White, P., & McTeer, W. (1994). Body talk: Male athletes reflect on sport, injury, and pain. *Sociology of Sport Journal, 11*, 175–194.

Part II

Pain Zones

Chapter 6

English Professional Soccer Players and the Uncertainties of Injury

Martin Roderick

Injuries have a number of well-understood meanings for English professional soccer players. For example, an injury might mean that they will lose their place in the team, and they may not be certain of regaining their position once the injury has healed (which may have financial consequences for them and significant others). Players may not be certain that the club physiotherapist or doctor has correctly diagnosed the injury, or possess a precise understanding of how long it will take to recover so that they are once again fit for selection. They may also fear the reaction of the manager, and those of other players, to their status as an injured player (Roderick *et al.* 2000; Young *et al.* 1994). There may even exist uncertainties in terms of assurances regarding future contracts at their present club and potential clubs in the future. Players become familiar with, and gain an understanding of, these fears and uncertainties in the course of their professional careers, as they observe the constraints within which other, more established players are bound up, and they talk to others about the consequences which may result from particular incidents. The inability of all injured players, from the inexperienced to notable veterans, to take part in the one activity which, above all others, sustains their positive self-images, may lead to the generation of guilt, depression, and frustration (Roderick *et al.* 2000; Young *et al.* 1994).

In the sociology of medicine literature, the concept of uncertainty has long been analysed as a central feature of day-to-day medical work, especially as it relates to the diagnosis and prognosis of a health problem (Adamson 1997; Calnan 1984; Davis 1960; Fox 1988; Roth 1963). Being ill and requiring medical

Sporting Bodies, Damaged Selves
Research in the Sociology of Sport, Volume 2, 137–149
Copyright © 2004 by Elsevier Ltd.
All rights of reproduction in any form reserved
ISSN: 1476-2854/doi:10.1016/S1476-2854(04)02006-0

treatment impacts the lives of people in varied ways and generates numerous types of uncertainties. All people debate inwardly about what the consequences being ill will have for them in terms of, for example, their employment potential and the way in which others will treat them (Adamson 1997; Conrad 1987). These aspects of uncertainty are central in relation to professional soccer as well. Thus, the objects of this chapter are, firstly, to identify the uncertainties experienced by English soccer players in the context of their occupation and, secondly, to understand the ways in which they try to cope during these indeterminate periods of time.

Research Methodology

This chapter is based mainly on semi-structured interviews with 19 current and 8 former professional soccer players. Of the current players, 6 were, at the time of the interview, playing for clubs in the Football Association (FA) Premier League, 6 were with clubs in Division One, 4 were with clubs in Division Two, while 3 were with clubs in Division Three.[1] Most of the former players had, during their careers, played for clubs in more than one division. The ages of the 19 current players ranged from 21 to 35 years. All 8 former players were over 35 years. Two players of the total number interviewed were of black African-Caribbean descent, though I was unable to explore social class, age, or minority group effects adequately. The interviews were tape-recorded with the permission of the players and the tapes were transcribed. For purpose of data analysis I worked from these transcriptions. All interviewees were given an assurance of confidentiality and were told that, insofar as it is possible, neither they nor the clubs for which they played would be identified.

The Sociology of Uncertainty

There are a number of categories of medical uncertainty found in the sociological literature (Conrad 1987). In the first instance, there exists the uncertainty of sensing that something unusual is going on. For example, a person may be suffering from soreness or a vague discomfort. In some cases, an attempt to deal

---

[1] There are four English professional soccer leagues. The top league is known as the FA Premier League. There are three lower leagues which are, in descending order, the Football League Division One, Division Two, and Division Three. It is possible to be relegated down, and promoted up, the leagues.

with this uncertainty may lead one to seek out medical advice; however, it is well established that responses to pain vary according to cultural experiences (Freidson 1970). The culture of professional sport is one such context in which responses to pain are well understood and normalised as an everyday feature (Messner 1992; Roderick *et al.* 2000; Young 1993). In the light of this point, one inexperienced Division Two player, who had suffered problems with the left-hand side of his groin, described why he continued to play in the following way:

> *Player*: I started feeling my groin on the left hand side, and I stared feeling it about the October time and I kept on playing with it, and eventually round about Christmas I went to see the physiotherapist.
> *Interviewer*: So you played through the pain?
> *Player*: Yes, I played through it for quite some time without telling anyone.
> *Interviewer*: How did you mask the pain at that time?
> *Player*: It's a funny thing really. You can get through games, but you don't really give it your all, you can't stretch for certain balls, that sort of thing. But you can definitely get through it. First of all I didn't say anything but then it got worse and worse and I told people gradually.
> *Interviewer*: Why didn't you tell anyone straight away?
> *Player*: Why, because I wanted to stay in the team. It's as straight forward as that.

This example was typical of the response of those players interviewed who developed a problem, such as a groin strain, which did not restrict mobility significantly in the initial stages, or was not observed first-hand. Many players spoke of their reluctance to seek medical advice in the first instance (that is, when sensing something was wrong), in part, because of what an injury could mean in terms of the fear of losing their place in the starting eleven. For many, playing soccer is the only job they have ever done, and the only job they know how to do.

The second category of uncertainty is referred to as medical or clinical uncertainty (Calnan 1984). In short, this uncertainty derives from medical encounters where doctors or other medical personnel are unable to formulate a reliable diagnosis. Moreover, they are unable to tell the patient precisely what is causing the discomfort. One veteran player, who had played in all four divisions, spoke of the period between "breaking down" and being diagnosed in the following way:

> The worst thing is, say you have an operation and you get back to fitness, and get back out playing and training and you break down. Then from breaking down until sort of finding out why you've broken down, you're just in limbo, and that is the worst time . . . But

> it's the time when nobody knows what's going on, that's the worst thing.

The impact of this type of uncertainty can end, or be reduced, when a player is diagnosed as having a particular injury.

A third category of uncertainty is broad and stems from the diagnosis itself. Among other names, it has come to be known as "existential uncertainty," and is central to the patient's experiences of their medical problem (Adamson 1997). Existential uncertainty refers to a privately experienced awareness by patients that their future is open and undetermined. The unpredictable trajectories of many illnesses both inside and outside of sport lead patients to ponder what it means to have a particular illness. From the interviews conducted it is clear that soccer players dwell on considerations concerning what the injury means in terms of their future playing career. How long will the injury take to recover? Will the injury heal and the body be as fit and strong as before? How will others treat them? Invariably these questions do not have simple or immediate answers for players and thus the uncertainties endure and are incorporated into, and become a central aspect of, the experience of being injured.

What is interesting about uncertainty, in all the forms identified, is how players manage it. This question has been addressed by a number of sociologists. Nixon (1992, 1993), for example, employs a "social network analysis" approach to examine the contexts that entrap elite athletes and constrain the range of alternative courses of action that they perceive are available to them. Applying a pro-feminist approach, Messner (1992), Sabo & Panepinto (1990), and Young *et al.* (1994) examine the risks of playing with pain and injury in terms of the way in which it leads to the validation of masculine and athletic identities. All of these studies, however, focus on the manner in which athletes normalise (Albert 1999; Curry 1993), rationalise, and legitimise their behaviour. They seek, that is, to understand the strategies developed by athletes in their attempts, in both the short and long-term (Young *et al.* 1994), to "restore" what constitute, for them, compromised and diminishing notions of self. The following discussion attempts to add to this literature, in a modest way, by examining further how professional soccer players come to construct a variety of time-orientated strategies to deal practically with the uncertainties of injury.

Coping with Injury

Soccer players conceive of their injuries largely in terms of "putting in time" (Roth 1963) rather than in terms of the changes which occur physically. When discussing their injuries, players tend to point out how long they were out for and how many matches they had missed. Thus, a young, Second Division player described a number of injuries in the following way:

> [With] the hernia, I was only out for four weeks. It was last year when we had the FA Cup run, and I'd been having problems with my groin for most of the season and we decided after the quarter-final game to get it done. I got back in four weeks. I was out for six games. My right knee, I did that this season and I missed eight games. My nose and my other knee I did when I was playing in the reserves so we didn't have to consider any first team games. My knee took about ten weeks at that time. And then my nose, I played the week after.

Conceptions of time, then, tend to predominate in the minds not only of players towards injuries, but also of medical personnel.

A young, First Division goalkeeper, for instance, described the emphasis which is placed on time and in most cases the general urgency to return to the playing squad as quickly as possible. This urgency is not only expressed by individual players, but by all club personnel who are connected with the "health" of team members. In the following example, the goalkeeper refers to the necessity to take advice from an appropriate surgeon and the differences such consultations can make. In his words, "some specialists are not particularly sports-orientated . . . They are not geared to dealing with sports people who really have got to get in, get it done and get back as quickly as possible." The point is that specialists who are not familiar with the time-related constraints of professional sport cultures are inadequate in terms of the particular needs of soccer players. The goalkeeper quoted above continued, asserting that:

> [some specialists] are on a different timetable, and their knowledge is not at the cutting edge . . . I mean, if you get the wrong specialist it can take twice as long as it would with the right specialist. I mean, we've had problems with people at the club where they just don't seem to have the appreciation that a sports person is not going to be able to muddle through [get by] for a year and wait for it to heal properly. If they make a mess of it then the chances are that the player will come back in to have it done again.

The central point is that medical specialists who deal with professional soccer players require a heightened awareness of timing in order to gain players' confidence. This orientation to their work is a consequence of the culturally-bound social situation in which players and physicians are tied.

Specific understandings of time-periods are gained through experience and by discussions with older players or players who have experienced similar injuries. One finds that for many common injuries such as, for example, "dead-legs," strained muscles and sprained joints, players have a clear understanding of how long it should be before they are ready to return to play. A First Division player suggested that "it's experience, it's just a matter of knowing your own body, right, because you naturally pick up those injuries through the career. You've had them before and you know how serious it is, and how long it'll take." Discussions among injured and fit players and physiotherapists regularly revolve round issues concerning how long they will be "out"; how long it will be before they can jog or kick or start training with the squad. Such discourse leads players to become increasingly familiar with particular types of recurring injuries, and one might even propose that some older players may see themselves, or may be viewed by others, as "mini-experts" (Waddington & Walker 1991). Their expertise, however, is connected in a narrow sense to a developed awareness of time, rather than an understanding of, firstly, the way in which one's body repairs any damage or, secondly, appropriate medical practices.

As they become increasingly familiar with particular injuries, players are able to generate timetables concerning when particular events should occur, such as, for example, when they will start to jog, sprint, begin ball-work, and so on. In an effort to define when certain things should happen, players develop time-related benchmarks which provide an indication of the passage to fitness. These benchmarks serve to focus the minds of injured players and make them aware of whether they are ahead of, or behind, the socially constructed timetable. In other words, players develop timetables in part as a method of gauging their own progress. So, one way in which all players tend to cope with the uncertainties generated when injured is to structure the time-period through which uncertain events occur. Even more complex injuries are also understood in terms of blocks of time. Consequently, the period of time spent receiving treatment and then rehabilitating from injury may become psychologically more manageable.

The Timing of Surgery

Within professional soccer clubs, encounters between players and club physiotherapists tend to be quite prolonged and their relationships can be highly personalised. For the most part, injured players are in contact with the club physiotherapist(s) daily and their progress is assessed and is a source of constant discussion. It is during these *focused* encounters (Goffman 1961) that players and physiotherapists negotiate and work out the details of treatment and rehabilitation timetables. However, as treatment progresses, both players and physiotherapists are better able to assess the speed of recovery and thus to re-interpret timetable benchmarks. The ability of players to negotiate with physiotherapists about their treatment and to step up the intensity of their rehabilitation is one of the more striking and distinctive features of this "doctor-patient" relationship. Taken as a whole, one might describe the injury "career" as a bargaining process (Roth 1962) in which players, especially first-team members, have a significant involvement in decision-making processes. It is not unusual for players to discuss future pathways with medical staff, or to be left with a choice of options in terms of the way their injury will be treated. This pattern of negotiation is conspicuously evident during discussions concerning the timing of surgery.

Compared with what might be termed "normal" timetabling of surgery, the scheduling of operations for soccer players might be said to be distinct. This distinctiveness is rooted in the fact that the people involved in deciding on the timing of surgery (usually players, club physiotherapists and doctors, surgeons and, possibly, managers) have different interests tied in with this decision-making process. For example the interests of a manager — particularly one whose tenure is under threat — may not necessarily be related to the immediate solution of the clinical problem or the long-term health of players. It is common practice for an operation to be postponed until the end of the season in order that the player can continue playing, carrying the injury, or he may request immediate surgery in order to be fit for a particular forthcoming match. In this way, players, in part, attempt to manage the uncertainties associated with injury.

One experienced, former England international player stated that he had had no fewer than sixteen operations in his playing career and that, as is common in professional soccer, he had continued playing with most of these injuries and had postponed the surgery — to his knees, groin and shoulder — in each case until the end of the season. He explained: "the injuries I was carrying weren't really interfering totally with my game ... so with my shoulder injury it was more painful at nights. Trying to sleep at night it had been very painful but I was getting through games with it." The player also noted that the decision to "get through games" in this manner was left to him and that he was happy to continue; there was, he argued, always an incentive to keep playing as the club was usually competing for a place in European competition for the following season, or was doing well in domestic cup competitions. For each of these injuries, then, the player, in conjunction with club medical staff, was able to put off the surgery and, if only in the short-term, alleviate any uncertainties which may have been generated.

Alternatively, players and medical staff may decide that in particular circumstances — perhaps with an important cup match pending, or maybe with the prospect of a relegation battle to come, or even in the early stages of a season — it is more appropriate either to undergo surgery immediately or for it to be timed for a particular break between important games. For example, a Division Two defender, who had been taking anti-inflammatory drugs and "resting" rather than training in order to get through games for most of this season, described the reason he decided to press for an operation to his groin: "Well, because we were having this FA cup run, I thought to myself, if I don't get something done about it [the groin] soon, it might get to the point where I might not be able to play in the bigger games later on. So I made the decision to go and get it done so it would allow me to get back for the semi-final." Describing a similar set of circumstances, another experienced Premier League player suggested that having a target date to aim for helped to focus his mind and gave him a goal to work towards. As he explained:

> I went over on my knee, and I thought I'd completely wrecked it...when they diagnosed everything they said that I'd been lucky...I went in [to hospital] on the Monday, Tuesday for an operation, and I was back playing within two and half weeks so it was quite pleasing really to play in the Cup Final. I think the Cup Final had a bearing on it because that gave me more of a compulsive attitude to want to be fit.

These two examples typify the central point being made; namely, that whether surgery is delayed until the end of the season or is timed in accordance with forthcoming cup or league matches, the uppermost consideration of players, managers and medical staff concerns availability to play, i.e. whether the player is "fit" for selection, rather than the healing of the clinical problem and the player's long-term health. The timing of surgery in this fashion enables players to play and offset, at least in the short-term, the uncertainties associated with the injury they are carrying.

While there may be some similarities between the pressures soccer players are able to exert on club doctors by comparison with the bargaining powers of "ordinary" patients, players appear, on the face of things, to have much greater latitude in relation to negotiating clinical decisions and treatment timetables. The patterns of behaviour identified in the course of this chapter may be understood more adequately if one thinks in terms of a culturally-bound time clock internalised by players. These strategies — the construction of treatment and rehabilitation timetables and the timing of surgery — might, then, be considered among the means by which players cope with the uncertainties associated with injury.

Second Opinions

The discussion thus far, which has focused on the way in which players cope with and manage uncertainties, has been underpinned by conceptions of time. For instance, injured players are concerned to get back to fitness in the shortest feasible time; a central characteristic of the culture of football, as it relates to medical practice, concerns a strong and ever-present constraint for club physiotherapists and doctors to "get players fit yesterday" (Waddington *et al.* 1999). All people involved in the management of injury in professional soccer are acutely aware of this constraint. Yet, from the interviews conducted, it is clear that from time to time players lose trust in their club physiotherapists. One Premier League player whose knee injury had "broken-down" a number of times in relatively quick succession described a clear example of this. He explained:

> I got to the stage where the physio was looking at me, he didn't know what to do and I was fed up being round the ground. People were looking at me if to say 'oh he's broke down again' and so I just went away. I went back to my former physio [at my previous club] who was top class and I stayed away from the club for about seven weeks and I just solely worked with him. The physio at this club doesn't know that, I spoke to the manager about it . . . and he said okay, I know the score with the physio here, go and get yourself sorted out.

The player in question, who had played for a number of teams in all four football leagues, described also how he lost trust with the expertise of his club physiotherapist and their relationship had "broken-down" too, which had motivated him to seek alternative advice.

Yet, as noted earlier, relations between players and club physiotherapists can be highly personalised. Players, whether injured or fit, have contact with their club physiotherapists almost every day. Over time, physiotherapists become familiar with most players at the club and, conversely, players get to know the mannerisms and working practices of their physiotherapists. However, there are pressures, especially on players, to be seen to be "good patients" when injured; in other words, to co-operate with the demands and expectations of the physiotherapist in deed if not in thought. While some players have complete confidence in their club physiotherapist, others, such as the player quoted above, have suggested that they do not trust their club physiotherapist to provide adequate medical support. Where this is the case, and players are uncertain whether they will receive accurate diagnoses and rehabilitation programmes, they have tended to seek second opinions. In order not to undermine the authority of their club physiotherapist, players tend to seek the advice of others without informing their club physiotherapist of their intention to do so. Seeking medical advice outside the club is often seen within the club as implying criticism of the club's facilities. Most players, however, said they felt guilty about "going behind the back of the club" and that they felt they were, in some sense or other, letting down their club physiotherapist. That said, every player interviewed had either sought a second opinion, or knew other players who had. Thus, seeking second opinions and receiving treatment outside the club is a very common pattern of behaviour in English professional soccer.[2]

One experienced Premier League player, who often sought outside assistance, explained this point vividly. When asked generally about meeting and getting to know physiotherapists at new clubs, he responded in the following way:

> You've got, like, your 'old school' physios and you've got your physios who know what the score is, and . . . it's just basically trying to suss the person out. I mean, I've been lucky really because I've been to a good physio in my career. I take him as a benchmark and I often go back to see him. He's okay, he takes me on, and he'll have a look at me, and I take more notice of what he says to me . . . if you trust the physio and he puts a bit of faith in your mind, you're half way there. You've got to believe in him. If you don't believe in him, there's no point in doing it.

My data indicate that players sought medical assistance from a variety of people whom they perceived as trustworthy and competent. The most common people among those to whom players turned — as the previous quote indicates — were physiotherapists from previous clubs.

A Division Three player described another common pattern of behaviour. When asked whether he knew of players who had sought second opinions without the consent of club physiotherapists, he replied that, "a lot of players, who don't live near the club, but who live where they've been at clubs before, and they know the

---

[2] Players are legally able to seek second opinions about, and treatment for, injuries. However, players who have sought treatment outside their clubs have experienced reprisals in terms of, for example, a distinct lack of "equal treatment" thereafter. Seeking advice and treatment outside the club can generate tension and unpleasantness in the relationship between the player and the club physiotherapist and/or doctor, which players attempt to avoid.

physio at that club, tend to go back to the physio that they know." Not all players retain contacts with previous physiotherapists in this manner. Chartered physiotherapists who worked in private practices had treated a small number of players. Other contacts with chartered physiotherapists were of a more "accidental" nature. For example, a Division Two player, who was undertaking a part-time degree course, had attended a number of guest lectures given by a chartered physiotherapist — with whom he retained contact — who worked full-time in another sport. Another Division Two player said that when dropping off and picking up his child from school, he had become friendly with a mother who worked as a physiotherapist in a local National Health Service hospital. He said that he often described the injuries he sustained to her — including the diagnosis of the club physiotherapist, who was not qualified to a chartered level — and the treatment he was receiving, and that they would then discuss both the diagnosis and the rehabilitation programme. It was not, he claimed, that he did not trust the club physiotherapist; he wanted merely to ensure that he was not "wasting time." There are enough examples described in the interviews to conclude that seeking second opinions is a common pattern of behaviour among professional soccer players in all four football leagues. Moreover, players may seek both advice and treatment and conceal this fact from their club physiotherapists.

In many of the interviews, players spoke in terms of "faith" and "trust" in accounts of medical relationships. In the sociological literature concerned with issues of trust in medical encounters, "good" doctors are effective communicators who "talk things over" and have the "ability to listen" (Lupton 1996). For professional soccer players, it is clear that while these skills are not dismissed as irrelevant, they do not appear to be central concerns. If players lose trust in their club physiotherapists, as seems to be the case from time to time, they may seek to take control of the uncertainties generated by engaging in what is known, in the sociological literature, as "consumerist behaviour" (Lupton 1996); for example, reading up about their injury, or consulting with different physiotherapists and doctors. Yet players do not seek out doctors in a manner similar to that of other consumers who exercise choice over, for example, hairdressers or restaurants; instead, they are constrained to move covertly back and forth between their present club physiotherapists and other medical personnel whose skills they have sought.

Conclusion

The purpose of this chapter has been to add to the sociological literature which examines the strategies developed among elite and professional athletes for coping with pain and injury. The strategies are employed such that, in this case, professional soccer players can make themselves available for selection as soon as possible; so they can alleviate the uncertainties generated that lead, in part, to a diminishing sense of self as professionals; but also so they may redress financial losses, for many have dependents who are affected by their non-playing status. Moreover, in a culture which emphasises the values of masculinity, active participation and victory (Messner 1992; Roderick *et al.* 2000; Young 1993), those who are not involved as players are denied the means necessary to sustain a meaningful and valued sense of self.

The uncertainties for soccer players discussed in this chapter may vary from one situation to another and may be related to factors such as the severity of the injury, the age and status of players,[3] the stage in the season and the importance of forthcoming matches, the orientation of managers towards injured players (Waddington *et al.* 1999), and the perceived competence of the physiotherapist. Yet there are clear patterns discernible in terms of how players cope with and manage these uncertainties. The strategies identified in this chapter include the construction of treatment timetables, the timing of surgery, and the seeking of second opinions. Of importance is the way in which conceptions of time tend to predominate in the minds not only of players and managers, but also of often highly qualified medical personnel. The time-related orientations of these people towards injuries leads them, on many occasions, to prioritise the short-term goal of getting players fit for selection for the first team, in spite of the consequences that this course of action may have for the players' long-term health.

References

Adamson, C. (1997). Existential and clinical uncertainty in the medical encounter: An idiographic account of an illness trajectory defined by inflammatory bowl disease and avascular necrosis. *Sociology of Health and Illness, 19*, 133–159.

---

[3] My data suggest that the contexts which bring professional soccer players to play with pain are, in part, related to their attitudes to their work: attitudes which can change over time as players become older and experience career and personal turning-points. In other words, the decision of players to play when injured may depend, in part, on whether, on balance, they view their work as a means by which to make ends meet and support dependents, or as a way in which they can fulfil their dreams and achieve occupational goals. For example, older players may decide to play when injured in order to secure future contracts so they may provide for their families. Other, usually older players, by contrast, have suggested that when they have sustained an injury in the early part of a season, they have chosen not to play and have, at times, exaggerate the full extent of their injury, in order to ensure that they are given enough time to recover fully. Other, usually younger players may decide to conceal an injury in order to play in an important forthcoming match that may help them in terms of establishing their credibility as reliable members of the first team.

Albert, E. (1999). Dealing with danger: The normalization of risk in cycling. *International Review for the Sociology of Sport, 34,* 157–171.

Calnan, M. (1984). Clinical Uncertainty: Is it a problem in the doctor-patient relationship? *Sociology of Health and Illness, 6,* 74–85.

Conrad, P. (1987). The Experience of Illness: Recent and new directions. In: J. Roth, & P. Conrad (Eds), *The experience and management of chronic illness: Research in the sociology of health care* (Vol. 6, pp. 1–31). Greenwich: JAI Press.

Curry, T. J. (1993). A little pain never hurt anyone: Athletic career socialization and the normalization of sports injury. *Symbolic Interactionism, 16,* 273–290.

Davis, F. (1960). Uncertainty in medical diagnosis: Clinical and functional. *American Journal of Sociology, 66,* 41–47.

Fox, R. (1988). Training for uncertainty. In: R. Fox (Ed.), *Essays in medical sociology: Journeys into the field* (pp. 19–50). New Brunswick: Transaction.

Freidson, E. (1970). *Profession of medicine: A study of the sociology of applied knowledge.* New York: Dodd Mead.

Goffman, E. (1961). *Encounters: Two studies in the sociology of interaction.* Indianapolis: Bobbs-Merrill.

Lupton, D. (1996). Your life in their hands: Trust in the medical encounter. In: V. James, & J. Gabe (Eds), *Health and the sociology of emotions* (pp. 157–172). Oxford: Blackwell.

Messner, M. (1992). *Power at play: Sports and the problem of masculinity.* Boston: Beacon Press.

Nixon, H. L., II (1992). A social network analysis of influences on athletes to play with pain and injuries. *Journal of Sport and Social Issues, 16,* 127–135.

Nixon, H. L., II (1993). Accepting the risks of pain and injury in sport: Mediated cultural influences on playing hurt. *Sociology of Sport Journal, 10,* 183–196.

Roderick, M., Waddington, I., & Parker, G. (2000). Playing hurt: Managing injuries in english professional football. *International Review of the Sociology of Sport, 35,* 165–180.

Roth, J. A. (1962). The treatment of tuberculosis as a bargaining process. In: A. M. Rose (Ed.), *Human behaviour and social processes: An interactionist approach* (pp. 575–588). Henley: Routledge.

Roth, J. A. (1963). *Timetables: Structuring the passage of time in hospital treatment and other careers.* Indianapolis: Bobbs-Merrill.

Sabo, D. F., & Panepinto, J. (1990). Football ritual and the social reproduction of masculinity. In: M. A. Messner, & D. F. Sabo (Eds), *Sport, men and the gender order: Critical feminist perspectives* (pp. 115–126). Champaign, IL: Human Kinetics.

Waddington, I., Roderick, M., & Parker, G. (1999). *Managing injuries in professional football: The roles of the club doctor and physiotherapist.* Leicester: Centre for Research into Sport and Society, University of Leicester.

Waddington, I., & Walker, B. (1991). Aids and the doctor-patient relationship. *Social Studies Review,* March, 128–130.

Young, K. (1993). Violence, risk, and liability in male sport cultures. *Sociology of Sport Journal, 10,* 373–396.

Young, K., White, P., & McTeer, W. (1994). Body talk: Male athletes reflect on sport, pain and injury. *Sociology of Sport Journal, 11,* 175–194.

Chapter 7

Risk, Pain and Injury:
"A Natural Thing in Rowing"?

Elizabeth C. J. Pike

In the 2000 Summer Olympic Games in Sydney, Australia, Steven Redgrave of
Great Britain achieved an unprecedented fifth gold medal in successive Olympics
in men's rowing. The British media hailed him as the greatest Olympian of all
time. However, in the year prior to the Games, one journalist reminded her readers
of what it had taken for Redgrave to achieve such success:

> A year away from the Olympic rowing finals and Steve Redgrave
> is preparing to become the most successful, the most impressive,
> the most respected, the most determined and probably the most
> arthritic British Olympic champion of all time . . . he is 37 . . . and
> the creaks and groans of protest that his back offers him in the
> morning, the regular stab of the insulin needle, the pills to keep
> his colitis in remission, the hole where his appendix used to be are
> all painful reminders that he has pushed his extraordinarily taxed
> body above and beyond any kind of normal, rational athletic duty
> (Mott 1999: 1).

While Redgrave may be the best known rower in Great Britain, it is evident that
he is not alone in experiencing rowing-related injury and illness. Categorising
rowing among a number of other water sports, the Sports Council (1991)
estimated one million incidents of injury per annum for this group in England
and Wales. A study of Senior British trialists found that 71% had taken time out

Sporting Bodies, Damaged Selves
Research in the Sociology of Sport, Volume 2, 151–162
Copyright © 2004 by Elsevier Ltd.
All rights of reproduction in any form reserved
ISSN: 1476-2854/doi:10.1016/S1476-2854(04)02007-2

of rowing with back pain (Edgar 1994) and, similarly, in a questionnaire survey of British club-level rowers, it was found that two thirds of the respondents had experienced rowing-related injuries (Pike 2000). In April 1994, the Amateur Rowing Association (ARA) established a working party to develop the nationwide "Injury Reporting System for Rowing," using what they termed a "yellow card reporting system." In the months between October 1994 and September 1995, 71 injuries were reported. Significantly, injuries were only to be reported if they "were likely to result in a reduction of training load or time off training" (Bernstein 1995: 24). In this way, the ARA also defined for athletes what it meant "to be injured" and any rower choosing to continue participation was defined as non-injured regardless of her/his physical condition.

Methodological Framework

This chapter will outline the main factors that appear to contribute to risk and injury in rowing, drawing upon an in-depth study of two women's rowing clubs in the south of England. It is argued that the symbolic interactionist framework is most relevant to an examination of experiences of risk, pain and injury. In particular, the work of Erving Goffman (1963, 1969) on stigma and impression management, is useful in understanding how people negotiate having "wrong face" when some information about them is inconsistent with their self-image. For example, it is often assumed that involvement in exercise equals being "fit," which in turn equals being "healthy" (Lupton 1997), and so an injured athlete, by definition, is not presenting an "appropriate" self. As a result, "the maladies of the body become the stigmatisation of the person" (Turner 1997: 223). If an injury challenges an athlete's sense of self-identity, it is possible that she/he may try to "save face" by, for example, training through her/his pain and risking further and more serious injury.

   The methods chosen for this study reflect the symbolic interactionist tradition of "sharing in people's lives while attempting to learn their symbolic world" (Silverman 1995: 48). Initially, I undertook a questionnaire survey of British rowers attending regattas during one summer season to identify some of the broad issues pertaining to the risk/pain/injury nexus in women's rowing. Questionnaires were left in the refreshment area at regattas, and rowers were also approached while they sat on the riverbank in between races and asked if they would complete one. I then became involved with rowers in two clubs through a two-year period of participant observation. In order to facilitate this, I negotiated various roles in the subculture from training partner to trainer-carrier, team photographer to tea-maker. In addition, I interviewed several of the rowers and their coaches. Recent research has made a strong case for the use of narrative studies in understanding the effects of illness and injury on self-identity (Brock & Kleiber 1994; Lupton 2000; Sparkes 1996, 1997). Interviews would also seem to be consistent with studying symbolic interactions in social settings (Denzin 1970), ensuring that "research interpretations are grounded in actual lived experiences" (Sparkes 1994: 173). The interviews were semi-structured, in keeping with the symbolic interactionist belief that since people are not "standard" so research techniques should not be standardised (Silverman 1995). Such a diverse and critical approach to research characterises what has been called the "fifth moment" of qualitative research methodology (Denzin 1997). In what follows, the findings from this multifaceted study are used to elaborate some of the injury experiences of rowers.

Introducing the Rowers

In order to contextualise the experiences of the rowers involved in this study, let me first give some background information on the subculture of rowing itself. The questionnaire responses indicated that the majority of the rowers were professional workers with university qualifications and, of the remainder, most were full-time students. For the purposes of anonymity, the names of the case study clubs and all interviewees have been changed. The first club, which will be called Rivertown, was traditionally a men's club which only took female members in the 1980s, and this with a good deal of resistance from the male members. In contrast, Bridgewater was specifically developed during the 1980s for the purpose of encouraging female participation in the sport, although the funding that was promised for this only lasted approximately six years. It is interesting to note that the development of women's rowing, including the issues of male resistance and inadequate funding in these two clubs, therefore reflects several of the social issues surrounding women's progress in sport and society generally. Women's rowing only really developed in the inter-war years when the absence of men gave greater access to facilities. However, their progress was not uncontested, and men maintained dominance over resources and power (Cooper 1989; Hargreaves 1994). As I explore the women's experiences of risk, pain and injury, so consideration will be given to such gender issues and their relevance for understanding how taking risks with their bodies is part of negotiating a dual identity as both "woman" and "rower."

It would appear that women's rowing is dominated by participants within a particular social class strata and, inevitably, those with access to a river or large lake (coastal rowing was not considered in this study), therefore limiting the overall number of participants. Roger, one of the rowing coaches at Rivertown who, in his 60s, was himself a veteran competitor, suggested to me that being a minority sport increased the chance of success and "then, of course, the pressure is to win." In such cases, it might be argued that athletes may be more likely to take risks to be remembered for their athletic achievement and the "symbolic reward of immortality" (Curry 1993: 287). In addition, it became evident that there is a status hierarchy within rowing. Most overtly is that rowers win points for success in regattas, and they are categorised according to the number of points held (from "novice" with no points, through "senior" ranks from Senior 4, the lowest, to Senior 1, and ultimately to "elite"). Less obviously, status was also determined by the position that the rower occupied in the boat. In crew rowing, seats are numbered from the bow (the front of the boat) which is number 1, through to the "stroke" which is the position in the rear of the boat and has the highest number. It was evident that the higher number seats were more highly valued. Julie, who was a Senior 2 lightweight rower at Bridgewater, told me, "I find it very hard to accept someone else rowing at 6 . . . you're in a power seat and you can influence the power of the boat, what kind of rating and how much work everyone is putting in." It became clear that part of many rowers' (over)commitment to training was to protect not only their crew selection but also their specific seat in the boat. Let us now turn our attention to these women's injury experiences.

Entering the Rowing Pain Zone

The majority of questionnaire respondents and interviewees had encountered some pain and injury during their rowing careers, to the extent that for many this was normalised as part of the sporting experience. For example, on a sample rowing club membership form (ARA 1998) some preliminary questions asking for name, contact details, and rowing standard were followed by the largest section of the form asking for injury and illness history. This assumption of injury risk in rowing has frequently been attributed to the technique of the sport (Edgar 1999; Redgrave 1999). Rowing (with one oar, as opposed to sculling where each athlete has two oars) necessitates a one-sided action. Janet, a Senior 2 rower at Bridgewater who was also training to be a physiotherapist, talked of her "muscle imbalance" due to rowing on one side, revealing that "I've got a slight curve in my spine." Max, one of the coaches, rationalised that this was a "natural thing in rowing." Other common injuries included tenosynovitis (inflammation of the tendons) in the wrist from the technique of turning the blade, knee injuries from the compression as the rower moves up and down the "slide" (the back and forward movement of the seat along its runners), and various injuries related to weight training. Pauline told me that the women at Rivertown, where she was a lightweight rower, were disadvantaged because the shoes in the boats were men's sizes and so there was a lack of foot support for women, indicating a direct effect of gender disadvantage on injury risk. Of particular concern was that many junior rowers also appeared to experience injury. A study of the British under-18 squad found that more than half attending a training camp were injured (Edgar 1993), while another study indicated that junior scullers had a tendency to lumbar spine curvature making it prone to disk damage (Carratu 1995). Some rowers felt that pain and injury were a desirable part of the rowing experience. For example, Julie told me that rowing training "can never hurt enough." Similarly, the majority of respondents (87%) to the questionnaire agreed that rowers should push themselves to their physical limits, and tended to rely on the principle of "no pain, no gain" (67%).

These attitudes were shared by some of the coaches. Max was one of the coaches at Rivertown and had previously competed at national standard. He told me that in order to become an elite rower "you've got to be able to overcome pain." This was perhaps most significant in the story of Nicky. Nicky was an elite heavyweight rower and sculler who, at 22 years of age, had a good chance of selection for the national squad. She had experienced pressure from her coach to change her technique to become a more effective rower, but in the knowledge that such technical "improvements" were causing her pain and could potentially injure her back: "I've been coached as a senior that the way I row is because I've been taught to protect my back and now part of my technique is being changed." As a result of this, Nicky's experiences of pain were framed in terms of technical efficiency taking precedence over personal safety (see also Brohm 1978), since she noted that she was not "really bothered about the pain I was in, it was just that I was annoyed that I couldn't sit properly." Such sacrifice of bodily protection to achieve more effective technique occurred in spite of the ARA Coaching Ethics recommendation that "coaches must place the well-being and safety of the performer above the development of the performance" (1998: 1).

Given that the likely causes of rowing-related injury are not shrouded in mystery, it is interesting to examine the preventative measures being taken. Stallard (1994) suggested that the predominance of back injury is most likely the result of performance improvement measures such as the use of "big blades," weight training, prolonged endurance training, ergometer work (the rowing machine), rowing style, and also insufficient warm up. Most of the rowers indicated that they knew the benefits of warming up and stretching to minimise these risks. For example, Pauline observed that she could have avoided many of her injuries "if I had stretched a lot and remained flexible." However, when asked if they did stretch, responses varied from "a token gesture" (Pauline) to a suggestion that warm up time was used for chatting to team mates, and the proclamation "the mouth is the only part of the body that gets exercise!" (Celia).

It appeared that there was almost a stigma attached to any injury-avoidance measures. Indeed, many rowers displayed physical signs of rowing-related injury as a symbolic display of their commitment to training, in this way presenting an appropriate self (Goffman 1976). Julie noted that if she did not have blisters on her hands she found this problematic "because it means that I'm not rowing," and Sarah, a novice in the sport, suggested that "I was really excited when I got my first callus, it was like 'look at my hand, I'm a rower.' " Identifying as "a rower" was central to many of the women's sense of self. I asked Janet why being a rower was so important to her, and she explained that "it conjures up the idea that you're really fit and you're really dedicated and I like that." In Goffmanesque terms, Janet liked to be "a person of action" (Goffman 1967), showing strength and activity. In most cases, this meant that rowing also dictated respondents' lifestyles. Most of the women would train four evenings a week and both days at the weekend, throughout the season. According to Alison, an elite sculler who was also in the national squad, "we live and breathe it." A resultant side effect for many of these women was that their social lives became dominated by rowing. Clare, an elite lightweight sculler who trained at Rivertown club twice daily, explained how non-rowing friendships became problematic: "the ones that don't row, it is difficult to fit in with them." Max took this a stage further to suggest that "rowers marry rowers because there's no time for anything else, and all of a sudden it becomes addictive." Max was married to one of the rowers in his squad! As noted elsewhere in this volume, this "all-or-nothing" attitude is indicative of an adherence to a sport ethic which carries a risk of injury if athletes are prepared to participate at any cost to maintain their lifestyle (Hughes & Coakley 1991). Furthermore, the inability to sustain friendships from outside the rowing subculture means that rowers are unlikely to receive messages challenging such a lifestyle (Adler & Adler 1991; Nixon 1992).

Negotiating the Rowing Pain Zone

Having received an injury, most of the women admitted to continuing to train with their injury, even though they were aware that they were risking further damage. Many felt that they were able to distinguish between pain and an actual injury, which Young *et al.* (1994) define as "disrespected pain." For example, Emma was a Senior 2 rower who had recently taken up sculling largely due to injury. She negotiated the "feeling rule" (Hochschild 1983) of normalising pain by stating that there was a difference between "the general masochistic agony each time you train . . . enjoyable pain" and "your body saying 'stop, something's wrong.' " For many of the rowers, training in pain was the result of being "worried about my place in the boat" (Nicky) or, as Sally, another heavyweight, noted, not wanting "to be dropped." The problem encountered by many injured athletes is that often an injury is not visible and may therefore be doubted (Scarry 1985). Brock & Kleiber (1994) suggest that the more dramatic an injury is, the more acceptable it is to significant others. In my study, it became clear that "invisible" injuries were considered particularly problematic to the women interviewed, especially when trying to explain them to crew members: "you get the feeling that they think you're faking . . . they believe it only if they can see it" (Emma).

In addition to the crew members, the coaches themselves complicated the process of negotiating an injury. Coaches talked of their own injuries from their days as competitive rowers, and appeared to act as role models displaying the necessary attributes required to succeed in sport (see Stevenson 1990). In symbolic interactionist terms, through interactions with significant others, athletes internalise the response of the "other," in this case the coach, and learn to train in pain (Curry 1993; Goffman 1976). For example, Mike, who coached at Bridgewater and was Julie's partner, told me of his back injury but stated that "it was bearable because I could train through it." Some rowers indicated that while coaches may not directly pressure the rower to train in pain, they might transfer the decision to the rower knowing that they would do so to display competency (see Goffman 1976). This is because, as Alison told me, "when you're in an atmosphere where everyone is training, it's more that you would want to carry on and you don't want to get behind." The process of coaches devolving responsibility to the athletes in this manner has been described in the literature as "risk transference" (Frey 1991; Nixon 1992). Many of these messages were even reinforced in the clothing that was worn. At regattas, rowers could be seen wearing T-shirts with slogans stating "if you can't cope, get out of the boat" and "row hard, no excuses." It has been suggested that use of such "props" serves to symbolically enhance credibility in the role being played by creating an appropriate image for the athlete in question (Casselman-Dickson & Damhorst 1993).

Ignoring pain (or what Young *et al.* 1994, term "hidden pain") was therefore seen as appropriate behaviour and, in this way, rowers demonstrated dramaturgical discipline (see Gallmeier 1987; Hochschild 1983; Snyder 1990). Examples of having to manage emotions were particularly evident in the stories of Pauline and Emma. Pauline talked of being "absolutely frustrated, fed up," while Emma told me that "not being able to get out (in a boat) was driving me nuts." The (male) coaches had also been forced to negotiate emotions due to their own injury experiences. Roger indicated feeling anything from "a bit down" to "very depressed" as a result of "enforced rest" due to pain and injury. This would seem significant in that the coaches were presenting role models to their athletes that they should be able to "put on the game face" (Gallmeier 1987; Snyder 1990); that is, to stage their pain and emotions so that they could continue with their sport.

Medical Implications of the Rowing Pain Zone

So far, we have only considered *pain and injury* related to participation in rowing. However, the women of Bridgewater and Rivertown also indicated that they had experienced forms of illness *per se*. Indeed, Emma, who had a recurring problem with bronchitis, told me that in rowing "illness (rather than injury) seems to be the major problem," and Max accepted that "illnesses are a part of sport." This is consistent with the findings of an ARA study which found occurrences of upper-respiratory tract infection, chest infections, asthma and gastro-enteritis among the rowers studied (Budgett & Fuller 1989). The lightweight rowers with whom I spoke indicated that they experienced specific problems related to their dietary restrictions (see also Chapman 1997); some would go on "sweat runs" and experience the effects of dehydration, and Clare talked of psychological ill-health. Clare struggled to maintain her lightweight status and described being "tetchy" because of diet and training-related tiredness. In some cases, training to the extent of causing illness was even considered to be a positive attribute. Klein (1995) describes how groups whose behaviour may be socially labelled as "deviant," respond to marginalisation by subverting the stigma to "wear it as an emblem of status or resistance" (p. 106). In Julie's case, this athlete demonstrated her commitment to her crew by telling me, "I'll give (them) everything, I'll puke for (them) tonight." Julie was 25 and had plans to commit to rowing in the following season to see if she could make the national squad. Her comment demonstrated an internalisation of an over-conformity to the sport ethic (Hughes & Coakley 1991), and it must be said that she appeared to take some pleasure in the deviant role. This is akin to what Goffman (1963) called "disaffiliation," or distinguishing oneself from one's peers by, for example, taking risks and training in pain.

Irrespective of whether the rower was injured or ill, it became apparent that a large number of the respondents did not receive any treatment or meaningful rehabilitation regime. This may be attributed to the widespread perceived inadequacy of general practitioners and hospital treatment (Lupton 1994). Pauline described her doctor as "atrocious" and "absolutely hopeless," while the views of Valerie, who was 19 and relatively new to rowing, were equally scathing: "they are incredibly incompetent." Many had stories to tell of misdiagnosis. For example, Helen, a Senior 3 rower who said she was cajoled into rowing by her partner who was also her coach, was incorrectly diagnosed with a gland problem for what turned out to be a displaced vertebrae in her neck. Where treatment was provided, a trend became apparent of the women being more likely to use selected forms of complementary medicine (59% of the female questionnaire respondents, compared with only 10% of the males). This may be as a result of the perceived "femininity" of treatments such as massage and aromatherapy which use fragrant oils and the like (Hardey 1998), and have a holistic approach to health, balancing body, mind and spirit. The choice of medicine may also mirror an attempt to present an appropriate self (Goffman 1976) as "woman" and "rower." Both of these identities are embodied and so any "fatal flaw" (Sparkes 1996: 463) to the body has the potential to disrupt this dual identity. It should not be surprising, therefore, that these women engaged in a form of impression management, by stating that despite having experienced such high levels of pain, injury and illness, they would continue to take risks, and that giving up rowing was "not really an option" (Helen).

Concluding Thoughts

In summary, it is apparent that rowing is a "situation of chance" (Goffman 1969), reflected in the fact that the ARA has felt it necessary to develop an injury-reporting system. Furthermore, injury and illness risk may be directly related to the minority status of the sport, since the perceived possibility of success makes the risk-taking worthwhile to the participants. The rowers also appeared to tolerate pain and injury in order to maintain their athletic self (Goffman 1976). As a result, it appears that performance efficiency has taken precedence over well-being (Maguire 1991). The resultant injury experiences have distorted the notion of this sport as healthy (Lupton 1997; Ogle & Kelly 1994). This has particular implications for *female athletes* whose sense of self is already complicated as they negotiate their dual (and potentially contradictory) identities (Young 1997). Injury to the body presents a stigma which has the potential to disrupt and threaten their embodied biography of self as both "female" and "athlete" (Goffman 1963; Shilling 1997; Sparkes 1996).

A study such as this is limited in its generalisability by virtue of focusing on a small population at a given time and place, which may not be representative of a broader population. However, it is suggested that the in-depth analysis of a critical case study such as this, along with the triangulation of methods, enables some moderate generalisation (Williams 1998) about identifiable aspects of the research situation. Having said this, it is important to recognise the relatively privileged position of the women in this study since, while they may have shared some experiences of gender oppression, they also experienced the benefits of their status as white, university educated, middle-class professionals.

On the basis of these findings, risk-taking in women's rowing appeared to be exacerbated by negligent coaching practices, and the athletes' suspicions of medical "care" which sometimes led to the avoidance of any medical support. It is evident that there is a need for more humanistic coaching practices that consider the development of human potential rather than being merely performance-oriented (Cross 1991). In addition, for those women who do get ill or injured through rowing (and other sports), the value of non-orthodox medical care appears to have value in presenting women with an opportunity to control their own health (Wilkinson & Kitzinger 1994). In this way, it may be possible to empower athletes to challenge the misconception that injury and illness are "a natural thing in rowing."

References

Adler, P., & Adler, P. (1991). *Backboards and blackboards: College athletes and role engulfment*. New York: Columbia University Press.

Amateur Rowing Association (1998). *A summary of coaching ethics*. London: Amateur Rowing Association.

Bernstein, I. (1995). *Injury reporting system in rowing*. London: Amateur Rowing Association.

Brock, S., & Kleiber, D. (1994). Narrative in medicine: The stories of elite college athletes' career-ending injuries. *Qualitative Health Research, 4*, 411–430.

Brohm, J. (1978). *Sport: A prison of measured time*. London: Ink Links Ltd.

Budgett, R., & Fuller, G. (1989). Illness and injury in international oarsmen. *Clinical Sports Medicine, 1*, 57–61.

Carratu, M. (1995). *Where do the seeds of back problems lie?* Unpublished report.

Casselman-Dickson, M., & Damhorst, M. (1993). Use of symbols for defining a role: Do clothes make the athlete? *Sociology of Sport Journal, 10*, 413–431.

Chapman, G. (1997). Making weight: Lightweight rowing, technologies of power, and technologies of the self. *Sociology of Sport Journal, 14*, 205–223.

Cooper, C. (1989). *Discrimination against women rowers at Cambridge University*. Unpublished BSc dissertation, Roehampton Institute, University of Surrey.

Cross, N. (1991). Arguments in favour of a humanistic coaching process. *The Swimming Times*, November, 17–18.

Curry, T. (1993). A little pain never hurt anyone: Athletic career socialization and the normalization of sport injury. *Symbolic Interaction, 16*, 273–290.

Denzin, N. (1970). *The research act in sociology*. London: Butterworth.

Denzin, N. (1997). *Interpretive ethnography: Ethnographic practices for the 21st century*. London: Sage.

Edgar, M. (1993). 1992 World junior rowing championships, Montreal, Canada: Physiotherapy report. *Physiotherapy in Sport, XVI*, 2.

Edgar, M. (1994, October). Back injuries in rowing: The physiotherapist's contribution. Paper presented at the Amateur Rowing Association Senior Rowing Conference, London.

Edgar, M. (1999). Rowing injury, A physiotherapist's perspective. *National Sports Medicine Institute Newsletter, 15*, 18–20.

Frey, J. (1991). Social risk and the meaning of sport. *Sociology of Sport Journal, 8,* 136–145.

Gallmeier, C. (1987). Putting on the game face: The staging of emotions in professional hockey. *Sociology of Sport Journal, 4,* 347–362.

Goffman, E. (1963). *Stigma: Notes on the management of spoiled identity.* Engelwood Cliffs, NJ: Prentice-Hall.

Goffman, E. (1967). *Interaction ritual.* New York: Doubleday Anchor.

Goffman, E. (1969). *Where the action is.* London: Penguin Press.

Goffman, E. (1976). *Presentation of self in everyday life.* Harmondsworth, UK: Penguin Books.

Hardey, M. (1998). *The social context of health.* Buckingham: Open University Press.

Hargreaves, J. (1994). *Sporting females: Critical issues in the history and sociology of women's sports.* London: Routledge.

Hochschild, A. (1983). *The managed heart: Commercialization and human feeling.* Berkeley: University of California Press.

Hughes, R., & Coakley, J. (1991). Positive deviance among athletes: The implications of overconformity to the sport ethic. *Sociology of Sport Journal, 4,* 307–325.

Klein, A. (1995). Life's too short to die small. In: D. Sabo, & F. Gordon (Eds.), *Men's health and illness: Gender, power and the body* (pp. 105–120). London: Sage.

Lupton, D. (1994). *Medicine as culture: Illness, disease and the body in western societies.* London: Sage.

Lupton, D. (1997). *The imperative of health: Public health and the regulated body.* London: Sage.

Lupton, D. (2000). The social construction of medicine and the body. In: G. Albrecht, R. Fitzpatrick, & S. Scrimshaw (Eds.), *The handbook of social studies in health and medicine* (pp. 50–63). London: Sage.

Maguire, J. (1991). Human sciences, sport sciences, and the need to study people 'in the round'. *Quest, 43,* 190–206.

Mott, S. (1999). Golden eye. *The Daily Telegraph,* September 11, Sport 1.

Nixon, H. (1992). A social network analysis of influences on athletes to play with pain and injuries. *Journal of Sport and Social Issues, 16,* 127–135.

Ogle, B., & Kelly, F. (1994). *Northern Ireland health and activity survey: Main findings.* Belfast: HMSO.

Pike, E. (2000). Illness, injury and sporting identity: A case study of women's rowing. Unpublished doctoral dissertation, Loughborough University, UK.

Redgrave, A. (1999). Rowing: An amateur sport for the masochist. *National Sports Medicine Institute Newsletter, 15,* 17.

Scarry, E. (1985). *The body in pain: The making and unmaking of the world.* Oxford: Oxford University Press.

Shilling, C. (1997). *The body and social theory.* London: Sage.

Silverman, D. (1995). *Interpreting qualitative data.* London: Sage.

Snyder, E. (1990). Emotion and sport: A case study of collegiate women gymnasts. *Sociology of Sport Journal, 7,* 254–270.

Sparkes, A. (1994). Life histories and the issue of voice: Reflections on an emerging relationship. *Qualitative Studies in Education, 7*, 165–185.

Sparkes, A. (1996). The fatal flaw: A narrative of the fragile body-self. *Qualitative Enquiry, 2*, 463–494.

Sparkes, A. (1997). Reflections on the socially constructed physical self. In: K. Fox (Ed.), *The physical self: From motivation to wellbeing* (pp. 83–110). Leeds: Human Kinetics.

Sports Council (1991). *Injuries in sport and exercise: A fact sheet*. London: Sports Council.

Stallard, M. (1994). Getting basic about backs. *Regatta, 66*, 15–16.

Stevenson, C. (1990). The early careers of international athletes. *Sociology of Sport Journal, 7*, 238–253.

Turner, B. (1997). *The body and society*. London: Sage.

Wilkinson, S., & Kitzinger, C. (1994). *Women and health: Feminist perspectives*. London: Taylor Francis.

Williams, M. (1998). The social world as knowable. In: T. May, & M. Williams (Eds.), *Knowing the social world* (pp. 5–21). Buckingham: Open University Press.

Young, K. (1997). Women, sport and physicality: Preliminary findings from a Canadian study. *International Review for the Sociology of Sport, 32*, 297–305.

Young, K., White, P., & McTeer, W. (1994). Body talk: Male athletes reflect on sport, injury and pain. *Sociology of Sport Journal, 11*, 175–194.

Chapter 8

Why English Female University Athletes Play with Pain: Motivations and Rationalisations

Hannah Charlesworth and Kevin Young

Although still very much in its infancy, the literature on women's experiences of sports-related pain and injury (Halbert 1997; Nixon 1994, 1996; Pike 2000; Rail 1990, 1992; Theberge 1997; Young & White 1995) is growing. Formerly almost exclusively male-centred, research has begun to focus upon what it means to be an injured female athlete and has helped to develop our sociological understanding of how women experience sports-related pain and how they feel about being injured. Importantly, this literature has begun to identify a number of clear overlaps with accounts of male athletes. Perhaps one of the most striking similarities, in this respect, is the willingness of athletes, regardless of gender or type of sport played, to repeatedly place their bodies at risk by training while they are in pain, competing while they are injured, or by returning to sport before they are fully recovered. Indeed, as Young & White (1995: 51) argue, "if there is a difference between the way male and female athletes . . . appear to understand pain and injury, it is only a matter of degree."

Injuries in sport are frequently seen as routine and uneventful by both male and female athletes, many of whom seem to believe that injury and pain are "part and parcel" of involvement in sport. Moreover, it has been shown that both male and female athletes may adopt similar techniques for neutralising pain including *hiding*, *denying*, and *disrespecting* it, as well as *depersonalising* its physical manifestations (Young *et al.* 1994; Young & White 1995). The fostering of a "no pain, no gain" ethic by male athletes has been well documented in the literature, with such an

Sporting Bodies, Damaged Selves
Research in the Sociology of Sport, Volume 2, 163–180
© 2004 Published by Elsevier Ltd.
ISSN: 1476-2854/doi:10.1016/S1476-2854(04)02008-4

attitude being explained, for example, in terms of the impact which dominant notions of masculinity have on the use of the male body in sport. Additionally, accounts have focused on the ways in which "social forces work upon male athletes in such a way that they become willing to subject their bodies to injury" (Young *et al.* 1994: 179). As Messner (1992) suggests, for example, male athletes may often comply with a "pain principle" and accept and tolerate pain because non-compliance may lead to their masculine identity being questioned. However, as with the sociological research more broadly, explanations as to why female athletes are involved in similar practices and likewise assume risk are somewhat scarce.

Since the sociological research on sports-related pain and injury to date has been unquestionably male-orientated, the aim of the following chapter is to begin to address this current imbalance by analysing the pain and injury experiences of female athletes, and in so doing to add to a developing body of work on this topic. More specifically, its sociological purpose is to contribute to our understanding of the range of overt and covert factors which may motivate female athletes to accept and tolerate pain, and to train and compete while injured.

Methodological Approach

The findings presented here represent the first stage of data collection in a largely qualitative study of the pain and injury experiences of female university athletes in England (Charlesworth 2004). For the purpose of the wider study, the principal method of data collection will be semi-structured interviewing, but the following chapter will be based upon the analysis of survey material; specifically, questionnaire responses obtained from 47 female athletes involved in a range of university sports including rugby, soccer, field hockey, track and field athletics, tennis, gymnastics, basketball, volleyball, and water polo.

The decision to examine athletes' experiences within a range of sports was not arbitrary but based upon a number of considerations and assumptions. Perhaps most importantly these choices were influenced by the notion that women are not a homogeneous group and that indeed that there is no one uniform "woman's experience" (Oakley 1981). The sociological purpose of studying a range of sport-types is, therefore, to account more fully for the diversity, contradiction, and ambiguity which research to date indicates is likely to be a central characteristic of women's sports-related pain and injury experiences.

Athletes were asked a number of survey questions that were geared towards developing an insight into how they experienced pain and injury. They were asked, among other things, to provide information about how often they suffered with pain or injuries because of sport, what kind of injuries they encountered, and how they felt while they were injured. Questions focused upon whether or not they had played through injuries and, if they had, what had motivated them to do so. Moreover, we were interested in which rationalising strategies were implemented and why.

Risk, Pain and Injury: The Experiences of Female Athletes

The data revealed that a range of injuries had been experienced by these female athletes. Most significantly, however, a majority of the sample had at some point sustained at least one significant injury as a direct outcome of participation in sport. Among the most serious of these injuries were several torn or snapped anterior cruciate ligaments, a fractured patella, a fractured eye socket and cheek bone, a broken collarbone, a dislocated knee cap, and a broken clavicle. A number of the injuries had required surgery and lengthy periods of hospitalisation, while nearly all had required ongoing physiotherapy treatment. For example, a female soccer player who, at the time of conducting the research, had been injured for 16 months with a medial and lateral meniscus tear, medial collateral ligament strain, and an anterior cruciate ligament tear, described how her injuries had required an arthroscopy, reconstructive surgery, painkillers and four months of intensive physiotherapy.

On the basis of the data generated from the survey it was, however, evident that regardless of the type of injury suffered, or the sport played, these female athletes quite frequently normalised and rationalised pain and injury as a necessary part of sport involvement. Additionally, the "no pain, no gain" mentality clearly identified as a central aspect of many male athletes' experiences was routinely reflected in the data. A majority of the respondents, for example, talked of pain as "just something you deal with ... something you just battle through" (Natalie)[1] and saw injury as "simply a result of playing ... part of the deal with most sports" (Claire).

In sum, when analysing the data it became clear that these athletes represented a group of women who were, more often than not, willing to rationalise injury and pain as part-and-parcel of their participation in sport. Moreover, consistent with studies of male sports environments (Curry & Strauss 1994; Nixon 1992; Roderick & Waddington 2000; Young 1993; Young *et al.* 1994), a range of overt and covert pressures appear to encourage female athletes to place their bodies at

---

[1] Pseudonyms are used in this chapter to protect the identities of the respondents.

risk by accepting injuries and tolerating pain. Since accounting for these factors is central to a more adequate understanding of female athlete's sports-related pain and injury experiences *per se*, the discussion that follows focuses on identifying the ten most frequent justifications for training while injured and competing in pain provided by this sample of athletes. While not based upon any precise quantitative measurement, the motivations/rationalisations presented here are ordered from the most often to least often cited.

Playing with Pain: Motivations and Rationalisations

Group Bonds and Team Commitments

When asked what motivated them to play while injured and in pain, the reason most frequently cited by these athletes was not wanting to "let down" fellow team mates. They had clearly forged extremely close friendship bonds with their athletic peers. Although these friendship groups were, on the whole, reported to be very supportive while an athlete is injured, the responsibility that these individuals felt towards their club or team may have inadvertently encouraged them to play with pain or return from injury too early. For example, Jenny indicated that not wanting to let down either her team mates or coaches was the main reason she continued to play in a rugby game with a fractured cheekbone and fractured eye socket:

> When I fractured my face, I played on for the rest of the game. Although it was really sore and I felt a bit vulnerable, it wasn't bleeding and I could still run and tackle. I felt it was more important that I stayed on so I didn't let my coach and team mates down. Our replacements that day, I didn't feel could have done as good a job.

Marie, a second year soccer player who had suffered numerous injuries including a snapped anterior cruciate ligament, gave similar reasons for continuing to play through injury: "I have played on while in pain many times because I don't want to let my team mates down. As long as the pain isn't unbearable, I will try to continue." Kelly, a rugby player, explained how her decision to play to the end of a game despite having a broken nose was influenced by the obligation she felt towards her team mates. She recalled that:

> We were short in defence so I made the effort to carry on in case I was needed to make a tackle. . . . Eventually, I was required to make

[one] which could have been important. Two serious injuries had already been suffered that afternoon and I noticed someone else was down when I was hit. Despite the bleeding I felt I could still contribute.

Forging extremely close bonds with individuals who share similar attitudes to risk and team commitment in sport may encourage athletes to accept pain and tolerate injury. Athletes may see denying pain as a sign of dedication to their team and, as Hughes and Coakley predict, "may do harmful things to themselves and perhaps others when motivated by a sense of duty and honour" (1991: 311).

Pressure from Significant Others

As demonstrated earlier in this volume, prior work (Curry & Strauss 1994; Nixon 1992, 1993, 1996; Young 1993) has shown that the pain and injury experiences of athletes may be best understood within the context of a network of social relationships which may "contribute to the willingness of athletes to play hurt and knowingly or unknowingly to risk greater pain, injuries, and possible long-term disability" (Nixon 1996: 34). Our data similarly suggest that pressure from significant others, in particular coaches and peers, may impact on athletes' decisions to either play while in pain or to return prematurely from an injury. Coaches, for example, appeared to be highly influential in this respect and were in some cases described as unsupportive of, even disinterested in, injured athletes.

As Nixon (1994) argues, coaches are "central figures in the athletic subcultures and social networks of athletes, and as central figures they may influence athlete's choices about taking risks with their bodies" (p. 80). Elizabeth's experience of injury within track and field provided a classic example of pressure being placed upon athletes by coaches who may, perhaps inadvertently, rank performance and success above the well-being of the athlete. Elizabeth explained that while suffering from a partial rupture of her achilles tendon, "One coach tried to persuade me to race despite the doctors advising me not to ... he wanted me to have a steroid injection which masks the pain and then to run regardless of the injury."

Similarly, a coach who was unsympathetic towards injury made it difficult for Lucy, a tennis player, to voice concerns about her injuries. Her experiences appear to be consistent with Roderick & Waddington's (2000) claim that athletes will often hide emotional responses because those "who demonstrate pain or remove themselves from competition because of injury run the risk of being stigmatised" for having the "wrong attitude" (p. 67). In Lucy's words:

> I just told my coach of a sore shoulder and he doesn't really
> understand players saying they are injured. He presumes it is an
> excuse or being soft, so I don't make a fuss about it. . . . He never
> believes you are injured so you feel pressured to play and keep quiet.

Not unlike Lucy, Catherine, a volleyball player, described how her coach was unsympathetic towards her when she was in pain and unwilling to discuss her injuries:

> Our coach doesn't take much interest in injuries — he just wants
> us back training. I saw the physio before a training session and was
> told I could do some light training that night. I told my coach and
> he replied 'you're damn right you're training.' This pressurised me
> into taking part in every drill and I was in a lot of pain during the
> session as a result.

As with the literature on male sports environments, Catherine's response indicated that coaches can make athlete's lives so difficult that some would rather train in pain than "be injured" and on the sidelines (Roderick & Waddington 2000). She noted, for example, that despite being injured her coach made her attend and watch every training session. In her words: "This was ok at first but, as we train twice a day, I became frustrated that I couldn't be involved and my attitude toward my injury became negative. I was tempted, therefore, to come back earlier than I knew I should."

Although most of these women described their team mates as being supportive and sympathetic while they were injured, on a number of occasions their responses indicated that along with coaches and trainers, athletic peer groups may often behave in ways which influence an athlete's orientations toward pain and injury. Debbie, a water polo player, for example, considered that she had perhaps returned from a shoulder injury too quickly because of the reaction of some of her team mates to the injury. In her words: "I felt some pressure from my team mates when I was injured — mainly to perform as well as usual and not to let the injury stop me from playing or affect me . . . some people actually accused me of faking the injury." Similarly, Belinda, a soccer player, described the pressure placed on her both by her coaches and team mates to continue to play despite suffering with ankle ligament damage:

> I was just told to strap it up and carry on, and for the . . . final I was
> told to strap it up really tightly and go to the hospital after. The
> second time I did it I refused to play, but that wasn't a very popular
> decision. . . . My team mates did pressure me, I didn't mind the first

time, but the second time I wanted to rest it properly, but I was made
to feel bad as we had a couple of FA Cup games that I missed.

In sum, it is evident that a network of significant others acted in ways which
influenced these women to tolerate injuries and ignore pain. They were often
willing to accept the risks associated with participating in their sport because
their "sportsnets" (or the networks of social relationships to which they belonged
— Nixon 1992) constructed such experiences as natural or worthwhile. For
example, in a Goffmanian (1968) sense, these women may have learned to manage
their bodies in a certain way (i.e. by hiding pain and tolerating injury) because
they realised that an "inappropriate" presentation of their body might have led
to their athletic identity being "spoiled" by the reaction of others. The data
indicated, however, that these athletes were very rarely, if ever, *forced* into playing
while hurt or returning to their sport too quickly after injury, but were more likely
subtly persuaded into hiding pain and concealing injuries by significant others and
audiences perceived to be critical (Young *et al.* 1994).

Body Confidence

Athletes' bodies acquire new meanings when they are injured, and injury is likely
to force new relationships between the athlete's body and self. The injured body
may be conceptualised as alien, and athletes may often feel out of place in, or
betrayed by, their new less efficient and less healthy bodies (Thomas & Rintala
1989; Young 1993; Young *et al.* 1994). For our respondents, time away from
sport as a result of injury brought about a number of unwelcome changes in body
size and shape. A number of athletes suggested that feeling less confident with
their body and less attractive while injured may have motivated them to return to
training and competing too quickly. Most of these women explained that while
the physical demands of their sport helped them to achieve their ideal body shape
(which typically meant being slim, toned and muscular), injury brought about a
number of undesirable changes that jeopardised this preferred physique. Several
athletes talked of feeling fatter, lazy, lethargic and more acutely aware of changes
in their body (most often loss of muscle tone and weight gain) while injured.

Samantha, a soccer player, noted the impact which injury had upon how she felt
about her body. Talking specifically about the comparisons she makes between her
"fit" and her "injured" body, she explained that:

> I feel better with myself knowing that I have an athletic body, strong,
> fit, little fat. When injured, I felt I wasn't training. Couldn't put my

excess energy into use. I felt I had to watch what I was eating for fear of gaining weight. This really affected me psychologically because I love food!

Mel, a track and field athlete, explained that she sometimes started training before being fully recovered from an injury because the changes to her body brought about by being injured and unable to train had such a negative impact on her confidence and self-esteem:

> I tend to feel a lot unhappier when I'm injured because I feel puffier. . . . I feel I gain weight quickly when I'm injured. I'm not used to being heavy, so it makes me extremely unhappy. I lose confidence when I'm injured and definitely feel less attractive, so if I can start training again, even if I am in some pain, I will.

Ruth noted similar feelings surrounding the impact that injury had on her body: "I was out of sport for about two years due to my injury and in that time all my muscles faded away and I put on weight. I felt unfit, untoned and unhealthy. This made me feel un-sporty, and much less confident with myself."

For male athletes who pride themselves on being healthy and strong, injury requires a great deal of physical and mental adjustment (Young *et al.* 1994). Changes in the body, including "decreasing mass and diminished fitness" can, for example, make male athletes feel "less attractive, less manly, and incompetent" (Young *et al.* 1994: 187). Our data indicate that sports-related injury can be problematic in similar ways for some women. Not unlike their male counterparts, when faced with injury problems, the female athlete's orientations toward her own body may change significantly. Quite often within the context of injury bodies become "disciplined," "lack desire" and cease to love themselves. Additionally, they may become "mirroring bodies" that seek to be desirable again and to recreate an image of a healthier body (Frank 1991). Changes in the relationship between body and self that are often experienced, for example, by chronically ill individuals, must, therefore, be taken into consideration when attempting to understand why female athletes often normalise pain and tolerate injury.

Ambition, Distinction and Striving for Success

Clearly, female athletes may often make the decision to play while experiencing pain or to return from an injury too early because they fear that not training will hinder their athletic development and lead to them falling behind the rest of their team mates or training partners. Additionally, several athletes explained that such behaviour is often motivated by a desire to reach specific goals and targets, or a fear of missing those targets When those who are involved in competitive sport believe that being a "real" athlete means striving for distinction, they may jeopardise health by ignoring injuries and tolerating pain. Jodie, a female field hockey player, for example, described how she frequently played with pain to the point where one of her injuries required hospitalisation and surgery. According to Jodie, progressing in her sport made these tests of endurance seem worthwhile (despite medical evidence to the contrary):

> I don't want to jeopardise my development and my training so I often keep playing when I am injured. The reason I needed surgery on my foot was because I played on it for so long with the inflammation and tried to ignore it. I have a bad habit of ignoring pain until it goes away . . . but it's better than not playing at all.

Zoe, an international level heptathlete, provided similar reasons for her decision to return to training before fully recovering from a hamstring injury. In her words:

> I felt everyone else in my sport was progressing and I was missing valuable time. The first time I injured my hamstring I questioned, whilst injured, if I'd ever be able to sprint properly again and I was scared it would happen again so I rested it for quite a while. The second time it happened I was worried about losing time, so I probably came back a bit too early.

According to Kim, a member of the British senior duathlon team, accepting injury and tolerating pain were simply prerequisites to being successful in sport, especially at the elite level: "In order to progress and maintain fitness levels, one has to experience pain. It is an everyday occurrence and is necessary in the plight to get fit and perform to the best of your ability."

Factors, then, such as ambition, distinction and striving for success may encourage female athletes to make sacrifices for their sport and accept no limits in the pursuit of athletic excellence. Indeed, the data indicated that for a number of these university and otherwise elite athletes a belief that "the true athlete seeks to improve, to get better, to come closer to perfection [and] are a special group dedicated to climbing the pyramid, reaching for the top . . . excelling" (Hughes & Coakley 1991: 314) motivated them to accept risking injury and even illness.

Team Status and Re-Selection

Fear of losing one's place in the team was a central concern for a number of these female athletes while they were injured. Some respondents suggested that feeling "useless" and of "little importance" motivated them to play despite being injured, while intense physical pain was often described as being accompanied by feelings of anxiety concerning re-selection. As Jo, a rugby player with a broken collar bone explained, for example:

> Although my coaches and team mates supported me when I was injured I was worried because someone else got to play my position and I was aware that I'd have to earn it back and that being injured might mean I'd lose it. . . . I worked really hard so I could get back as quickly as I could.

Similarly, Jane, a soccer player with ankle ligament damage, described how her previous experience of being dropped from her team because of injury had impacted her decision to train through injuries in the future:

> I was bitter because I was playing well at the time and resented that other people were playing in my position and playing well . . . it was a real struggle to get my place back. I have an ankle injury now and shouldn't play tomorrow, but I will. I wouldn't want to lose my place on the team.

Lindsay's experience of injury (a torn cruciate ligament and cartilage in her right knee) confirmed why athletes are often justified in their concern about being able to secure a place in their team while injured. In her words:

> After I got injured, I no longer had any ability or status in the team, no one seemed to care any more, I was on the scrap heap at eighteen. Although team members felt sorry for you, I always felt they excluded me . . . some of them just didn't want to know.

Additionally, the treatment Claire received from her coaching staff illustrated that even athletes who are well established within their club or team risk losing their place while injured. She explained that despite being a well-respected and regular netball player within her squad, after getting injured three days before the netball World Cup she was promptly dropped by her national team coach:

> I was totally devastated in the days that followed as I was dropped
> from the squad and asked to move out of the team block. . . . I felt
> useless. As soon as I was injured I was dropped and I was no longer
> an important part of the team.

The data, then, underline that female athletes are often willing to "pay the price" to stay involved in their sport. When athletes value highly their place on a team or squad they may compromise their health by taking excessive risks with their bodies. As Young (1993) has shown is the case at the professional level, athletes learn from their own experiences, and those of others, that they are dispensable commodities who, when injured, may be easily replaced.

Routine Pain

Since many athletes suffer with pain on a daily basis, they may often devise a number of coping techniques or mechanisms. Athletes often hide pain from themselves and their coaches, show a lack of respect for pain, and depersonalise it by objectifying body parts that are injured (Young *et al.* 1994). Indeed, hiding and ignoring pain were strategies adopted by a number of these female athletes because injuries were such a pervasive and routine feature of their lives. When asked the question "Have you ever continued to participate in sport while injured or in pain?", field hockey player Natalie explained that, "I have played on when my knee hurt lots of times because it so often hurts. If I didn't, I wouldn't play. You don't want to admit you are hurt. As long as you are playing, it's ok." Since pain was such a frequent accompaniment to her canoeing career, Gemma found that ignoring pain and training through her injuries was a necessary part of participation in the sport. In her words:

> I always paddle when my back is sore, I just put up with the pain
> and it's so often sore it meant that I would never have trained. I
> would still race even if injured . . . you don't normally feel the pain
> during a race anyway, just after.

Ruth, a 100m runner, described how she simply got used to "running through injuries" because the pain from her ankle ligament injury was so constant. She explained: "Pain is what we had all the time in some form . . . you have to [train with injuries]. If you stopped running every time you were in pain, you would hardly train or race at all."

As the data presented here suggest, many athletes adopt a nonchalant and blasé attitude to pain because it is such an ordinary feature in their lives. Moreover, "because pain is present wherever athletes push themselves to peak performance, it is often minimised or ignored" (Nixon 1993: 184).

Team Camaraderie

While injury and pain are traditionally conceptualised as essentially physical phenomena, responses gleaned from this sample of female athletes support the notion that they should instead be viewed as simultaneously physical *and* social experiences. Indeed, a number of athletes indicated in their responses that their reaction to injury and decision to play despite being in pain was influenced far less by the physical or sensory experience of pain than by factors in their social environment. Some athletes explained, for example, that one of the things that appealed to them most about the sport they played was "being part of a team" or "being a member of a training group." When injured, however, they felt isolated from the social network of athletes and consequently disassociated from their sport. Indeed, some suggested that the worst thing about being injured, for them, was "not being part of a team." Cara, for example, a rugby player injured at the time the research was conducted, explained how problematic being unable to train and play was for her:

> I feel like I've missed out on 'the bond' that you get from playing in the team. Despite the fact that I go and watch training and matches and go to all the socials and am still good friends with the club, I feel like I'm not as much a part of it as the people who play.

For Angela, a track and field athlete, injury presented similar worries:

> Being injured is lonely as many of my friends are athletes and you experience quite intense emotions with them, such as pain, disappointment, dread, joy. It's therefore quite a jolt to be removed from that . . . not seeing my training partners was the biggest issue, it was very hard to be suddenly detached from such a significant group of peers.

On several occasions, respondents noted that feelings not unlike those described by Cara and Angela may have encouraged them to return to their sport prematurely. As Jane, a soccer player, reported: "I felt pressure to play even though I wasn't properly fit because I didn't want to lose touch with the whole social network."

In sum, and as Hughes & Coakley (1991) argue, "being separated from those few others who truly understand what it means to be an athlete can be a frightening experience" (p. 314); nevertheless, this is a real possibility for those who are injured. When the desire to "maintain their membership in the special and elite athletic fraternity" (p. 314) is critical to an athlete, she/he may again compromise her/his health by accepting pain and tolerating injuries.

Questionable Medical Advice and Support

When speaking about the treatment that they had received for their sports-related injuries, a number of athletes' responses indicated that the medical advice they had been given was inadequate, frustrating or untrustworthy. Several athletes explained that doctors were unsympathetic to injuries sustained through sport, while hospitals either misdiagnosed injuries or were unable to detect their cause (see Chapters 6 and 10). For these reasons, some athletes trained unaware of the full extent of their injuries, and in several cases now suffer repeatedly with them as a result. Gemma's encounter with an unsympathetic GP, for example, led her to race with a back injury that now causes her frequent pain:

> I re-injured my back while racing abroad. I sought medical advice when I got home. They said no permanent damage would be done so I took painkillers, iced it and raced . . . the GP was insulting and rude and didn't seem to understand. He stated that someone of my age couldn't have a problem with her back. I was angry and upset . . . now I have quite a lot of pain with my back after every training session.

Similarly, lack of specialist advice about her sports injury meant that Fiona, a lacrosse player, trained while carrying a painful knee injury:

> After my initial cruciate ligament injury I continued to play for about eight months, as I didn't know what I had actually done. I went to the doctor but he just told me that it was ligament strains. . . . I was in pain every time I played.

Additionally, soccer player Carrie described how she continued to play with serious ligament damage because doctors were unable to diagnose her injury accurately:

> I suffered some serious ligament damage to my ankle playing football in 1998. I went to the hospital repeatedly because the

swelling just wouldn't go down. Each time I was just told to rest and ice it. Eventually, after several hospital visits later I was told that it should have been in plaster!

Sports-related injury experiences are clearly likely to be shaped by the quality of medical support and advice available to athletes. Athletes may be unaware of the true extent or seriousness of their injuries and, therefore, unable to make informed decisions about participation if they are subject to insufficient or inadequate help. Importantly, this is often the case for female athletes who are arguably less likely to have access to specialist sports medical support than their male counterparts (Theberge 1997; see Chapter 10).

Financial Incentives

Athletes are often more likely to conform to a sport ethic which encourages them to accept no limits in the pursuit of possibilities, make sacrifices for their sport, accept risks, and play through pain when conformity to such an ethic increases the likelihood of being funded or sponsored (Hughes & Coakley 1991). Indeed, this appeared to be the case for Cara, a British Under-20 javelin thrower, who explained that, among a range of other factors, financial incentives motivated her to compete while carrying a shoulder injury:

> I was not fully recovered when I competed at the European Juniors . . . I still competed as I had been preparing so hard for it and wanted to prove myself. Also I knew that if I competed and did well it would boost my lottery funding status.

Maintaining funding for her involvement in sport was partly the reason why Kim, a duathlete, was motivated to compete with a serious foot injury. Here, she describes the incident:

> I competed in the 1998 World Duathlon Championships in severe pain for 70% of the race, but I was going well and was motivated that my result would help lottery funding. . . . I ended up coming third, which secured funding for the following year.

While women are competing in more sports and at higher levels than at any other time in history, their involvement in sport remains, undeniably, a product of contestation and negotiation (Donnelly 1988; Hargreaves 1994; Hollands 1984; Whitson 1984). At the elite level, where financial support is vital, struggle is even more likely to be a central characteristic of their involvement. As the data here suggest, women involved in top-level sport may on some occasions feel it necessary to take risks with their bodies to secure funding which, in and of itself, is likely to be relatively scarce for female athletes. In this respect, pain and injury in the lives of female athletes need to be understood in the wider context of gender equity issues (see Chapter 2).

Disrupted Routines

Accompanying injuries that prevent participation in sport is a period of adjustment in which athletes must adapt to "disengagement" from their sport (Young *et al.* 1994; Young & White 1995). Just as illness more generally limits everyday physical and social activities, sport injury is often highly disruptive to an athlete's everyday schedule. Being injured, therefore, can be particularly problematic for the athlete who must deal with interference to their ordinarily intense training routines. Indeed, a number of women talked of having "too many hours in the day" to reflect on their injury and missing routine. Getting back to training as soon as possible, often perhaps before properly recovered from injury, was a major priority for athletes concerned with returning a sense of structure and organisation to their lives usually facilitated by sport participation. Elizabeth, a track and field athlete, noted, for example, that her life felt disjointed while she was injured:

> When I was competing I was much more organised in all areas of my life because I had to be if I wanted everything to fit in. Injury disrupted my regular pattern and even though I had more time on my hands I did not get as much done. . . . I just wanted the routine back.

When asked to reflect on the worst thing about being injured, Zoe focused specifically on the disruption which a shoulder injury had brought to her previously highly disciplined training programme. In her words: "The worst thing about being injured is having too much time. With no training to do you seem to have too many hours in the day . . . when I'm injured I just think about training all the time and want to get back."

While a small number of athletes less seriously involved in sport were able to reflect upon the *positive* aspects of being unable to train or compete (more time to socialise and to study, for example), in the main being injured and not training was *seriously problematic* for most of the female athletes in this sample whose lives ordinarily revolved around (fairly to very) regimented training regimes.

Summary

Although this list and discussion of the "top ten" motivations to play through injury and pain is clearly not based on any quantitative scale or exact measuring device, it undoubtedly represents the most frequently cited rationalisations among this particular group of women. While likely unrepresentative of women athletes' experiences across the full spectrum of abilities and playing levels, data derived from the preliminary stages of a study of English female university athletes hopefully make a number of modest contributions to the wider sociological literature on sport, pain and injury, and gender.

Firstly, the data invite us to consider the fact that while pain and injury are likely to be linked to gender socialisation processes, they may also be a product of socialisation into sport culture per se. Since there are clear parallels between how male and female athletes experience as well as talk about sports-related pain and injury, it seems apparent that these experiences may be shaped by a distinct culture that fosters a specific attitude toward risk (see Chapter 3); a culture which may teach athletes, regardless of their gender, to tolerate pain and accept injuries. Of course, there are likely differences between specific sport (sub)cultures and even playing positions with respect to the pressures imposed on female or male athletes to play through pain, but this is yet to be shown conclusively. Additionally, these data indicate that motivations for playing through pain are likely to be both internal and external. While overt pressures (such as pressure from coaches and peers, fear of losing team status, and securing financial rewards) may shape an athlete's orientation towards injury, equally important is the pressure which athletes place on themselves to perform and reach goals. In this respect, the athlete's experience of sports-related pain and injury may be conceived of as both a determined and determining experience; a product of physiology on the one hand and of both human agency and social structure on the other. To be sure, our data also indicate the overwhelming need for a more in-depth qualitative analysis and exploration of the sports-related pain and injury experiences of female athletes at a number of different levels.

References

Charlesworth, H. (2004). *Sports-related injury, risk and pain: The experiences of English female university athletes*. Unpublished Doctoral Dissertation, Loughborough University, UK.

Curry, R., & Strauss, T. (1994). A little pain never hurt anyone: A photo-essay on the normalisation of sport injuries. *Sociology of Sport Journal, 11*(2), 195–208.

Donnelly, P. (1988). Sport as a site for popular resistance. In: R. B. Gruneau (Ed.), *Popular cultures and political practices* (pp. 69–82). Toronto: Garamond Press.

Frank, A. W. (1991). For a sociology of the body: An analytical review. In: M. Featherstone, & B. Turner (Eds), *The body: Social process and cultural theory* (pp. 36–102). London: Sage.

Goffman, E. (1968). *Stigma: Notes on the management of spoiled identity*. Harmondsworth: Penguin.

Halbert, C. (1997). Tough enough and woman enough: Stereotypes, discrimination and impression management among women professional boxers. *Journal of Sport and Social Issues, 21*(1), 7–37.

Hargreaves, J. (1994). *Sporting females: Critical issues in the history and sociology of women's sport*. London: Routledge.

Hollands, R. G. (1984). The role of cultural studies and social criticism in the sociological study of sport. *Quest, 36*(1), 66–79.

Hughes, R., & Coakley, J. (1991). Positive deviance among athletes: The implications of overconformity to the sport ethic. *Sociology of Sport Journal, 8*(4), 307–325.

Messner, M. A. (1992). *Power at play: Sports and the problem of masculinity*. Boston: Beacon Press.

Nixon, H. (1992). A social network analysis of influences on athletes to play with pain and injury. *Journal of Sport and Social Issues, 16*(2), 127–135.

Nixon, H. (1993). Accepting the risks of pain and injury in sports: Mediated cultural influences on playing hurt. *Sociology of Sport Journal, 10*(2), 183–196.

Nixon, H. (1994). Coaches' views of risk, pain and injury in sport, with special reference to gender differences. *Sociology of Sport Journal, 11*(2), 79–87.

Nixon, H. (1996). The relationship of friendship networks, sport experiences and gender to expressed pain thresholds. *Sociology of Sport Journal, 13*(1), 78–86.

Oakley, A. (1981). Interviewing women: A contradiction in terms. In: H. Roberts (Ed.), *Doing feminist research* (pp. 30–61). London: Routledge & Kegan Paul.

Pike, E. C. J. (2000). *Illness, injury and sporting identity: A case study of women's rowing*. Unpublished Doctoral Thesis, Department of Physical Education, Sports Science and Recreation Management, Loughborough University, UK.

Rail, G. (1990). Physical contact in women's basketball: A first interpretation. *International Review for the Sociology of Sport, 25*(4), 269–285.

Rail, G. (1992). Physical contact in women's basketball: A phenomenological construction and contextualization. *International Review for the Sociology of Sport, 27*(1), 1–27.

Roderick, M., & Waddington, I. (2000). Playing hurt: Managing injuries in professional football. *International Review for the Sociology of Sport, 35*(2), 67–82.

Theberge, N. (1997). "Its part of the game": Physicality and the production of gender in women's hockey. *Gender and Society, 11*(1), 69–87.

Thomas, C. E., & Rintala, J. A. (1989). Injury as alienation in sport. *Journal of the Philosophy of Sport, xvi*, 44–58.

Whitson, D. (1984). Sport and hegemony: On the construction of the dominant culture. *Sociology of Sport Journal, 1*(1), 64–78.

Young, K. (1993). Violence, risk and liability in male sports culture. *Sociology of Sport Journal, 10*(4), 373–396.

Young, K., & White, P. (1995). Sport, physical danger and injury: The experiences of elite women athletes. *Journal of Sport and Social Issues, 19*(1), 45–61.

Young, K., White, P., & Mcteer, W. (1994). Body talk: Male athletes reflect on sport, injury and pain. *Sociology of Sport Journal, 11*(2), 175–194.

Chapter 9

Normalising Risk in the Sport of Cycling

Edward Albert

> Pro cycling is not for the nervous. Crashes are part of the daily
> routine. Yet these men of single determination recover only to do it
> all over again ... Fortunately, serious injury is comparatively rare
> despite the competitiveness of the sport ... (Bromley Television
> Production 1996).

In this voice-over to a cycling video, British sports commentator Phil Liggett
theorises features of the sport of cycling, providing details of the normative order
while, at the same time, helping to constitute it. Here, he formulates a crash
sequence as "routine," not serious enough to interfere with the expectation that one
will "do it all over again." In this way, danger is construed in ways that neutralise
its threatening character. The process of routinising danger is one in which cyclists
employ a number of normatively sanctioned methods that create a place for risk
and help constitute what it means to engage in the sport in the first instance. This
chapter examines some of those methods.

Theoretical and Methodological Considerations

Recent scholarship has addressed the acceptance of risk, injury, and violence
in sport from a number of theoretical perspectives, including psychoanalytic,
functionalist, and feminist approaches (Hunt 1995). From a social constructionist
perspective, risk-taking behaviour has also been viewed as constitutive of the
culture of sport (Curry & Strauss 1994; Frey 1991; Hunt 1995; Lyng 1990; Nixon

Sporting Bodies, Damaged Selves
Research in the Sociology of Sport, Volume 2, 181–194
Copyright © 2004 by Elsevier Ltd.
All rights of reproduction in any form reserved
ISSN: 1476-2854/doi:10.1016/S1476-2854(04)02009-6

1992, 1994; Williams & Donnelly 1985). Paying special attention to recreational sports involving few extrinsic rewards, this tradition, closest to my own interests, asks if the acceptance of risk and risk-taking behaviour by participants can be understood as part of the work of doing sport in general and the sport of cycling in particular. Thus, is the risk of potential injury a feature of the social production and understanding of the very activity itself, no less constitutive of the sport than, for example, are the formal rules of racing, and can the omnipresent possibility of injury from crashes be seen to provide participants partial grounds for making sense of riding behaviour in the first place (see Donnelly & Young 1988; Hunt 1995; Williams & Donnelly 1985; Young *et al.* 1994)? It is to these relatively informal and avocational involvements — what Stebbins (1982) refers to as "serious leisure" — that the current research is directed.

In the subculture of climbing, risk is essential; the sport simply would not be climbing without it (Williams & Donnelly 1985: 4). This formulation is also reflected in Lyng & Snow's (1986) use of Hunter Thompson's notion of "edgework," which they apply to the sport of skydiving. Edgework is the "intentional participation in life-threatening or anomie producing activities ... (providing) an opportunity to 'take it to the limit' ... " (p. 169). The present work asks both whether the acceptance of risk and risk-taking behaviour can be construed as an integral part of the work of doing the sport of cycling, and if risk and injury "talk" can be seen as a form of "membership talk," establishing participants' identities, and representing an iconic version of the community of cyclists.

Specifically, this case study addresses the social world (Crosset & Beal 1997) of the serious recreational and racing road rider, drawing occasionally from the related sport of mountain biking. Data were collected from four main sources: (i) the cycling publications *VeloNews*, *Bicycling*, *Winning*, *Bicycle Guide*, and *Road Bike Action*. Informal content analysis was undertaken on 1995–1997 volumes; (ii) unstructured interviews related to risk were conducted while riding and socialising with members of a road cycling club (referred to as the TRC) located in suburban New York City. Composed of serious recreational and racing cyclists, participants were predominantly white professional males ranging in age from their mid-twenties to mid-fifties; (iii) materials were gathered from a website called the "Cycling Accident Data Base" (CADB) on which visitors posted accounts of cycling accidents in which they had been involved. It logged 323 entries from 1996–1997 including 35 women, 276 men, and 12 of undetermined gender; (iv) the research also relied on a store of insider knowledge accumulated as both a researcher and participant in recreational cycling and racing (see Albert 1984, 1990, 1991).

Producing and Managing the Orderly Character of Risk

There were 750 "pedalcyclist" deaths and 51,000 bicycle-related injuries in the United States in 1999 (U.S. Dept. of Transportation 1999). Cyclists understand that these risks derive from a number of sources including motor vehicles which, because of their lethal potential, are central to cyclists' construction of the where, when, and how of "the ride," the context of riding in compact groups, and the presence of road/trail obstacles including rocks, roots, drop-offs, glass, animals, road cracks, parked cars, gusts of wind, etc.

Serious riders often ride in groups which take the form of ad hoc assemblies created on the road, planned rides with friends, club or racing teammates, or "unofficial" rides that acquire a permanency with fixed start time, place, route, and name with large numbers of riders taking part. Such rides provide a sense of camaraderie for the hours spent on the bike, distribute the work involved in riding by allowing riders to share the effort of breaking through air resistance (see Albert 1991), give the protection of numbers and aid in case of trouble, and provide an opportunity to sharpen one's group riding skills, and to train at an intensity resembling actual racing. Newcomers to group rides will be scrutinised with a view to establishing their "bike handling" skills and knowledge of the rules of riding.

Rules of the Ride

Although group riding minimises certain risks, at the same time it increases the chance of colliding with road hazards in that riders adopting forward positions oftentimes block a clear view of what is approaching. Thus, there is an expectation that companions will provide warnings of potentially dangerous situations. These warnings are continually invoked but obscured by what riders happen to be actually discussing. Such warnings are subject to an ongoing group assessment of risk with the emergence of a constantly changing group norm. The appropriate use of the risk management strategies detailed below also serves the latent function of certifying competence.

A rider at the front of a group will often point to obstacles on the ground that might impede riders directly behind. When deemed necessary, the gesture will cascade down the line, each rider in turn pointing the warning to the rider following. Novices frequently vocalise these warnings yelling such things as "hole!" or "rock!," learning by imitation — or eventually being told — that pointing to the hazard is sufficient. Experienced riders will react with bemusement upon hearing each obstacle met with its name called out, sometimes resulting in a steady stream of cautions, e.g. "hole . . . rock . . . stick . . . etc." Only when an obstacle is seen to pose an inordinate threat (e.g. a large hole that appears in the middle rather than at the edge of a field of riders) will an experienced rider view calling out a caution as appropriate. Alternatively, riders who fail to point to a road hazard will be instructed to do so either directly or, in a more general way, as when a rider, speaking to the group as a whole, exclaims "point it out!" following a narrowly missed hazard.

Leading riders are also expected to "call out" warnings of upcoming hazards such as "car up!" (indicating an oncoming car), "runner right!" (indicating a runner approaching on the inside curb), "heads up!" (for some unspecified danger), "car right!" (indicating a parked or stopped car), "light!" (indicating a stoplight in the red position) or, alternatively, "clear!" (indicating it is safe to proceed through a dangerous intersection). Following riders — from the back and cascading forward — will warn of approaching hazards from the rear. The call of "car back!" indicates an approaching vehicle that will soon pass the group. The TRC group often shortened this cry to "back!" Such warnings, however, are never straightforward, but subject to considerable informal taken-for-granted, practices. For example, calling out a warning over and over on a heavily trafficked road, or on a very wide road with a shoulder would not be done. In these contexts riders would assume that the risk had already been recognised, or that is was minimal.

The Motor Vehicle/Bicycle Connection

Road riders often see their relationship with motor vehicle drivers as contentious and adversarial. Every experienced rider has a stock of stories about encounters with drivers who passed too closely, swerved into them, turned into them, etc. The cycling press often recounts the worst case scenario of intentional acts resulting in a cyclist's injury or death:

> . . . the car that hit her . . . had passed a rider who had been dropped from the group. The car's occupants screamed at the cyclist and threw stuff at him. So it was a presumably deliberate act when the car . . . swerved into the bike lane at (her) and her friends . . . (I)t slammed into (her), catapulting her more than 150 feet . . . (*VeloNews* 1998, *27*(2), 78).

Novice riders often cite the motor vehicle/bicycle nexus as the reason for not pursuing the sport further, or taking up mountain bike riding instead. One TRC rider, speaking about a forthcoming move, lamented his leaving a place that offered "great training routes" on untravelled roads for one where there was just "no place to ride." He elaborated that the area to which he was relocating had few roads without heavy automobile traffic.

Encounters with cars become occasions for such accounts. A conversation with another TRC member began with "I almost got killed yesterday." The comment had a matter-of-fact quality and was seamlessly embedded in the ongoing conversation. In fact, "I almost got killed yesterday," is common usage. In this particular case, its accompanying story, once completed, received no further attention.

Anticipating the Inevitable

Rationalising the risks expected with riding is a consistent element in articles in the cycling press. The following excerpts taken from various cycling publications exemplify this practice of attributing an expected, taken-for-granted character to past and future accidents:

> But mostly I hate injuries because they remind me that, when I'm riding, I'm one errant car from The Big One . . . (*Bicycling*, September, 1995: 103).

> In the last few years I've developed a disturbing familiarity with the local emergency room personnel . . . Fact is . . . crashes typify the accidents most of us experience . . . Try this simple exercise: Recount every crash you've ever experienced . . . (*Bicycling*, May, 1996: 18).

> Bobke's 10 commandments[1]
> I *THOU SHALT CRASH AND LOOK LIKE A FOOL
> SOONER OR LATER* . . . (*VeloNews* 1996, 25(6), 110).

> I don't get injured often . . . Sure, I've taken the occasional dive off the mountain bike into the sagebrush or the long, skin-melting slide across pavement in crit corners. But somehow I pop back up . . . (*Bicycling*, September, 1995: 103).

---

[1] Bobke is a penname for the American ex-professional rider Bob Roll. This example is taken from one of his humorous columns where he characterises the sport.

That we have all had/will have crashes is assumed in the above, leaving no room for alternative formulations. Such references can be seen to encourage readers to recognise their own past or future experiences in these accounts, seeing themselves as part of the subculture of cycling.

When Risk turns to Injury

> You know you're a rider when . . . the first thing you ask when you regain consciousness is "How's my bike?" (*Bicycling*, October, 1997: 32).

Riders commonly use variants of the phrase "how's the bike?" It is not uncommon to hear the question voiced by a fallen rider still lying on the ground. The concern for the bike is ironic and underlines the fact that every rider understands the significance of equipment. In attributing greater importance to the condition of the bike rather than the rider, one hears both an encouragement and commitment to resume riding again as soon as possible.

Several layers of meaning inform the passage quoted above. First, it was presented as part of a list of humorous characteristics with which those who know they are riders will identify. The fact that one identifies with such statements serves to make of them membership-producing devices. On the one hand, the question "How's my bike?" signifies that one is alright but, on the other, the ironic concern for the bike is a gloss for the ways in which accidents represent a vulnerability that is discomforting at best. Further, if one is injured, concern for the bike both produces and announces one's commitment to the sport. It attests to an awareness that crashes serve as rights of passage into the sport, as symbolic affirmations of one's claims to membership, and as assertions of one's intent to ride again. A variant on this is found in the exclamation "to hell with you, how's the bike?" This apparent insensitivity by other riders for the condition of a fallen companion is, again, rather an affirmation of the other's status as a bike rider for whom there can be no question but that they will return to riding as soon as possible.

"Ready to Hit the Road"

> My helmet is cracked, so I guess I hit pretty hard, but I sacrificed my body to save the bike (ha, ha) (CADB 1996).

Concern for "the bike" does the work of affirming the commitment to ride again. This is a consistent theme of website crash accounts which often conclude with such testaments. These were found to take two general forms:

(1) Crash accounts that conclude with explicit descriptions of an actual or intended return to riding:

> They x-ray'd (sic) my neck, ribs, and kneecap, and said I was extremely lucky. Scrub the wounds, take pain killers, more head checks, and I'm ready to hit the road (CADB 1996).

(2) Crash accounts that conclude with the ride resuming:

> My friend lost the seat of his favourite (sic) bib shorts as well as a bit of the underlying skin. My handlebar slightly dented my top tube, and my jersey and handlebar tape were destroyed. The adrenalin must have been flowing, because both of us instantly got back on our bikes and hammered the last 20 kms home. The pain hit that evening (CADB 1996).

Similarly, in races, accidents are to be "ridden through":

> This was in a training criterium: I was just getting caught after several laps alone off the front... As I looked back, I forgot to turn... I slid into a chain link fence... I got up and took a free lap... and finished the race (CADB 1996).

Such crashes are occasions to exemplify core subcultural values that include cycling at whatever cost, and enduring the pain of the sport. These values are repeatedly enacted in racing where, regardless of the severity of a crash, the race goes on. Published race accounts treat pile-ups as normal. For example:

> But on the final lap, Shaklee's Brian McDonough crashed after the first turn and Klasna got caught behind the ruckus. Horner crossed the line alone, with Eddy Gragus of the U.S. Postal Service right behind... (*VeloNews* 1996, *25*(8), 112).

It is also the case that crashes are treated as an opportunity for "bike-riders" to display commitment to continuing the race. An incident involving a masters amateur is illustrative:

> Sixty-three-year-old Monsalve . . . suddenly took a turn too wide and dropped four feet off the edge of the road . . . Monsalve's mishap occurred directly in front of the Mavic support vehicle piloted by Bill Woodull . . . "Is he all right?" yelled the EMT from down the road. "Of course he's okay," yelled . . . Woodull. "He's a goddamn Colombian. He's too tough to be hurt.". . . Monsalve wiped off some of the blood, quickly remounted his Masi and charged off down the road (*VeloNews* 1995, *24*(15), 22–24).

Similarly, this demonstration of commitment can be seen in the following account of a women's race:

> Late in the women's road race, someone ran over a piece of wood in the road. The chunk of 2-by-4 flew into Shaklee racer Louisa Jenkins' bike, bounced up and nailed her teammate Molly Renner right on the jaw . . . Looking like someone had slugged her on the chin, Renner was racing the next morning. That's an example, by no means rare, of the terrific resiliency of bike racers. Awful stuff happens to them — deep cuts, major bruising . . . brutal head-banging crashes. But they're chasing the field as soon as someone straightens their bars and replaces their pretzeled wheel. Broken bones and skull fractures may mean DNF today, but they're back on their bikes tomorrow . . . (*VeloNews* 1996, *25*(9), 110).

As noted, cyclists routinely manage circumstances relating to risk. When that potential is realized, the resultant injuries provide an occasion, however unwelcome, for reasserting one's identity as a cyclist and one's membership in the subculture of cycling. Such expressions have been observed to take several forms including an almost ironic concern for the bike rather than for the injury, the immediate resumption of the ride in spite of any injury, and/or the assertion that one will, as soon as possible, ride again.

Managing Causal Attribution in Accidents and Injuries

In the subculture of cycling, crashes, close calls, injuries and the like are formulated as stories in and through which they are made sense of. However, close calls will frequently engender stories of superior bike-handling skills and crash stories will carry with them the risk of stigmatisation, i.e. of being a "bad bike-handler" and potentially a danger. Thus, it is a matter of interest to those not directly involved to establish blame and, for those involved, to re-establish their credentials and minimise culpability.

James, a lawyer in his mid-thirties and a novice racer among a group from New York City, had a reputation for often crashing. He would frequently appear, following a weekend race, with extensive "road rash." There was talk of staying away from him for reasons of safety. His reputation as a "squirrelly" rider stayed with James for years, in spite of the fact that his bike-handling improved over time and he no longer crashed regularly.

Similarly, a group of recreational riders from suburban New York City talked about Bob, an insurance executive in his fifties who, having recovered from a broken collarbone received in a fall resulting from touching wheels with Hank, crashed again, cracking his wrist. Bob's companions expressed misgivings about riding with him, playfully suggesting to him that "maybe he should take up a safer sport." Later, in private, one of these riders expressed serious unease about riding with his friend, whom he characterised as a "bad bike-handler." The first crash had been formulated as not necessarily Bob's fault, the second was accountably his. The analysis of Bob's riding was not limited to his usual companions. A small group of TRC riders had come upon this group immediately following Bob's first crash and they stopped to assist. It was related to me that Hank, the rider whose wheel Bob had "touched" appeared to blame himself for the crash. The TRC riders expressed dismay for Hank in that, after all, "Bob had to watch out for himself. Maybe he had overlapped wheels." In the expression "maybe he had overlapped," responsibility, although left unsaid, firmly shifted to Bob who should have been experienced enough not to do that. Upon hearing of his second crash, TRC riders unequivocally shifted responsibility for both incidents to him.

When a crash occurs it is construed so as to make it accountably somebody's or something's crash. At one extreme, crashes are theorised as ordinary occurrences. For example, the expression "that's bike racing" may warrant a crash that occurs in a "bunch sprint" finish producing it as normal for such circumstances. Hunt (1995: 441) calls this finding of the sport itself accountable "normal risk." At the other extreme, responsibility may be attributed to intent on some rider's part. Intent, if identified, can result in disqualification or relegation to a lower position. In the accusation "he hooked me," a rider is accused of intentionally crossing their rear wheel over another's front wheel, often resulting in the following rider crashing. The intent implicit in being seen to have "thrown a hook" does not, however, necessarily carry the stigma of "bad bike handler" – a "dirty" rider, yes, but a skilled and aggressive one. Far more common is the attribution of a responsibility that does not carry the implication of intent. Here a crash comes to be formulated as the result of unavoidable circumstances, a riding mistake so stupid that it could not possibly reflect one's real ability, or bad bike-handling.

Unlike during races, training or recreational rides will stop when crashes occur and talk will almost immediately begin to formulate how the crash could be seen to have occurred. For example, during a TRC training ride a rider "went down" on a steep descent. Several others, ahead of the crash, were told by riders coming down the hill of the crash behind. After trying unsuccessfully to determine who had fallen, the group went back towards the accident. As these riders climbed, a consensus emerged producing the cause of the crash as a crack in the pavement that each had been forced to negotiate while descending the hill. As the cluster of riders surrounding the crash came into sight, the fallen rider's identity, now established, was formulated in "Not Jay! He's an incredible mountain bike rider." This account, intended to preclude a stigma, formulated Jay (a man in his thirties) as a good mountain bike rider who must be a good bike handler since his skills exceeded those needed to negotiate the crack (see Hewitt & Stokes 1975: 3; see also Scott & Lyman 1968). Thus, the crash was now explainable as not his fault. Reaching Jay and finding him holding his arm protecting what appeared to be a "normal" broken collar bone, talk turned to his cracked helmet, the condition of his bike, how well his expensive wheels had held up, crashes others had experienced, and how to get his bike home after the ambulance arrived.

Ironic Reconstructions and Self-Esteem

Retrospectively, crashes are often related in ironic ways that deflect accountability and preserve a rider's self-esteem and reputation. The following quotes are illustrative:

> Rolling country road. 30 mph. Dog playing chicken tries to make it through the group. Does not. Dog ok. Rider trip to emergency room . . . (CADB 1996).

> Cause of Accident: A curb. Bad Curb!!!!!! (CADB 1996).

> Cause of Accident: A golfer! During a magnificent break on my part, I was suddenly struck in the chest by a golf ball driven from a tee not too far away. I must admit though, the golfer drives much better than myself (CADB 1996).

These accounts make light both of the vulnerability to which each accident attests, and the relative impossibility of preventing their occurrence. In this way, they manage risk so as to make it less threatening. "Bad Curb!", in its absurd attribution of intent, also mitigates responsibility by suggesting that things happen regardless of cyclists' attempts to keep them under control. A member of the TRC group told of running into the side of a deer standing in the road at the bottom of a hill. As if on cue, someone asked, "how was the deer?" Not put off by the question and its apparent lack of concern for his own condition, he replied that, of course, the deer took off unscathed leaving him lying on the ground. How could it have been otherwise?

Reaction Accounts as Warranting the Unattributable

Who actually caused a crash sometimes remains undetermined. For example, riders will sometimes bunch up due to a slow-down at the front resulting in the equivalent of a traffic pile-up. Such chain reactions can be attributed, for example, to the sudden unexpected braking by a rider who may be warned to "stay off the brakes!" by those following. More often, however, pile-ups are unattributable and result in a round of reaction accounts where each rider explains her/his behaviour as a reaction to others. If fault is to be found, however, it is not uncommon for it to fall on the rider deemed least competent, permitting the more experienced to save face.

This dynamic was present following a relatively minor crash involving the author and two TRC riders. Riding single file, Ken (a research consultant in this mid-forties and the least experienced rider of the three) led, I followed, and Adam (a mid-forties chemical industry worker) came last. Adam touched my rear wheel, lost control and crashed. Although on our way again within minutes, the issue of the crash lingered. Adam took responsibility for his fall in that, as discussed above, the rider behind is expected to avoid "touching a wheel," but he clearly did not believe that he was at fault. When alone, he and I talked and "agreed" that Ken was to blame although we never told him so. Months later, riding again at the front of a group, Ken made a sharp move forcing those following to swerve. Adam said to Ken that "he was doing it again" and that he had caused the previous crash. Ken responded that he never realised he had been responsible. Adam told him he shouldn't worry about it. I concurred, saying that yes, he had been the cause, and that Ken shouldn't make such abrupt moves. The issue here is not whether or not he actually was the cause, but rather that his inexperience could be viewed to warrant such an attribution. In short, his precipitous riding move enabled the reconstruction of an earlier, unconcluded event.

The Group Caused It

References to the idiosyncratic dynamics of a group may, on occasion, be retrospectively used to help account for the cause of a crash. Participants may formulate a group ride over its course in various ways. Thus, a ride may be typified as "a hammer-fest," "a hard ride," "a killer," "scary," or "an accident waiting to happen." Following some mishap within a large group of riders or field of racers one will hear riders invoking formulations such as "I knew something bad was going to happen," or "the group was riding crazy," or "I had a bad feeling about this ride." Small groups of riders will cluster around affirming such a seen-to-be-already-held-belief and, in so doing, make the crash accountable and exempt themselves from responsibility. Such self-exemptions are rationalised by the observation that I (we) saw the craziness and, thus, was (were) not part of it.

Conclusions

The larger research from which these excerpts derive set out to examine, from a social constructionist perspective, the ways in which athletes produce the experience of risk and injury as a feature of the activity of doing sport. This approach to risk-taking behaviour suggested that far from being merely an inconvenient, even peripheral element in sport, danger and risk-taking are better understood as constitutive of participation in the first place; part of the lived experience of sport, especially in a sport like bicycle racing.

Observations indicated that serious cyclists create a subculture similar in many respects to other sport subworlds that have been characterised as forms of edgework (Lyng & Snow 1986). Such worlds construct normative practices that give order and place to danger and risk, normalising their occurrence as taken-for-granted features of participation. Serious recreational and racing cyclists were seen to invoke such practices to manage the everyday physical risks associated with the sport, making such common occurrences as falls, crashes, near-misses, and pile-ups accountably routine. Risk management practices were employed prospectively, concurrently during "the ride," and retrospectively. Cyclists took risk into account when deciding where and how to ride, were routinely guided in anticipating and formulating risk in cycling-related publications, invoked risk management practices and related risk and injury experiences while riding, and reconstructed dangerous and/or injury-producing events in ways that served to show, and re-establish if necessary, one's credentials as a "bike rider." Although it might be argued that objective data suggest that cyclists, especially road cyclists, place themselves unduly at risk of significant physical injury, cyclists do not court risk for its own sake. Rather, due to the unavoidably risk-laden nature of the activity, the subculture of cycling has incorporated the dangers of riding in ways which inextricably link them to the very enactment of that life, the bike-life. Cycling's constitutive activity — "the ride" — is produced over its course around minimising risk while, at the same time, using it as a feature bound up with what it means to be a "bike rider" in the first instance.

References

Albert, E. (1984). The role of equipment as warrant for membership in the sport of bicycle racing. In: N. Theberge, & P. Donnelly (Eds), *Sport and the sociological imagination* (pp. 318–333). Fort Worth: Texas Christian University Press.

Albert, E. (1990). Constructing the order of finish in the sport of bicycle racing. *Journal of Popular Culture, 23*(4), 145–154.

Albert, E. (1991). Riding a line: Competition and cooperation in the sport of bicycle racing. *Sociology of Sport Journal, 8*(4), 341–361.

Bromley Television Production (1996). *The Sean Kelly story: An Irish cycling legend.* London: Bromley Video Entertainment.

Crosset, T., & Beal, B. (1997). The use of "subculture" and "subworld" in ethnographic works on sport: A discussion of definitional distinctions. *Sociology of Sport Journal, 14*(1), 73–85.

Curry, T. J., & Strauss, R. H. (1994). A little pain never hurt anybody: A photo-essay on the normalization of sport injuries. *Sociology of Sport Journal, 11*(2), 195–208.

Cycling Accident Data Base, 1996–1997. http://duke.usask.cal~yeo/your_accident.html.

Donnelly, P., & Young, K. (1988). The construction and confirmation of identity in sport subcultures. *Sociology of Sport Journal, 5*, 223–240.

Frey, J. H. (1991). Social risk and the meaning of sport. *Sociology of Sport Journal, 8*(2), 136–145.

Hewitt, J. P., & Stokes, R. (1975). Disclaimers. *American Sociological Review, 40*(1), 1–11.

Hunt, J. C. (1995). Divers' accounts of normal risk. *Symbolic Interaction, 18*(4), 439–462.

Lyng, S. G., & Snow, D. A. (1986). Vocabularies of motive and high risk behavior: The case of skydiving. In: E. J. Lawler (Ed.), *Advances in group processes* (Vol. 3, pp. 157–179). Greenwich, CT: JAI Press.

Lyng, S. (1990). Edgework: A social psychological analysis of voluntary risk taking. *American Journal of Sociology, 94*(4), 851–886.

Nixon, H. L. (1992). A social network analysis of influences on athletes to play with pain and injuries. *Journal of Sport & Social Issues, 16*(2), 127–135.

Nixon, H. L. (1994). Coaches' views of risk, pain, and injury in sport, with special reference to gender differences. *Sociology of Sport Journal, 11*(1), 79–87.

Scott, M. B., & Lyman, S. M. (1968). Accounts. *American Sociological Review, 33*, 46–62.

Stebbins, R. A. (1982). Serious leisure: A conceptual statement. *Pacific Sociological Review, 25*(2), 251–272.

U.S. Department of Transportation (1999). *Traffic safety facts 1999*. http://www.fhwa.dot. gov/safety/fourthlevel/pdf/PedCycle99.pdf.

Williams, T., & Donnelly, P. (1985). Subcultural production, reproduction and transformation in Climbing. *International Review for the Sociology of Sport, 20*(2), 3–17.

Young, K., White, P., & McTeer, W. (1994). Body talk: Male athletes reflect on sport, injury and pain. *Sociology of Sport Journal, 11*(2), 175–194.

Chapter 10

Scars on the Body: The Risk Management and Self-Care of Injured Female Handball Players in Denmark

Lone F. Thing

> The scars remind her of it. The scars remind her of a life she could have had, which she does not have now. It is those scars that have changed her entire existence. That is how it is. That is the harsh reality. (Words spoken by the mother of a young female handball player in Denmark who underwent surgery on her cruciate ligament).

Sociological research on the risk and management of sports injuries is scarce and relatively new (Roderick 1998; Roderick *et al.* 2000). The more recent research shows how primarily male players, both on English professional football teams and in North American college sports, accept playing with pain and injury. But even though sports injuries affect men, and although some injuries may perhaps have more extensive and long-lasting consequences for men than for women in sports as they are currently played (White & Young 1999; Young & White 2000), sports injuries are obviously not an unknown phenomenon in women's sports (Young 1997). Like their male counterparts, today's young sportswomen are also involved in risky sport activities (Rail 1992; Thing 2001, 2002). Instead of focusing on how the sports environment brings about injuries through ideology

Sporting Bodies, Damaged Selves
Research in the Sociology of Sport, Volume 2, 195–209
Copyright © 2004 by Elsevier Ltd.
All rights of reproduction in any form reserved
ISSN: 1476-2854/doi:10.1016/S1476-2854(04)02010-2

and value standards,[1] this study observes injured female athletes outside of their sport, after the injury has occurred. Specifically, the case illustrates encounters between female Danish handball players and the medical treatment system in Denmark.

Women who participate in recreational club handball just below the First Division in Denmark are not paid to perform, and they are not offered assistance from club physicians or therapists if they suffer bodily injury. Rather, they are forced to seek treatment themselves outside the sports system. The argument made in this chapter is that rehabilitation of sports injuries in such non-professional contexts and below the elite level in Denmark is subject to broader and significant individualising processes (Beck 1997; Lupton 1999; Petersen & Lupton 1996). Quite simply, the non-professional female athlete who trains 3 to 4 times per week deals with her injuries on her own. It is she who is held responsible for rehabilitation and, even in a Nordic welfare state, she must navigate her own way through the healthcare system in order to do the appropriate things to heal the scars on her body.

Research Context and Methodological Considerations

This chapter is based on a larger sociological study of the rehabilitation of female Danish handball players with a particular kind of knee injury. The purpose of the study is related to the broader question of public health and may be classified as a part of the field of sociological research on evaluating medical technology.[2] A principal idea is that the embodied experiences of laypersons[3] be prioritised as a focus for research and be compared to experts' views of the body. Arguably,

---

[1] This chapter does not attempt to examine the risk-tolerant culture of sports, the normalisation and rationalisation of injuries and pain (Howe 2001; Roderick *et al.* 2000; Waddington 2000; Young *et al.* 1994), processes of "biased social support" (Nixon 1994), stigmatisation processes or hegemonic masculinisation processes (Messner 1992; Young *et al.* 1994; Young & White 2000), although I implicitly make use of research on these issues.

[2] It should be added, however, that the concept of risk is not seen as an individual and optional property, as some in the public health tradition define it. The key monitoring strategies in the public health project, such as epidemiology, statistical surveys, and the calculation of risk probabilities (Castel 1991) will not be found in this chapter. "Scars on the Body" is part of the new critical epistemological discussion of the concepts of health and disease (Gannik 1999; Lindqvist 1997; Petersen & Bunton 1997). The need for fresh new concepts of disease and treatment and for developing science that incorporates the *social context* of health and disease is considered.

[3] There are various creative ways of experiencing and dealing with the injury process but, having said that, it has been found that patients also have some common experiences with ACL injuries. These experiences appear to cross all boundaries of class, gender, ethnicity, sexual orientation, etc. In this chapter, I am attempting to stress the similarities of what appear to be *individual* injury processes.

there is too little knowledge of the layman's perspective (Lupton 1997b: 103; Williams & Calnan 1996: 14), which could reveal how patients experience the use of bio-medical technology. Moreover, there is a lack of knowledge as to how patients handle technology in contemporary sports medicine.

All of the women in the study had suffered from an anterior cruciate ligament (ACL) injury and had undergone reconstruction, meaning that they had had surgery to implant a new, artificial ACL. This difficult process involves a new ligament being taken from the thigh and attached using channels drilled in the femur, frequently with various forms of surgical sutures and screws (Jørgensen 1999). ACL injury is the most common form of serious sports injury in Danish women's handball. The injury is serious in the sense that, in the best case, the athlete can be rehabilitated in six months (undergoing rehabilitation treatment several times a week) and, in the worst case, she may never again participate actively in handball, even after years of treatment and help. Thus, ACL injury is potentially career-ending, but it is also an injury that changes the athlete's social life in general.

The study is based on a series of prolonged observations of rehabilitation involving female patients with ACL injuries at a private physical therapy clinic in Denmark. Patients with reconstructed cruciate ligaments undergo rehabilitation at the clinic, on average, three times per week, one hour each time for at least six months. Along with observational studies at the clinic, in-depth qualitative interviews were conducted with the patients.[4] The focus was on the women's *experience* with their injury (Denzin 1984; Giorgi 1985; Kvale 1997; Valle & Halling 1989). Thus, the project does not examine the question of *why* injuries arise. The focus and aim of the project are to reveal *how* the patient with a sports injury experiences the injury as well as to examine her encounters with the treatment system. The women's accounts and views were compared to the observational studies and, taken together, they form the starting point and empirical basis for the chapter and for the aforementioned broader study.[5]

---

[4] The interviews were recorded on tape and transcribed in their entirety.

[5] With regard to the sample, the interviewees were respondents selected at random. Patients were selected as they arrived for treatment for sports-related injuries. A relatively heterogeneous group was desired, including both elite athletes and representatives of the broader masses of players, as well as patients who were at various stages of rehabilitation, and people of various ages and levels of education. The point of contact was a physical therapy clinic known as one of the most active and prominent such clinics in Denmark (Thing 2000). The study group includes 17 female handball players ranging in age from 19 to 33 years. The fieldwork at the clinic lasted one year. The problems faced by the injured female handball players are interpreted with respect to 3 main topics: *identity, self-mastery,* and *emotions.* The interpretation is guided by a hermeneutic interest in meaning. The phenomenology of the body was also prioritised in the interviews by seeking *concrete* descriptions of narratives rather than explanations of the injury event (Frank 1995).

Women's Handball and the Administration
of Injury in Denmark

The total number of sports injuries in Denmark is difficult to assess. There is no central registry and, since the injuries are divided among a great number of diagnostic groups, hospital record systems cannot easily classify or quantify the injuries (Jakobsen 2000). Today, however, when the greater part of the Danish population is involved in some type of exercise, as many as a million sports-related injuries are expected annually (Jakobsen 2000).[6] For context, this figure may be compared to the mere 5 million people living in Denmark.[7] The elite organization, Team Denmark, which handles the national teams, has physicians, physical therapists, and massage therapists attached to all elite centers throughout the country. However, these centers offer treatment only for injuries sustained by athletes who belong to Team Denmark, which means non-elite athletes and top players from the individual professional clubs must turn to the public health system of the welfare state for assistance. Here, sports medicine is still an under-prioritised area. As an example, Danish physicians are still unable to specialise in this field (Bak 2001).

The former Danish government's public health program for 1999–2008 states that people's involvement in sports shall be improved, quantitatively as well as qualitatively (Regeringens Folkesundhedsprogram 1999: 53). The government stresses that the aspects of sports that are injurious to health shall be reduced and this shall include preventive measures against sports injuries. This problem has also been cited by The World Health Organization (WHO) (Wedderkopp *et al.* 1999). WHO calls for an effort to prevent injuries; damage to the body is an unintended but significant matter that can no longer be ignored by the politicians. As indicated above, statistics on sports injuries are scarce, but recent Norwegian research indicates that injuries at both the elite and recreational levels are a problem, particularly among women. Female handball players have 2 to 5 times as many knee injuries (including ACL lesions) as men (Myklebust *et al.* 1997, 1998).[8]

---

[6] A total of 70% of the adult Danish population have indicated that they were regularly involved in sports or exercise *in the last year*. Interest in sports and exercise among the Danish people has risen steadily since the 1960s. In 1975, 29% said they participated in sports or exercise, and in 1998 the figure was 51% (Fridberg 2000: 150).

[7] Uffe Jørgensen, Chief Physician of the Sports Medicine Function of Copenhagen County, estimates that, on average, a knee injury costs 130,000 Danish kroner from the time the patient is injured until the patient is completely functional again.

[8] A similar type of injury rate is also found with other types of injuries in American studies on basketball, volleyball, and football (Aagaard 2001).

It may be argued, however, that Danish women's handball is a "success story" with regard to participation and results. Among contact sports, handball is the one that attracts the most women in Denmark. As many as 75,000 women play organised competitive handball, a participation rate which surpasses that of men, who have approximately 67,000 participants in Denmark.[9] The gender-based division of labour between football-playing boys and handball-playing girls is a traditional pattern in the Danish team-sport context. Throughout the twentieth century in Denmark, handball became an activity in which women participated as a supplemental alternative to Danish gymnastics (Skjerk 2001). Thus, Danish women's handball has a long history, which is also reflected in the level of play. Although, again, Denmark has only 5 million inhabitants, the Danish women's national team has done well, winning medals such as the Olympic gold medal, gold in the World Championship, and gold in the European Championship. Clearly, the degree of national performance and tradition in the sport indicate that the level of play in the Danish divisions is high. Training is extensive and serious, and even though only a few play at the professional level, the level of competition is high. Girls begin training at approximately age nine and may develop an eye toward a career on an elite team later in life.

Individualisation and the Athlete's Duty to be Active and Autonomous

Parsons (1975) describes how the role of "patient" implies a minimal level of activity on the part of the person involved. He maintains that even if active participation in the treatment is required, the social role of the patient involves a release from daily obligations and expectations (1975: 262). This view of medical treatment is frequently discussed in medical sociology, where it is said that the role of patient is generally seen as less active, as being free from the burdens of daily life, free of responsibility, so as to avoid placing demands on those around the patient (Holstein *et al.* 1997: 18). However, based on empirical observations of patients with sports-related injuries being treated in Denmark's present healthcare system, this description of the course of illness appears rather inadequate. Indeed, on the contrary, it seems that the obligation for the patient to be active and autonomous permeates the entire treatment process where sport

---

[9] As an example of the popularity of women's handball in Denmark, during the 2001 World Championships held in Italy, 1.4 million Danes watched the television broadcast of the women's quarter final match against Angola.

injury rehabilitation is involved. In the words of one 27-year old handball player (herself a physiotherapist) who was injured in a tournament:

> The emergency room doctors, they don't have any specialisation at all, at least I didn't see that they did, and like I said I was treated by no fewer than four doctors from the time I came to the ER for the first time until I came to this doctor who said, 'There is something wrong here . . . we will have to send you for an MRI'. That was actually the first time I felt there was anyone who actually did something about it. I felt it was a lot like, 'Now we will pull a little here and there, tear a little there and we see a little bit there and, well, we didn't find out anything there', and then just 'Go home'. So I felt it was very frustrating during that period, when I didn't have anything to go by, since I didn't know what it was, other than that I had an idea myself, 'Well, it was probably the meniscus!' (Maj Britt)

In an effort to rethink the notion of the patient as passive and uninvolved in the process of rehabilitation, I have adopted theoretical ideas from risk sociology as well as the sociology of the body and the emotions.[10] Subsequently, the empirical data that follow are interpreted especially in the light of risk sociology (Beck 1997, 1999; Lupton 1999). The idea of a "risk society" is a new form of "reflexive modernity," where risks are seen as being the result of the technological development of a fundamentally industrial society. According to Beck, risks can no longer be estimated and, thus, they are seen as an irreversible threat. In Beck's view, current threats differ from pre-modern dangers in that they are uncompleted events of a non-localisable nature, with potential, incalculable long-term effects. I believe that this view of risk is applicable to the understanding of sports-related injuries. According to Beck, the scientific tradition of knowledge has lost its authority, due to the unpredictability of risk and the difficulty of analysing it. Thus, the concept of risk is also linked to a process of reflexivity, since the fear of risk raises questions, surprises, and political reactions concerning social practice (Lupton 1999: 66).

The Body in the Clinic

In many ways, being an injured athlete is a painful and risky experience. Physically, the body is injured, it hurts, and it does not work as it normally does. But

---

[10] I have been greatly inspired by Lupton's work on risk sociology as it applies to the body and the emotions (cf. 1997a, b, 1998, 1999, 2000).

it is not only the physical body that notices the change acutely or lastingly, since health and well-being are related to the body, the psyche, and society *as a whole*. The pain over being unable to participate in sport sparks a number of thoughts and feelings of anxiety, anger, and sorrow. There is often doubt and uncertainty with regard to the future and, consequently, the athlete must reflect on the level and content of her favourite sports activity. Questions arise after the injury. What will it be like not being able to participate in sports? What meaning will life have without exercise and club camaraderie? Let us now take a look at the complex experiences some injured women athletes encounter on their way through the rehabilitation period.

We visited the clinic in central Copenhagen. At the rehabilitation facility, which simply consists of one large room, the atmosphere is one of intensity and concentration. Three female patients stand facing a mirror, focusing on co-ordinating their body movements. Facing the patients, in front of the mirror, the trainer stands and guides the rehabilitation exercises for their knees. The male physical therapist demonstrates how the exercises are done properly and corrects the patients when they make mistakes. From the observer's bench, it is frightening and even paradoxical to see highly trained young female athletes using all their physical resources to make basic movements. They no longer take for granted even the simplest task. The basic forms of motion, such as walking, running, jumping, squatting, standing on one leg, or perhaps bending slightly at the knees, are activities that must be relearned and retrained. After just a few knee bends, the sweat is visibly running down their faces. Free bodily movement is put on hold for a time. The players accept their condition and work systematically to regain their bodies' natural status. The "absent presence" of the body (Leder 1990) is a mere dream, hovering in the distance. The body hurts. Fear and uncertainty are expressed in the players' eyes. The challenge is no longer to produce the best sports results, but to face the body's limitations — the pain and fear that are produced simply by lifting the heel.

About the injury and the non-control over the body, 21-year old Nina commented:

> Well, first of all, I have never experienced pain like the pain of a cruciate ligament injury. The pain was horrible and . . . well, I really had nightmares after that wrench in my knee and the uncertainty during those months afterward, since my leg just disappeared out from under me. I think that was really awful. It wasn't that painful, but just not knowing, OK, can I count on my right leg now, will it hold if I just turn around or if I go out dancing, or if I go out running or something. It was like I didn't really have control over my body or control over my leg.

In making these observations and in describing her fears, Nina was underlining the fact that when the body's dimensions change (Burkitt 1999; Damkjær 1998a, b; Frank 1991; Shilling 1993; Turner 1992; Williams & Bendelow 1998), the identity is also affected and, thus, the relationship between one's identity and surroundings is changed in the short- or long-term. Let us now look at how the injured body is not just an object, but is also interwoven into social mechanisms, and at how risk management is experienced.

Risk Management: Injury as a Lonely Journey

Ordinarily, we do not think about our body. It is almost a sort of 'stowaway' in our lives. But when an injury occurs, a keen bodily awareness enters the scene and, for the athlete, who usually seeks to perfect physical skills, the injury is a biographical disruption (Bury 1982; Giddens 1996: 135). In the same interview with Nina, for example, this athlete described the disruptive effects of her injury:

> When I first found out it was a cruciate ligament injury, I thought that just *can't* be right. I was the one on the team who had trained the most, I mean strength training and all that over the summer holidays. So it felt so unfair that this should happen to me. So I just thought, 'Oh, that is just nonsense'. And, I believe you are really isolated . . . I mean it is so hard, it is tough to deal with, both because you have to go through the whole process, but also because it is not the same. I mean, you can go to the gym and watch the team play and practice, but you are not a part of it. Even if they do something to keep you from feeling too down, you are not a part of it, I mean you are not part of the game. That is really tough, I believe.

Twenty one year old Lene had similar reflections to offer on her ACL diagnosis and her experiences with coming to terms with her injury and her "disrupted" body:

> I really feel a lot like I have been on my own the whole way, I believe. Especially with the diagnosis and what would be done, or from when the injury occurred until the operation. I think it is really frustrating. Because you are told, now it is halfway torn and now it is completely torn, and you don't really know what that means. You could say you could ask more questions, but you don't really know what it is you should ask!

The injured knee is not an insignificant matter for the sports-injury patient. As Damkjær noted (1998b: 141; 2000), the body is the nucleus of the person's identity formation process, and the individual with a sports-related injury lacks bodily skills, specifically with regard to the aspect of motion. We have a body (Turner 1992) which we tend to regard as something apart from ourselves, as something we possess; but the body is unique, it cannot be replaced. One's own body is the link between the self and the external world (Leder 1990: 6). Twenty six year old student teacher, Lisbeth, also experienced a problem with her identity, but her problems were more connected to the identification with the sport in itself:

> Another thing is that you have just played handball all the time. I mean, I have never tried to do without it, and now I have to. Everybody identifies me with handball, not with my studies or anything else. Just Lisbeth, the one with the handball, this or that. And just like that, that was no longer me. That was really strange. I have learned a few things about myself since then. What can I be if I can't be 'handball-Lisbeth'?

Motion skills, such as crawling, walking, running, and dancing, are no longer "givens" and may still be painful. The knee suddenly appears as an existential part of life and as a necessity. The motion skills of the body are also crucial to forms of social interaction (Goffman 1967). Frequently, the camaraderie of the club and fellow club members have been the athlete's primary social contacts outside the family. When the body is injured and player is forced to look on from the sidelines, her social identity is challenged. This change may be accompanied by profound changes in the athlete's concept of her body and of her self as well as by changes in her social situation. For example, 19 year old Tina had been injured with knee problems since the age of 16, and remarked that all of her present friends knew her only as "Tina with the knee," thus indicating that her identity was linked to being an injured athlete. With regard to her lengthy period of rehabilitation, she noted:

> I see myself as a person who is totally different from the others, since suddenly I am no longer the ordinary girl I was before. I am just a bit of an outsider with the others. And that is tough, I mean it was really tough. Half a year is a long time to live with defeat. I really felt every day was a defeat, since every day I had to sit and watch other people doing what I couldn't do. That, in itself, was a major defeat for me.

The potential loneliness of the injury experience was also illustrated by another patient, 20 year old Line:

> Being injured has been really rough on me, because I am not able to play handball and actually have not been able to for 2 years now. It meant so much. Before I was injured, I liked to train 3 or 4 times a week, and then there were the matches. I had school and I had my handball and I don't have that any more. In the fall, when I was injured the second time, everything went wrong. I went into almost total depression, because I thought this was a bad joke, that I had to go around waiting to be operated on. I was no longer part of the team.

However, the risk management of the injury process is not a lonely journey just because the athletes feel abandoned by their club and their friends. The feeling of loneliness is far broader. The injury narratives from my research show that many of the women have felt alone and isolated with their problems with respect to the medical industry. They feel that they have had to struggle to get a reliable diagnosis and have shouldered the responsibility to learn about ACL injuries and possible treatments. In other words, they have been very active in the illness process. When I asked Bente, one of the older handball players at 29, about her illness process, which had lasted for over three years, she observed:

> Yes, it has been just me all along, through the whole thing. I go up to the doctor and say, 'You know, there is something wrong'. You know, you can always tell with your knee that there is something wrong. It is also easy to tell the difference with what is going on in your knee. You go up to the doctor over and over again and he just turns you away, you know, sends you home again. 'There's nothing wrong with you'. So you have to go in, go in, and go in on your own the whole time, that's the way it has been through the whole thing. And that's how it is now with the physical therapists, that you have to go to them yourself the whole time, if there is something wrong.

As such, the loneliness and frustration of the experience mean that the battle for dignity can be a major factor. Tina, for instance, talked about how she handled her treatment at the physical therapy clinic in terms of her self-doubt and her self-concept:

> I am constantly going to rehab where I actually manage to twist it again and again, but I don't tell him (the trainer). I remember being

ashamed of it. So, I don't like to say that some exercise he makes up, and then suddenly I rush out, because it hurts like *hell* and I just pretend like nothing has happened . . . I think somehow, I tell myself it can't be anything. It's just you doing the exercise wrong or something.

Tina said nothing about the pain and how she felt about the treatment and being injured for fear of being considered "soft" and for fear of not being able to continue her handball career and return to her friends. Thus, even though the non-professional female athletes stand alone in some respects, the culture of risk (Waddington 2000; Young & White 2000; Young *et al.* 1994) in sports is probably significant in terms of how these women express themselves during treatment. Even if the athletes are not pressured or helped back into the sport, the culture of injury is clearly an influence. Afterall, the women have a difficult time showing their feelings during treatment and they do not want to be considered "soft."

Summary

This chapter illustrates the individualising effects of the sport injury event by providing examples of how the non-professional female injury patient experiences and handles injury and pain. It shows that, in Denmark, sports injuries are increasingly seen as problems on a personal rather than a social level, despite the government's attempts to optimise sports medicine resources and facilities. Even though many athletes who have sustained sports injuries have been supported by voluntary organisations and clubs for many years, the fact of the matter is that once these athletes are injured they must bear the responsibility of the injury alone. Female athletes must themselves seek knowledge of treatment for their injuries and struggle through a not always helpful medical process for diagnoses. They deal alone with their change of identity, since rehabilitation focuses exclusively on the physical body and not on the body, the psyche, and society *as a whole*. The injury process for women at the non-elite level can be described as a lonely journey, one for which the traveller cannot pack lightly. Unassisted, she is required to "carry the luggage" of reflexivity, knowledge, and skills. At present, self-mastery in treatment and knowledge is an ability that is absolutely essential to female Danish athletes.

The consequences of risk management are multifaceted. On the one hand, the individualising tendencies of the injury experience create active agents who, despite opposition, remain capable of acting knowledgeably. On the other hand, the risk management creates problems with the patient's actions, in the form of uncertainty, searching, and anxiety over what will happen should the management fail. There is clearly a need for sports organisations to formulate and develop thoughtful *injury policies* for the benefit of athletes — this does not exist in Denmark today. Aspects such as emotions and the consequences of the injury for the person's relationships with respect to such things as identity, education, work, and family are downplayed in treatment in favour of bio-medical considerations about anatomical and physiological knee functionality (Thing 2004). There is also a need to distinguish between the short-term and long-term consequences of sports injuries (Roderick 1998), a topic that is almost completely neglected in current treatment in Denmark.

The conclusion from this Danish case is that current social conditions guide the patient to active self-mastery. In other words, the patient is left to take care of matters for herself — in effect, to become her own administration office (Beck 1997). The female athlete is confronted with far more than simply the pain she experiences when she is injured on the court. The rehabilitation process in itself is a long, complicated, and painful personal experience. Pain is not just a physical problem (Howe 2001), but a social phenomenon, a key part of which becomes the athlete's ability to deal with loneliness and uncertainty on a number of levels.

References

Aagaard, P. (2001). Korsbåndsskader og faren ved kreatin. *Puls.* Nr. 2 — årgang 12, 23–25.

Bak, K. (2001). Idrætsmedicinsk uddannelse af Læger. *Puls.* Nr. 2 — årgang 12, 15–16.

Beck, U. (1997). *Risiko Samfundet: På vej mod en ny modernitet.* København: Hans Reitzels Forlag.

Beck, U. (1999). *World risk society.* Cambridge: Polity Press.

Burkitt, I. (1999). *Bodies of thought: Embodiment, identity & modernity.* London: Sage.

Bury, M. (1982). Chronic illness as biographical disruption. *Sociology of Health and Illness, 4,* 167–182.

Castel, R. (1991). From dangerousness to risk. In: G. Burchell, C. Gordon, & P. Miller (Eds), *The Foucault effect: Studies in governmentality* (pp. 281–298). Chicago: University of Chicago Press.

Damkjær, S. (1998a). Kroppens sociologi og den biologiske organisme. København: *Dansk Sociologi* — Nr. 4/9.

Damkjær, S. (1998b). Patient og sygeplejerske — et møde mellem kroppe. In: H. P. Hansen (Ed.), *Omsorg, krop og død. En bog om sygepleje* (pp. 136–159). København: Gyldendal.

Damkjær, S. (2000). Dimensions of the body. In: D. E. Gannik, & L. Launsø (Eds), *Disease, knowledge, and society* (pp. 105–123). Frederiksberg: Samfundslitteratur.

Denzin, N. K. (1984). *On understanding emotion.* San Francisco: Jossey-Bass Publishers.

Frank, A. (1991). For a sociology of the body: An analytical review. In: M. Featherstone, M. Hepworth, & B. S. Turner (Eds), *The body: Social process and cultural theory* (pp. 36–102). London: Sage.

Frank, A. (1995). *The wounded storyteller: Body, illness, and ethics*. Chicago: University of Chicago Press.

Fridberg, T. (2000). Sport og motion. In: *Kultur- og fritidsaktiviteter 1975–1998* (pp. 143–154). København: Socialforskningsinstituttet.

Gannik, D. E. (1999). *Situationel sygdom: Fragmenter til en social sygdomsteori baseret på en undersøgelse af ryglidelser*. København: Samfundslitteratur.

Giddens, A. (1996). *Modernitet og selvidentitet: Selvet og samfundet under senmoderniteten*. København: Hans Reitzels Forlag.

Giorgi, A. (1985). *Phenomenology and psychological research*. Pittsburgh, PA: Duquesne University Press.

Goffman, E. (1967). *Interaction ritual*. New York: Pantheon Books.

Holstein, B. E., Iversen, L., & Kristensen, T. S. (1997). *Medicinsk sociologi*. København: Foreningen af danske lægestuderendes forlag.

Howe, P. D. (2001). An ethnography of pain and injury in professional rugby union: The case of Pontypridd RFC. *International Review for the Sociology of Sport, 36*(3), 289–303.

Jakobsen, B. W. (2000). Behandling af idrætsskader i Danmark. *Dansk Sportsmedicin, 3*(4), årgang, 25–27.

Jørgensen, U. (1999). Rekonstruktion af forreste korsbånd — operativ teknik, postoperativ behandling, årsager til funktionssvigt og kvalitetskontrol. *Dansk Sportsmedicin, 4*(3), årgang, 6–10.

Kvale, S. (1997). *Interview. En introduktion til det kvalitative forskningsinterview*. København: Hans Reitzels Forlag.

Leder, D. (1990). *The absent body*. London: The University of Chicago Press.

Lindqvist, R. (1997). *Medikalisering, professionalisering och hälsa. Ett sociologiskt perspektiv*. Lund: Studentlitteratur.

Lupton, D. (1997a). *The imperative of health*. London: Sage.

Lupton, D. (1997b). Foucault and the medicalisation critique. In: A. Petersen, & R. Bunton (Eds), *Foucault, health, and medicine* (pp. 94–110). London: Routledge.

Lupton, D. (1998). *The emotional self*. London: Sage.

Lupton, D. (1999). *Risk*. London: Routledge.

Lupton, D. (2000). *Medicine as culture: Illness, disease and the body in western societies*. London: Sage.

Messner, M. (1992). *Power at play: Sports and the problem of masculinity*. Boston: Beacon Press.

Myklebust, G., Maehlum, S., Engebretsen, L., & Solheim, E. (1997). Registration of cruciate ligament injuries in Norwegian top level team handball: A prospective study covering two seasons. *Scandinavian Journal of Medicine & Science in Sports, 7*, 289–292.

Myklebust, G., Mæhlum, S., Holm, I., & & Bahr, R. (1998). A prospective cohort study of anterior cruciate ligament injuries in elite Norwegian team handball. *Scandinavian Journal of Medicine & Science in Sports, 8*, 149–153.

Nixon, H. L., II (1994). Social pressure, social support, and help seeking for pain and injuries in college sports networks. *Journal of Sport and Social Issues, 18,* 340–355.

Parsons, T. (1975). The sick role and the role of the physician reconsidered. *Health and Society, 53,* 257–278.

Petersen, A., & Lupton, D. (1996). *The new public health: Health and self in the age of risk.* London: Sage.

Petersen, A., & Bunton, R. (1997). *Foucault, health, and medicine.* London: Routledge.

Rail, G. (1992). Physical contact in women's basketball: A phenomenological construction and contextualization. *International Review for the Sociology of Sport, 27,* 1–27.

Regeringens Folkesundhedsprogram 1998–2008 (1999). København: Sundhedsministeriet.

Roderick, M. (1998). The sociology of risk, pain, and injury: A comment on the work of Howard L, Nixon IIa. *Sociology of Sport Journal, 15,* 64–79.

Roderick, M., Waddington, I., & Parker, G. (2000). Playing hurt: Managing injuries in English professional football. *International Review for the Sociology of Sport, 35*(2), 165–180.

Shilling, C. (1993). *The body and social theory.* London: Sage.

Skjerk, O. (2001). *Dameudvalgets inderlige overflødighed. Kvindehåndbold i Danmark 1900–1950.* København: Institut for Idræt, Københavns Universitet.

Thing, L. F. (2000). Et greb med hænderne. *Sport & Psyke,* Nr. 23–24: 25–30. Tidsskrift for Dansk Idrætspsykologisk Forum.

Thing, L. F. (2001). The female warrior: Meanings of play-aggressive emotions in sport. *International Review for the Sociology of Sport, 36*(3), 275–288.

Thing, L. F. (2002). Er kvinders boldspil en tavs social kritik? *Sociologisk Tidsskrift. Journal of Sociology.* Årgang *10*(2).

Thing, L. F. (2004). Risk bodies. Rehabilitation processes in the physiotherapy clinic. Under review in *Nursing Inquiry.*

Turner, B. S. (1992). Kroppen i samfundet. Teorier om krop og kultur. København: Hans Reitzels Forlag.

Valle, R., & Halling, S. (1989). *Existential-phenomenological perspectives in psychology: Exploring the breadth of human experience.* London: Plenum Press.

Waddington, I. (2000). *Sport, health, and drugs: A critical perspective.* London: E & FN Spon.

Wedderkopp, N., Kaltoft, M., Lundgaard, B., Rosendahl, M., & Froberg, K. (1999). Prevention of injuries in young female players in European team handball: A prospective intervention study. *Scandinavian Journal of Medicine & Science in Sports, 9,* 41–47.

White, P., & Young, K. (1999). Is sport injury gendered? In: P. White, & K. Young (Eds), *Sport and gender in Canada* (pp. 69–85). Don Mills, Ontario: Oxford University Press.

Williams, S. J., & Bendelow, G. (1998). *The lived body: Sociological themes, embodied issues.* London: Routledge.

Williams, S. J., & Calnan, M. (1996). *Modern medicine: Lay perspectives and experiences.* London: UCL Press.

Young, K., White, P., & McTeer, W. (1994). Body talk: Male athletes reflect on sport, injury, and pain. *Sociology of Sport Journal, 11*, 175–194.

Young, K. (1997). Women, sport, and physicality: Preliminary findings from a Canadian study. *International Review for the Sociology of Sport, 32*(3), 297–305.

Young, K., & White, P. (2000). Researching sports injury. Reconstructing dangerous masculinities. In: J. McKay, M. Messner, & D. Sabo (Eds), *Masculinities, gender relations, & sport* (pp. 158–183). London: Sage.

Chapter 11

Risk and Injury: A Comparison of Football and Rodeo Subcultures

James H. Frey, Frederick W. Preston and Bo J. Bernhard

Rodeo riders and football players can be acknowledged as exhibiting or representing what White & Young (1997) have called "dangerous masculinities," or a social construction of masculinity that supports a normative acceptance of violence in sport to the extent that bodies can be severely damaged. White and Young's injury data show that men in certain sports are injured at a much greater rate than women, making gender a predictor of injury.

Traditionally, the use of prevention or safety measures has been viewed as reflecting a lack of commitment to the norms of masculinity associated with the sport — even though it would appear to be more prudent to wear such devices. The resistance to safety measures, such as in the form of protective equipment, reinforces the participants' anti-feminine and often homophobic views of self and social world. This view accepts and demands physical toughness and a high pain tolerance. In fact, injury may even be welcomed as a confirmation of an identity that demonstrates the character and strength to withstand injury and the pain associated with it. Playing with pain and demonstrating one's willingness to take risks is often rewarded and celebrated in society (White & Young 1997).

This view is supported by what Nixon (1993, 1994) has called a culture of risk, pain, and injury (see Chapter 3). This cultural configuration is generally reinforced by an "assumption of risk" maxim that suggests that the risk of injury is normal in sport, and that athletes generally accept this risk when they commit to participate (Nixon & Frey 1996). As Messner (1992) has noted, despite their worries, athletes will play hurt, and this characteristic is seen as central to athletes' interpretation of masculinity and playing with pain.

Sporting Bodies, Damaged Selves
Research in the Sociology of Sport, Volume 2, 211–221
© 2004 Published by Elsevier Ltd.
ISSN: 1476-2854/doi:10.1016/S1476-2854(04)02011-4

The extent and nature of risk associated with any activity is a social construction, sensitive to cultural and social evaluations. This is true, for example, of skydivers as well as for football and rodeo participants (Douglas 1985; Frey 1991; Miller & Frey 1997). Perceptions of risk and the acceptability of risk (in this case the possibility of injury) are hence bound by cultural considerations. What the general public might deem dangerous, others would either assess as safe or define the risk as reasonable given the potential benefits, such as recognition, thrill, income, and character development. Risk of injury is often neutralised as a justifiable component of the game or by the false sense of control that athletes may feel over the possibility of being injured.

Risk-seeking behaviour, including playing with injury or knowing the potential for injury, has also been called "edgework" (Lyng 1990). In edge work, participants deliberately seek out dangerous activity, and this is a socially constructed motivation that responds to mechanistic and bureaucratic characteristics of other realms of social life. The concept of edgework has not been extensively applied to athletes, although the compensation notion is prevalent in leisure research. Quite obviously, one could easily translate athletic participation into the concept of edge work; after all, athletes push the envelope of pain in order to continue to experience the thrill of participation, while at the same time meeting the subcultural expectations of masculinity. In this sense, risk-taking is a measure of masculine commitment to the subculture.

Rodeo

Rodeo has been called a folkloristic performance of American western culture. It is a distinctly western phenomenon first performed over a century ago to display the working skills of the cowboy. The cowboy is a romanticised figure representing a set of values very consistent with mainstream and traditional American ideology (Stoeltje 1989). Notably, these values are both lived and consciously presented as athletic performance. Rodeo participants live and perform according to what they often term the "Cowboy Code." This code directly and indirectly reflects rural and Judeo-Christian values of honour, honesty, individuality, hard work, a positive attitude, and courage. Rodeo reminds us of country and farm, of small towns and a simple life (Preston *et al.* 1999; Wooden & Ehringer 1996).

Whether it is seen as an athletic act or a lifestyle, it is clear that rodeo is dangerous. Elite rodeo participants exhibit an injury rate of 11.7% while college riders are injured at a 39.6% rate (Nebergall 1992: 86). Virtually all cowboys have substantial injury histories. Most compete with injuries (e.g. shoulder separation) that would likely sideline other athletes. This is due in large part to economic need:

rodeo participants are independent contractors who pay their own entry fees and travel expenses. Significantly, rodeo athletes do not have "guaranteed contracts" and hence must perform to receive compensation. Few have sponsorship contracts and fewer still become wealthy. The average annual income of a rodeo cowboy competing at the highest levels is approximately U.S. $30,000. Ironically, the cheapest event to participate in is also the most dangerous: bull riding, which requires that the contestant purchase only the rope that they cling to during the course of the seconds-long ride.

The Justin Sports Medicine Program has been implemented at the elite levels to serve the medical needs of rodeo participants. One "Justin Healer," a medical doctor and former physician to a professional football team, claimed that rodeo athletes were the "toughest" athletes he had ever encountered, adding that hockey players and American football players from a generation ago were the only groups who came close.

Protective equipment (such as gel vests, braces, and even helmets) has also been developed for riders as a preventative measure and to make it possible to ride while injured. Older cowboys often express that these developments portend a sort of "feminisation" of rodeo. In reference to a former bull riding champion who chose to wear a helmet, one retired rider commented, "He's not a cowboy. He's *(pause)* . . . something else."

Rodeo cowboys know the risks, yet like athletes in other dangerous sports, they believe that meticulous preparation gives them a significant degree of control over their bodily harm. Tippette (1972: 20) notes that, "Like everyone else involved in a dangerous sport, (the cowboy) likes to believe that, by preparation and foresight, he can reduce the odds until he is actually in control of the situation." Rodeo athletes also believe that knowledge (about a given bull's bucking tendencies, for instance) can help them gain control over the dangerous physical situations that present themselves to the rider.

Rodeo's subcultural emphasis on masculinity is exemplified by the term "cowboy up," which refers to the ability to persevere in the face of pain and adversity. Disregarding an injury and continuing to compete is a classic manifestation of this norm. This tendency is part of the cowboy mystique, an aura that some claim simply reflects a celebration of masculine patriarchy and feminine subordination (Kimmel 1987). Support for this view of rodeo was not absent in this research. As one participant said in reference to barrel racing (the only event for women in the National Finals), "It's an opportunity to see fifteen great horses." Others wondered why the research team would even display an interest in female rodeo participants.

Today, rodeo is an increasingly commercial enterprise. The Professional Rodeo Cowboys Association (PRCA) is the dominant organisational and regulatory arm of rodeo. Collegiate rodeo, governed by the National Intercollegiate Rodeo Association, or NIRA, also holds a national championship. Even in these collegiate rodeos, participants can earn prize money because rodeo is not sanctioned as an official National Collegiate Athletic Association sport.

Football

Football is the one American athletic activity that is most often associated with the culture of risk and the expression of masculine values and character predispositions. This is the basic argument of Nelson's (1994) interesting treatise on the fascination of men with football. Nelson claims that football is one of the few athletic endeavours where "male muscle matters" (p. 6). Others have noted that athletics in general and football in particular "verif(y) masculinity" (White & Young 1997).

The aggressive and violent nature of football needs little empirical verification. Journalistic accounts abound with graphic descriptions of paralysing tackles and crippling blocks (see, for example, Telander 1989). These acts receive little or no condemnation from the football establishment, the media, or fans since they are viewed as a manifestation of the aggressive tendencies inherent to the game.

Athletics in general and football in particular "verifies masculinity" (White & Young 1997). This view persists even in the face of potential death. In fact, a total of eleven professional, college and high school players died while participating in pre-season drills in the fall of 2001. A good portion of these drills was conducted under conditions of extreme temperatures and humidity. The following comments from a player and coach illustrate this mentality:

> John Lawson, an offensive tackle at Virginia, hooked up to an intravenous drip after practice to replenish fluids. During a 13-day stretch of two-a-day practices, Lawson received 33 IVs. "It's all about being a man, Being tough." (*Las Vegas Review Journal*, September 8, 2001: 2B).

> You have to be physically tough on them. You have to push them to the brink, and either they are going to break or they are going to stand up and be a man. That's how you change young boys into being men. You have to be willing to inflict pain on others, and you have to be willing to push yourself or have someone push you beyond normal boundaries. (Quote from high school coach, *Las Vegas Review Journal*, September 8, 2001: 2B).

Performance enhancing drugs sometimes augment football players' aggressive tendencies, but these tendencies are also encouraged by the football and sport subculture. Football athletes acknowledge the violent nature of their sport — and in most cases, even embrace it as a distinctive element of their activity — but few spend a great deal of time worrying about it. Recently, American media outlets have questioned whether training practices that lead to deaths on the field are appropriate, but these questions have not led to any challenges to the basic nature or structure of the sport itself.

Hence, football players are in a very real sense the current-day gladiators of American sport. In the US, football represents the sport culture's ultimate pageant. The commercial presentation of football has served to promote a culture in which physical toughness and the potential for bodily harm are part of the sport's allure. In the current research, the football respondents serve as a useful point of contrast for rodeo discussions, because of the relative familiarity of the former sport's masculine subculture and the relative anonymity of the latter one.

Methodology

The purpose of this research was to determine how rodeo and football athletes perceived "playing with pain," and to examine their self-perceptions of masculinity and toughness. It was our prediction that these athletes would neutralise pain and reinforce the subcultural expectation that playing with pain was normal and an indicator of masculinity or toughness.

We utilised self-administered questionnaires consisting of 25 questions requiring 65 responses. The instrument included a mix of structured, closed-end questions and several open-end or qualitative questions calling for elaboration on previously selected alternatives. The questions on both the rodeo and the football questionnaires asked about the respondent's experience with injuries in their sport (e.g. the nature and extent of the injury, the impact of the injury on subsequent competition, the views of teammates regarding injuries, and the responses to a doctor's or trainer's advice to stop competing). In addition, the respondents were asked about their perceptions of toughness, and responded to the Bem Sex-Role Inventory (BSRI), a measure of gender role orientation. The BSRI includes subscales of femininity and masculinity, and assumes that respondents have internalised, and then view as socially desirable, the traits society associates with gender categories (Bem 1974). Respondents are asked to record their responses on a 1–7 scale, with 7 representing "almost always true" and 1 representing "never true." A 30-item version with the same parameters has been developed, and it is this condensed version (Kolbe & Langefeld 1993) that was used in the rodeo

Table 1: Perceptions and experiences of injury among rodeo contestants and football players.

Variable	Rodeo Contestants	Football Players	Significance Level?
Ever competed while injured?	97% yes	86% yes	0.05
Tougher than average person?	76% yes	96% yes	0.001
Are participants in your sport tougher?	85% yes	89% yes	No significant difference
Do you consider what others think?	20% yes	53% yes	0.001
Has a doctor told you to stop competing?	41% yes	24% yes	0.05

and football questionnaires. T-tests were run to determine statistical significance. The BSRI has been used extensively since its development, and evidence for its reliability and validity has been established. Before it was taken into the field, the questionnaire was pre-tested on the University of Nevada, Las Vegas collegiate rodeo team.

A majority of the successful rodeo interviews were obtained from contestants in the National Finals Rodeo (NFR) between 1995 and 1999. The research team received permission to enter locker rooms and gathering areas to administer the questionnaire before or after an event. Additional respondents were participants in

Table 2: BSRI variables among rodeo contestants and football players.

BSRI Variable	Rodeo Contestants	Football Players	Significance Level?
Warm	5.2	4.7	0.05
Sensitive	5.6	5.0	0.001
Conceited	2.9	3.8	0.01
Jealous	3.1	3.7	0.05
Moody	4.2	4.8	0.05
Truthful	6.5	5.9	0.001
Secretive	4.0	4.8	0.05

Table 3: Masculine, feminine, and androgynous scales among rodeo contestants and football players.

BSRI Variable	Rodeo Contestants	Football Players	Significance Level?
Masculine scale	5.9	6.0	No significant difference
Feminine scale	5.2	5.0	No significant difference
Androgynous scale	5.0	5.1	No significant difference

regional PRCA rodeos. The total number of respondents was 94. The majority of the football respondents were Division I collegiate football players, but a different sample of professional Arena football players contributed to an overall N of 84. When necessary, researchers trained by the research team administered the football questionnaires.

It should also be noted that one of the study's authors (Preston) took "participant observation" to an intriguing level by signing on as an academic advisor (and later as a coach) for the university's rodeo team. This level of participation allowed the research team insights perhaps unattainable via other methodologies; for instance, these athletes were observed in both "front stage" and "back stage" mode (see Preston *et al*. 1999).

Results are summarised in Tables 1, 2 and 3.

Results and Discussion

Rodeo and football athletes differed significantly in their injury history: almost all of the rodeo participants (97%) participated while injured, while 86% of the football players competed while injured. The most common rodeo injuries were broken bones, shoulder separations, and ankle and knee sprains. Lost fingers were hardly rare; as one participant put it, rodeo cowboys were expected to "learn how to rope with two fingers." In rodeo, injuries are normalised in a way that is not as common in other sports. In the locker room, stories abound in which rodeo cowboys awoke in ambulances (or, as in one instance, apparently hopped out of an ambulance to get back to the event). During television broadcasts, announcers occasionally revel in the often-spectacular injuries that are incurred. After one rider was bucked into the metal railing of a rodeo arena, one announcer barked, "Ooh! Look at that! Bonk!" After another rider was knocked unconscious, blood was clearly visible, leading to the following comment: "It just knocked him out! Got him a new shavin' scar too!" Another commentator remarked that the animal had "kicked him (the cowboy) clear off TV!" and provided the following commentary on a further vivid accident: "Boom! There's a concussion for ya!" While not all rodeo fans are as demonstrative in their devotion to the sport's violence, the sheer frequency of injuries suggests that these injuries are an expected part of the sport.

Football injuries were slightly less severe, and centred around predictable body areas: ankle, knee and shoulder injuries were most prominent, followed by bone injuries to hands and fingers. Despite the severity of these injuries, many of the participants in both sports displayed a stubborn willingness to continue playing. Notably, 41% of the cowboys and one-fourth of the football players competed against medical advice to desist. When asked about their willingness to play through pain, respondents in rodeo tended to point to economic factors (such as "you only get paid if you ride"), while football players invoked more general subcultural factors (such as "learning to play with pain" or "blocking out" injuries). In general, rodeo cowboys interpreted the relation of injury to competition in economic terms, while football players responded in more ideological terms. The following field description of a bareback rider captures the nature of these injuries and the reasoning behind continued performance:

> One of the contestants says to "excuse me for not getting up," but please sit next to him. He looks no older than I am (25 at the time), but his hands are gnarled into shapes that are more animal than human. One hand is missing a finger, which gives him a cartoonish four-finger look. He unwraps his right knee, which has numerous torn ligaments. He says he keeps participating because you have to in order to make money, and this is the richest purse of them all (Bernhard 1996).

Both football and rodeo participants were of the overwhelming opinion that they were "tougher than the average guy" and that participants in their sport were "physically" tougher than athletes in other sports. However, the groups differed significantly on the former variable: 96% of the football players and 76% of the rodeo riders felt they were tougher than the average person. Hence, football players deemed themselves and their fellow players "tougher" than rodeo contestants did.

The authors speculate that the primary explanation for this difference is once again cultural in nature. Rodeo athletes are expected to be humble, and that expectation is reflected here. Several rodeo participants even hesitated to fill out the surveys, claiming that they "did not want to brag" about their athletic background.

One participant, who had undergone facial reconstruction surgery earlier that year, remarked that "pain is a personal thing. Most other people aren't all that interested in hearing about it" (Preston 2000).

The anticipated response of teammates often becomes a source of pressure to continue playing through pain. On this variable, dramatic differences were observed. With football players, over half (53%) felt that their fellow competitors would have lower opinions of their character if they did not play through pain. On the other hand, this was not the case with rodeo cowboys, where only 20% felt that they would be criticised by others for not competing while injured. Football players explained their thinking in the following sorts of terms:

- "Just couldn't let my teammates down"
- "You should play with pain"
- "They might think you are a punk"
- "I'm looked at as weak"
- "Unwritten rule: play with pain"
- "Desire to compete overruled pain; felt like team needed me"
- "Because the team needed me and the coach pressured me"

Rodeo athletes again tended to cite economic factors more than a perceived stigma (though obviously stigmatisation plays a role with this group as well). While part of this is no doubt due to the more team-oriented nature of football, rodeo players also rely heavily on fellow competitors (to ride alongside the participants during roping events, and to "scout" the tendencies of animal participants), and in any case adhere to a subcultural norm that usually de-emphasises any kind of interpersonal antagonism.

Bem Sex Role Index Items and Conclusions

The portrait that emerges from this research is hardly a unidimensional one. One of the most striking paradoxes in rodeo is the almost invariable politeness, and even sensitivity of its participants. As one African American rodeo veteran put it, "rodeo cowboys are gentle persons in an aggressive sport." The BSRI results show rodeo riders to be sensitive while participating in a sport that is dangerous and male-dominated. At the same time, the sport's code certainly adheres to masculine norms of toughness, courage, aggressiveness, and individuality. Rodeo riders scored somewhat lower on the masculinity items than football players did, and higher on the femininity items than do their football counterparts, though neither of these scores show a statistical significance (the difference on the feminine scores was significant at the 0.1 level). As noted in the tables, rodeo athletes are more likely than football players to perceive themselves to be warm, sensitive, and truthful. They are less likely than football players to perceive themselves as conceited, jealous, moody, or secretive. As would be expected, there seem to be both cultural and structural explanations for these apparent differences.

Rodeo subculture exhibits less interpersonal antagonism among competitors than does football. Even though they are competing against each other, rodeo athletes often help each other with knowledge about stock. In this context, the adversary is not another rider or roper, but an animal (Preston *et al.* 2001). Football players exhibit a form of "antagonistic cooperation," which is the outcome of competing for playing time and recognition within the team, while competing against another team for money and glory. Additionally, as previously discussed, the encompassing rural culture of rodeo strongly demands adherence to the iconic values of the old West.

Interestingly enough, the football players' average scores on the "femininity" items are also higher than what might be expected, since all fell above the middle values (or towards the "feminine" side of the scale). This might be partially explained by social desirability of these responses, but some variation can be accounted for by the fact that players may subordinate real feelings to what they perceive to be cultural expectations. Thus, what Messner, White and Young and others say about the cultural prohibitions of sport on male personality may be correct, in that the culture forces many to adopt what might be uncomfortable character profiles. This is less of a problem for rodeo riders, who both claim to be less sensitive to what others think of their actions, and come from a traditional, old west, and perhaps more compassionate and cooperative cultural configuration.

References

Bem, S. L. (1974). The measurement of psychological androgyny. *Journal of Consulting and Clinical Psychology*, *42*, 155–162.

Bernhard, B. J. (1996). Field notes.

Douglas, M. (1985). *Risk acceptability according to the social sciences*. New York: Russell Sage.

Frey, J. H. (1991). Social risk and the meaning of sport. *Sociology of Sport Journal*, *8*, 136–145.

Kimmel, M. S. (1987). The cult of masculinity: American social character and the legacy of the cowboy. In: M. Kaufman (Ed.), *Beyond patriarchy: Essays by men on pleasure, power, and change* (pp. 235–249). New York: Oxford University Press.

Kolbe, R. H., & Langefeld, C. D. (1993). Appraising gender role portrayals in TV commercials. *Sex Roles*, *28*, 393–417.

Lyng, S. (1990). Edge work: A social psychological analysis of voluntary risk-taking. *American Journal of Psychology, 95,* 851–886.

Messner, M. A. (1992). *Power at play: Sports and the problem of masculinity.* Boston: Beacon Press.

Miller, W. J., & Frey, J. H. (1997). Skydivers as risk takers: An examination. *Humanity and Society, 20,* 3–15.

Nebergall, R. W. (1992). Rough riders: How much risk in rodeo? *The Physician and Sports Medicine, 20,* 85–92.

Nelson, M. B. (1994). *The stronger women get, the more men love football.* New York: Harcourt Brace.

Nixon, H. L. (1993). Social network analysis of sport: Emphasizing social structure in sport sociology. *Sociology of Sport Journal, 10,* 315–321.

Nixon, H. L. (1994). Social pressure, social support, and help seeking for pain and injury in college sports networks. *Journal of Sport and Social Issues, 13,* 340–355.

Nixon, H. L., & Frey, J. H. (1996). *A sociology of sport.* Belmont, CA: Wadsworth Publishing Company.

Preston, F. W. (2000). Field notes.

Preston, F. W., Bernhard, B. J., & McGinnis, T. (1999). Frontstage and backstage in American rodeo. In: F. W. Preston (Ed.), *Sociology: Approaches, issues and everyday life* (pp. 167–172). Needham Heights, MA: Pearson.

Preston, F. W., Bernhard, B. J., & Shapiro, P. (1999, August). The cowboy subculture. Paper presented at the annual meetings of the Pacific Sociological Association, San Francisco.

Preston, F. W., Bernhard, B. J., & Shapiro, P. (2001, April). The rodeo athlete and their non-human competitors. Paper presented at the annual meetings of the Pacific Sociological Association, San Francisco, CA.

Stoeltje, B. J. (1989). Rodeo: From custom to ritual. *Western Folklore, 48,* 244–255.

Telander, R. (1989). *The hundred yard lie.* New York: Simon & Schuster.

Tippette, G. (1972). *The brave men.* New York: Macmillan.

White, P., & Young, K. (1997, April). Sport and dangerous masculinities. Paper presented at the annual meeting of the Pacific Sociological Association, San Diego, CA.

Wooden, W. S., & Ehringer, G. (1996). *Rodeo in America.* Lawrence, KA: University of Kansas.

Chapter 12

Pain and Injury in a Youth Recreational Basketball League

Rhonda L. Singer

The Westland Youth Recreational Basketball League (WYRBL) provides the girls and boys of this small, American college town and surrounding communities an opportunity to play organised basketball from second grade through early high school. With over a thousand children playing in the league each season, it is possible to observe how the intersecting identities of athleticism, gender and age shape players' team-situated experiences of pain and injury. In this case study, I will show how children collectively create team-appropriate responses to pain and injury, which then work to reproduce asymmetrical gender hierarchies between boys and girls as well as hierarchies of masculine status among boys.

My research began in November 1996, with participant observations of four youth basketball teams in the WYRBL: one fourth/fifth grade co-ed team, one fourth/fifth grade girls' team, one fifth/sixth grade co-ed team and one fifth/sixth/seventh grade girls' team. The co-ed teams were generally all boys, with the exception of Yvonne, a fourth grade girl on the fourth/fifth grade co-ed team. In addition to interacting with the children as they practised and played games, I video-taped some of their activities and talked with all but three of the players in 60–90 minute, semi-structured interviews at the end of the season in late Spring.

The kids with whom I worked accepted pain and injury as inevitable, if not ideal, outcomes of playing basketball. Most of the players recounted stories of past injuries, replete with details of how the injury came about, and how they and

Sporting Bodies, Damaged Selves
Research in the Sociology of Sport, Volume 2, 223–235
Copyright © 2004 by Elsevier Ltd.
ISSN: 1476-2854/doi:10.1016/S1476-2854(04)02012-6

their peers responded to it. Sometimes players would give an account of a variety of bruises and scars, or recount a list of past injuries. Ted, a sixth grader, sat in the chair across from me and pointed to the numerous scratches, sores and bruises that covered his legs and arms, stating with some pride that he got them all at a regional three-on-three tournament. Lyn, a seventh grade girl, told me about a split lip she had, in which, in her words, "there was a lot of blood, yeah." Sixth grader Heather kept rotating her ankle so I could hear the clicking sound it made as a result of a sprain she received in basketball. Sometimes a player and I would exchange sport injury stories, his broken finger for my chipped ankle, her sprained ankle for my concussion. Scars, bruises, bumps and cracking ligaments served as visible badges of honour, symbols of distinguished service in sport.

Yet, behind these stories lie a complex process by which players negotiated with their team-mates on what was seen as appropriate responses to pain and injury. This team-situated vocabulary of pain[1] was formulated in concert with a hierarchy of injuries that designated the relative seriousness of injuries. Together, these standards were used by players to distinguish between injuries that were serious enough to "act hurt," and those that were no big deal. When I asked a fifth grade boy why he didn't sit out when he hurt his ankle, he told me, "... because it wasn't like a serious injury. It wasn't exactly like I sprained it or anything, or I broke it... it hurt a lot, but I knew it wasn't something like really serious." Kids' experiences of pain and injury were filtered through the context of the team's prevailing hierarchy of injury.

A team's vocabulary of pain and hierarchy of injury reflected the gender and age of the players. Overall, boys had more restrictive standards of appropriate responses that reflected the masculine ideals of toughness, aggressiveness and strength. While girls did not want to be seen as "wimps" by others, their incorporation of the "feminine ideals" of compassion, kindness and friendliness into their team culture allowed for more latitude in responses to injury. Within gender categories, older players were more restrictive than younger players, reflecting a developing association between an ability to manage pain and social competence. By successfully managing their responses to pain and injury to fit with team standards, players were able to find support for their gendered and age-appropriate identities. Kids who failed risked losing status relative to their team-mates and other peers.

---

[1] A vocabulary of motives (Mills 1940) delineates a set of responses determined as appropriate given the definition of the situation. As suggested by Young, White and McTeer's (1994) discussion of vocabularies of motive in reference to pain and injury, a vocabulary of pain is a specific set of responses to pain that is situationally appropriate.

In the remainder of this chapter, I present a comparison of two of the teams that I worked with: the sixth/seventh grade co-ed team and the sixth/seventh/eighth grade girls' team. In each case, dominant ideals of athleticism, gender and competence played an important role as kids worked out the meaning and experience of sports injuries. Among boys, deviant gender labels were fundamental as sanctioning devices, simultaneously reproducing hegemonic masculinity, status hierarchies and what Curry & Jiobu call the heroic ethic of sport (1984). While girls co-opted some of the labels used by boys — like "wimp" — they modified the heroic ethic to avoid the types of responses they associated with boys.

Responses to pain and injury often served as a primary gender boundary between boys and girls and as a justification for sex-segregation in the league. Girls felt that boys were generally too casual about injuries, and boys felt that a fundamental aspect of being a guy (and not a girl) in basketball was not to make a big deal out of injuries. Consequently, both players and league adults argued that as a rule, girls and boys should be allowed to play on sex-segregated teams. Ironically, sex-segregation created environments where gender-specific constructions of pain and injury could take place. These same-sex environments narrowed boys' opportunities to modify the heroic model while expanding girls' opportunities. In addition, sex-segregation contributed to the reproduction of patterns of status production and gender asymmetry within the league.

The Sixth/Seventh Grade Co-ed Team

Underlying the sixth/seventh grade boys' constructions of a vocabulary of pain and hierarchy of injury were the multitude of messages boys heard about what it meant to be a man. Team-appropriate responses to pain and injury demonstrated that a guy was tough, strong, serious and aggressive. More importantly, these responses were recognised as evidence that a boy was not a "wus," "wimp," "cry-baby," "girl" or "faggot." Boys who lived up to this team version of the heroic ethic were able to differentiate themselves from girls, who they tended to believe were neither as serious or aggressive, nor as willing to "throw their bodies around" as boys. Perhaps most significantly, the sixth/seventh grade boys' version of the heroic ethic helped to perpetuate the idea that the sport domain was masculine.

Earning Honour

For older male players, the honour associated with injuries was only bestowed after a player had proven that he was "tough" by appropriately managing pain, even in the case of broken bones. Sam, a sixth grader, broke his middle finger playing informal basketball about mid-way through the season:

> Sam arrives at the bench just after the second half of the game begins. Some of the kids know about his finger, others don't, and he has to explain what happened . . . I look up and ask to see his finger. In a finger splint, it is bruised and very swollen. I express sympathy, and shudder from how bad it looks and must have hurt. I comment that it must have really hurt. Sam says, 'not really'. I don't believe him, and reply, 'yeah, right'. Sam says, 'no, really, it didn't hurt that bad, I didn't even cry'. Sam seems to stand a little taller, perhaps proud about his ability to control his emotions or to withstand pain. Tim interjects in support, 'he didn't (cry)' [Author's observation notes].

Later, in my interview with Sam, I asked him what it was like when everyone wanted to see his injury and talk about it. He told me, "yeah, it was pretty cool." He then went on, elaborating on his story of the injury:

> Like when I get hurt, I don't show I'm hurt. I don't go out and start crying, I just keep it to myself. Like when I broke my finger, I didn't tell anybody, I just thought it was really jammed. And my finger got really fat, and I was just sitting in the classroom trying to do work, and my teacher noticed I wasn't really saying anything, and the teacher asked what was wrong. And told me to go to the nurse.

Sam was concerned with maintaining a particular image of himself in our conversation, hence his emphasis on not crying. But, unlike his stories to his team-mates, he also shared with me the reason why he kept his injury to himself:

> I don't know, it kind of makes you feel like a wimp, and it doesn't really hurt after a while. It hurts for like a couple of seconds, and then you hold it, and squeeze on the hand, and then it goes a way, but then it still hurts, and you don't want to show it.

Sam was proud of the fact that he didn't give in to the pain of his injury. It would have made him feel like a wimp if he had let it get to him and made him cry. It was also "pretty cool" to gain the admiring attention of his peers. But his story suggested that that attention came not just from the injury itself, but from how he managed it.

Challenging Claims of Injury

On this team, peers frequently challenged claims of injury. For example, when I asked about the injuries that took place over the course of the season, I received responses such as this:

> He was such a wimp. Sometimes if he gets hit in the leg, like just gets kicked, he'd be like, 'oh, I broke my leg'. He kept saying that and he'd be bouncing up and down, but he wouldn't be like crying. He'd just be like, 'I broke my leg', and shaking it . . . (a wimp is) someone who exaggerates a lot. Like if they get hit, they can't take it [sneer in his voice].

These challenges reflected the important role played by the heroic ethic of sport in the construction of competitive male hierarchies on boys' teams. Not only were boys able to earn higher status on their team through their appropriate management of pain, they could also achieve status by putting down other boys whose responses to injury and pain could be seen as questionable. As Eder *et al.* (1995) found in their study of eighth grade boys, "causing others to lose their cool or be humiliated was an acceptable means of demonstrating superior status" (p. 79).

Getting Mad not Sad

For the sixth/seventh grade boys, anger was a strategy of managing pain and presenting the basketball-playing self as mature and masculine. I saw many of these boys expressing anger after an injury by yelling, slamming their fists onto things, and pushing people away. But this went beyond the flash of anger that any one of us might experience spontaneously after striking our head or stubbing our toe. I observed the latter at all age levels. Rather, the anger expressed by the older boys appeared to be more deliberately produced to displace "inappropriate" emotion and serve as an announcement of the player's seriousness as an athlete.

This was certainly the case when Ted jammed his fingers at practice. Impulsively, he cried out, grabbed his fingers, no doubt stunned by the pain stimuli streaming into his brain. But now he was left with the task of managing the pain in a manner appropriate for an athletic boy his age. Part of that task involved what Hochschild (1983) has called "emotion work," in this case the evocation of anger and suppression of an emotion he called sadness. During the interview, I asked Ted about the anger he expressed following the injury:

> Ted: I get mad when I get hurt. I don't get sad, I get mad.
> Rhonda: You did, you looked mad.
> Ted: I'm not in pain. I'm just mad.
> Rhonda: You're just mad that you're hurt?
> Ted: Yeah.
> Rhonda: Because I was afraid to come talk to you at first.
> Ted: I get mad 'cause I have to get tooken [taken] out, and then I have to wait.
> Rhonda: So you get mad because you have to get taken out (of the game). But there must be some pain there, 'cause you went off the court.
> Ted: Yeah, but, it feels bad, but then a little bit after, it feels fine. And then, they are, like, putting in another person, and it takes a long time to get back in. And you're just sitting there. When you probably just got in.

It is interesting that during the interview, Ted told me that the injury did not cause pain so much as made him mad while, at the time of the incident, he let me know that his fingers hurt quite badly, and there was clear evidence of tears in his eyes.

Through his talk after the fact, Ted redefined his experience in such a way as to negate the identity-threatening presence of pain and injury. There was no doubt that he was angry that he had to leave the court as a result of the jammed fingers. But his explanation also served as an account that made sense of his initial response to the injury and helped sustain his desired identities. Anger was a far more acceptable emotional response for a boy than being sad or in pain, and could even help explain the tears I witnessed. Furthermore, anger was a way that boys on Ted's team demonstrated their seriousness about playing basketball. Ted wanted me to know he wasn't expressing pain; he was expressing his seriousness by being angry about not being able to play. In the end, Ted was managing both his experience of pain (which, in retrospect, he said he didn't have), as well as the impression he gave to others.

Ironically, very few boys successfully managed to fully live up to the very narrow, restrictive vocabulary of pain and hierarchy of injury constructed within their team. The only injury I witnessed that was not disputed or made fun of at any point was when Tim sprained his finger. In this case, the honour associated with injury was fully and uncritically given when Tim stood impassively as his finger was treated, focusing only on the game and shrugging off any suggestion that he might be hurt. By playing through the injury, he proved his masculinity, athleticism and maturity.

Ambivalence and Acquiescence

While all of the sixth/seventh grade boys participated in the construction and enforcement of their teams' vocabulary of pain and hierarchy of injury, some expressed ambivalence and resistance to the control these expectations had on their own behaviour. For instance, while Sam told me he didn't want to feel like a wimp when he hurt his finger, moments later he told me that he didn't care that his team-mates think he's "got to be weak" since he gets injured so often: "Yeah, it doesn't really bother me. I mean, I don't care if they think I'm a wimp or something like that." Or consider Max, a seventh grader. On the one hand, he told me that he might be concerned about being called a "wus" for letting someone know he's hurt. On the other, he remarked, "When I'm hurt, I'm going to express it. I'm not going to hold it up inside." In the interview situation, these boys challenged the hegemony of the heroic ethic on their team, while at the same time defending their own masculine status by telling me that they did not let the teasing and insults of others get to them. Nevertheless, whether they liked the team's version of the heroic ethic or not, they knew that when they did not measure up to it, there were very real consequences for their relative status and the integrity of their athletic, gender and age-related identities.

The Sixth/Seventh/Eighth Grade All-Girls' Team

There was no question that the heroic ethic contributed to the sixth/seventh/eighth grade girls' team vocabulary of pain and hierarchy of injury; many of the players were very much involved in the management of pain and injuries. They played through pain and they discounted injuries that were not perceived as "serious." Some girls talked about not wanting to be seen as a wimp because they let an "insignificant injury" keep them from playing in a game. While such a label did not call a girl's gender into question, it certainly had the potential of making her athletic identity problematic. Girls constructed vocabularies of pain and hierarchies of injury that reflected their understanding that people playing sports need to be able to deal with some level of injury and pain.

The Possibility of Challenges

Unlike the two co-ed teams, only a couple of the players on this girls' team expressed criticisms concerning specific team-mate's injuries, and they tended to be quite vague: "I think sometimes people overreact too. You know, they fall and they're like, 'oh!' and then they're up five minutes later" (Beth, eighth grade). While Beth believed that some people overreacted, she did not mention anyone in particular, nor could she imagine anyone on her team getting teased for crying because they were hurt. Many of her team-mates agreed with her, saying that there was little concern that someone might get teased for acting injured, and that harassing an injured team-mate would just "be rude." As for myself, I never saw a player on the sixth/seventh/eighth grade girls' team get teased for claiming an injury. On the contrary, what I did see were expressions of concern and sympathy.

Despite the relative absence of teasing and challenges to injured status, girls' behaviours were guided by the possibility of these responses. When I asked Heather, a sixth grader, whether she worried about what people might think if she let on that she was hurt, she commented: "Well, yeah, sort of. I didn't worry about it like crazy. I just didn't tell people. They'd be like, 'oh, you're faking' or something like that." Negative responses remained a possibility for the girls due to the predominance of the heroic ethic in the larger discourse of sport and their own experience with this ethic in basketball situations outside the league. For instance, Darbi commented on how there was much more pressure to carefully manage pain and injuries on the playground, where girls play with boys, than when on the all-girls team:

> Rhonda: Have you ever seen in your league anybody giving some-body a hard time for being a wimp?
>
> Darbi (sixth grade): Not really in a league, but in a school there's more of that. Like if somebody gets hurt they don't want to cry or anything.

The possibility of negative responses, and the "heroic ethic" it represents, was mediated through its relevance and practicality to the girls' group.

Pain, Injury and the Definition of the Situation

When girls played on teams outside of the all-girls' division, they often participated in sport cultures that promoted a more extreme version of the heroic ethic. In this different environment, girls adapted their responses to injury and pain, as well as their presentation of the athletic self. A comparison of two girls' accounts of injurious incidents illustrates the degree to which gender and behaviour were shaped by context and the definition of situation.

Darbi, a sixth grader, told me about when she got hurt at a regional basketball tournament that Spring: "Last year at [the tournament], I fell down and I got a gash about this big [uses her fingers to suggest a length of several inches] in the middle of the game. I didn't even go fix it until after the game was over." Darbi remembered presenting herself at the tournament as a tough, dedicated athlete by ignoring her wound. Consider how different her story would have been if, after she fell, she had got up and ran off the court, or if she had screamed when she saw blood. As a participant in a tournament known for its competitive, street-ball style environment, Darbi found honour not just in the injury itself, but in how she appropriately responded to it. As a regular spectator of the annual tournament, I knew the value of Darbi's injury as she had managed it, and I found myself confirming the validity of her "badge of honour."

Lyn, the seventh grader who described in detail the blood coming from her split lip after a fall during a league game, had a somewhat different experience: ". . . And I just sacked out or something and then I started crying I think, yeah, and cried because it really hurt, like I didn't notice it 'til like two seconds after, I'm like, 'Oww!' I'm like (screeches)."

Like Darbi, Lyn was presenting herself as a particular kind of athlete. She used her stories of injuries as testimony of her place within the culture of sport, where injuries carry heavy symbolic weight. But unlike Darbi, Lyn did not ignore her injury. Rather, she cried, which, she suggested, was a reasonable response given how much the injury hurt and how much it bled. Her team-mates' responses of concern and compassion did not challenge this view. The coaches were quick to "sub" her out of the game, making sure that she was okay, and with the help of other adults, getting ice and helping her with the bleeding.

In comparing Darbi and Lyn's injuries, it can be seen that the nature of each event, the attitude of the other participants and the type of sport culture being emphasised led to very different responses to injury and presentations of the athletic identity. The tournament that Darbi played in was characterised by the tacit understanding among many of the participants that aggression was the norm and fouls should only be called in the most extreme cases. In contrast, Lyn's incident occurred while playing in the girls' division of the town league that tries to de-emphasise "unhealthy" competition and overt aggression and where expectations concerning resilience in the face of pain and injury were considerably lower than those faced in the male dominated tournament Darbi participated in. Both Darbi and Lyn considered their behaviour appropriate. And each girl carried her injury as a badge of honour, a symbol of her status as a "real athlete." Yet the type of situation each girl was in, and the vocabulary of pain found there, led to very different ways of announcing and gaining support for their identities as competent female basketball players.

The Pros and Cons of Modifying the Heroic Ethic

It is here that we can see both the benefits and costs of girls' constructions of modified versions of the heroic ethic in all-girl teams. On the one hand, they were able to create a more supportive, less punitive, and perhaps less physically risky environment of sport. In doing so, they both explicitly and implicitly challenged the hegemony of the masculinised heroic ethic. But, on the other hand, such environments are treated by league participants and outsiders as separate from the "real" sport played by men (Theberge 1997), and the identities constructed there were somewhat trivialised. In addition, many of the girls accepted the idea that boys played a more real, more valued style of basketball. Ultimately, sex-segregated teams and girls' creations of alternative vocabularies of pain and hierarchies of injury reproduce the very same structures and ideologies of gender asymmetry that led them to construct alternative models of sport in the first place.

Conclusion

The prominence of the "heroic" orientation of sport has contributed to the practice of treating "acts of violence" upon the body (Messner 1990) as badges of honour. Sport celebrates and rewards the selfless athlete willing to sacrifice his or her body for the good of the team and competition (Coakley 1994; Curry & Jiobu 1984; Messner 1992) and injuries have become part of the criteria "for defining what it means to be a real athlete" (Hughes & Coakley 1991: 308). Consequently, "injury in sport becomes endowed with a unique symbolic meaning" (Curry & Jiobu 1984: 244) that can be used to shore up or challenge identity claims in the sport context.

Appropriate responses to, and therefore meanings of, sport-related injuries are not inherent to a particular physical condition. Rather, appropriate responses are determined through a process of "social interpretation" (Curry & Jiobu 1984: 244), in which dominant idealisations of the heroic ethic are filtered through the situated experiences of sport participants. Intersecting player characteristics, such as athletic identity, gender and age, made the heroic ethic more or less salient for each team.

It has been argued that sport is one of the last areas in social life where men can be assured of their difference from, and superiority to, women (i.e. Klein 1990; Messner 1990, 1994; Willis 1994). This assurance arises in part from the willingness of male athletes to assert their toughness and power through violence against both the opponent and their own body (Messner 1992; Whitson 1994). Thus, when a male player talks about his injuries, he is not only making announcements about his athletic identity, but his masculine identity as well. To be a good athlete is also to be a good man.

But where does that leave female players? I have suggested that there is a lack of fit between idealised notions of femininity and sport, in large part due to the isomorphism of sport and masculinity. Yet, female players who clearly identify themselves as female are also active in using accounts of sports-related injuries to make claims of an athletic identity. In my own observations and interviews, I found girls to be quite active in the negotiation and management of injuries in light of this culture. Like boys, they used injuries to substantiate their athletic identities. Just the same, success in making claims to the athletic identity could potentially make female players' gender identity problematic.

The girls negotiated the tension between the identities of athlete and female by adopting attributes of the ideal athlete while at the same time maintaining a differentiation between males and females.[2] As athletes, the girls enacted and valued certain levels of physicality, aggressiveness and an ability to withstand pain. At the same time, they are able to maintain the differentiation between males and females by utilising both cultural and structural arrangements that don't expect girls to be as "tough" as boys. The girls saw the violence and the "macho" attitude about injuries that girls observed in boys' play as inappropriate, unnecessary and undesirable. As a result, the girls constructed vocabularies of pain that enabled them to be more flexible and less critical than boys in their responses to pain and injuries. While this alternative model of sport had the potential to challenge the narrow, masculinised heroic ethic of sport that set the standard of athleticism in the league, it instead served as evidence of the girls' difference and therefore inferiority in comparison to boys.

Theberge's (1997) and Young & White's (1995) work with elite athletes show that some women have embraced the culture of sport that normalises pain and injury. In this sense, elite female athletes may embrace what could be called a "male" model of sport that values traits associated with masculinity and devalues those associated with femininity (Blinde *et al.* 1994; Young & White 1995). As my research suggests, girls can and do create vocabularies of pain and hierarchies of injury that reflect a rigorous heroic ethic, often in highly competitive, if not masculinised, situations. In doing so, they may be in a better position to find support for their athletic identities although they may be "called into account" for their gender identities (Crosset 1995; West & Zimmerman 1987). Yet, as Young

---

[2] Crosset (1995) discusses this same strategy among women professional golfers. Theberge's (1997) interviews with elite adult women hockey players suggests that they also actively differentiate men from women in sport, even as they argue against efforts to differentiate women's hockey from men's (see p. 75).

and White (1995) point out, the potential of girls' and women's participation to challenge the potency of the heroic model as well as the isomorphism between sport and masculinity is limited when they embrace the "male model" of sport. Instead, the masculinised model of sport is reinforced, leaving hierarchies of gender and athleticism intact.

The constructions of pain and injury among youth basketball players in WYRBL were a microcosm of the larger practices of gender in sport, and to some degree, society at large. As these players negotiated their experiences and meaning of pain and injury, they simultaneously created and enforced definitions of age-appropriate gender displays. Subsequently, dominant ideals of gender, the reproduction of status hierarchies, the maintenance of gender boundaries and the perpetuation of asymmetrical gender relations were all instrumental in, and reinforced through, team responses to pain and injury.

References

Blinde, E. M., Taub, D. E., & Han, L. (1994). Sport as a site for women's group and societal empowerment: Perspectives from the college athlete. *Sociology of Sport Journal, 11*, 51–59.

Coakley, J. (1994). *Sports in society: Issues and controversies* (5th ed.). St. Louis, MO: Mosby.

Crosset, T. W. (1995). *Outsiders in the clubhouse: The world of women's professional golf.* New York: State University of New York Press.

Curry, T. J., & Jiobu, R. M. (1984). *Sports: A social perspective.* Englewood Cliffs, NJ: Prentice-Hall.

Eder, D., Evans, C. C., & Parker, S. (1995). *School talk: Gender and adolescent culture.* New Brunswick: Rutgers University Press.

Hochschild, A. (1983). *The managed heart: Commercialization of human feeling.* Berkeley, CA: University of California Press.

Hughes, R., & Coakley, J. (1991). Positive deviance among athletes: The implications of overconformity to the sport ethic. *Sociology of Sport Journal, 8*(4), 307–325.

Klein, M. (1990). The macho world of sport — a forgotten realm? Some introductory remarks. *International Review for the Sociology of Sport, 25*(3), 175–183.

Messner, M. A. (1990). When bodies are weapons: Masculinity and violence in sport. *International Review for the Sociology of Sport, 25*(3), 203–216.

Messner, M. A. (1992). *Power at play.* Boston, MA: Beacon Press.

Messner, M. A. (1994). Sports and male domination: The female athlete as contested ideological terrain. In: S. Birrell, & C. Cole (Eds), *Women, sport, and culture* (pp. 65–80). Champaign, IL: Human Kinetics.

Mills, C. W. (1940). Situated actions and vocabularies of motive. *American Sociological Review, 5*, 904–913.

Theberge, N. (1997). "It's part of the game": Physicality and the production of gender in women's hockey. *Gender and Society, 11*(1), 69–87.

West, C., & Zimmerman, D. H. (1987). Doing gender. *Gender and Society, 1*(2), 125–151.

Whitson, D. (1994). The embodiment of gender: Discipline, domination, and empowerment. In: S. Birrell, & C. Cole (Eds), *Women, sport, and culture* (pp. 353–371). Champaign, IL: Human Kinetics.

Willis, P. (1994). Women in sport in ideology. In: S. Birrell, & C. Cole (Eds), *Women, sport, and culture* (pp. 31–45). Champaign, IL: Human Kinetics.

Young, K., & White, P. (1995). Sport, physical danger, and injury: The experience of elite women athletes. *Journal of Sport and Social Issues, 19*, 45–61.

Young, K., White, P., & McTeer, W. (1994). Body talk: Male athletes reflect on sport injury and pain. *Sociology of Sport Journal, 11*, 175–194.

Chapter 13

Welsh Rugby Union: Pain, Injury and Medical Treatment in a Professional Era

P. David Howe

The game of rugby union has traditionally been a breeding ground for masculine identity (Dunning & Sheard 1979; Nauright & Chandler 1996). As such, pain and injury issues connected to rugby may have been dismissed as a by-product of identity formation by scholars who focused upon the social-historical importance of the game. Because physical contact is part of the game of rugby, injury and medical treatment play a fundamental role in the environment of the elite rugby club, especially in an age of professionalism. Once it is injured, the body of a rugby player must be repaired as rapidly as possible if the professional club for which he plays is going to receive "full value" from his contract. While this chapter examines these issues using ethnographic methods (particularly participant observation), it also builds upon research done by social scientists of sport who have used other methods for the examination of pain and injury (Nixon 1992, 1993a, b; Roderick *et al.* 2000; White *et al.* 1995).

The essential purpose of this chapter is to provide a sample of data on injury and medical treatment collected within the particular cultural setting of one rugby club in South Wales — Valley Rugby Football Club (VRFC).[1] These data are theorised using the notions of embodiment adopted from the work of Foucault (1979) and Bourdieu (1977, 1990, 1993). Specifically, Foucault's conceptual

---

[1] The name "Valley" is a pseudonym; it refers to an actual town with an actual professional rugby club in South Wales.

Sporting Bodies, Damaged Selves
Research in the Sociology of Sport, Volume 2, 237–248
Copyright © 2004 by Elsevier Ltd.
All rights of reproduction in any form reserved
ISSN: 1476-2854/doi:10.1016/S1476-2854(04)02013-8

ideas about discipline and Bourdieu's concept of habitus are used as an underlying theoretical framework on which the research has been grounded. Leder's (1990) notion of absence is also employed. This suggests that the body only reveals itself to the social actor in times of pain.

An Ethnographic Research Approach

Researchers who are interested in the cultural world of sport have been using ethnographic methods increasingly in recent years. For instance, work by Armstrong (1998), Foley (1990), Sugden (1996) and Wheaton (1997, 2000) highlights how this collection of methods is a useful "tool-kit" with which to explore the sporting social world. Ethnography is a methodology that enables a diachronic (that is to say, a longitudinal) understanding of pain and injury, since the participant observer may be present at the point where injury occurs. The point of getting hurt is only the start of lengthy processes surrounding pain and injury, but it is an important stage from which to begin to understand these concepts. Ethnography allows an exploration of pain and injury to be undertaken throughout the full cycle of injury from the point of onset of pain to the medical treatment of injury and the rehabilitation that follows, as well as intervening periods of wellness. As a result, the ethnographic method helps to illuminate the relationship between the injured player and the expectations of his/her sporting environment.

The research on which this chapter is based was undertaken over a period of two and a half years beginning in the Spring of 1994. Throughout this time, I was resident within the community of Valley. The social importance of the professionalisation of sports medicine was the main focus of the research. A key consideration was the way in which the sporting community, including players, medical team, club committee and supporters in Valley, dealt with the ambiguous nature of pain and injury. The players were all elite performers in the game of rugby union, aged between 18 and 38, and worked largely as skilled labourers or teachers. Participant observation was undertaken through general "gopher" duties such as helping out in the treatment room and acting as "water boy" during matches. This access enabled me to observe, and informally discuss, pain and injury in the treatment room, at training, during matches, on tour and generally anywhere I came in contact with those involved with the club.

Pain and Injury at Valley RFC

Injury is generally accepted within the culture that surrounds the game of rugby. In the specific context of the South Wales, where rugby is supported with an almost religious fervour (Smith & Williams 1980; Williams 1991), injury to star players can have a great impact on community identity. For example, part of the habitus of VRFC is constituted through the notion of "underdog" which is articulated in relation to arguably more vibrant regions and clubs in Wales. As a result, when one of the club's key players is sidelined with an injury the impact is felt within the community at large. In fact, support for the club is often greater when it is cast in the "underdog" role, which is often the case when key players are missing from the squad due to injury.

The rate and type of rugby injuries can vary depending on a number of factors including game position and field conditions during both games and training sessions (Howe 2004). At VRFC, there was no shortage of injuries to study. Perhaps the most interesting detail about pain and injury at VRFC was the manner in which athletes reported their injuries. Generally, there was a desire by my informants to talk of the injury only if it was related to training or to the goal of becoming a better player. If the pain and injury were a result of what could be seen as physical inadequacy on the part of the athlete, then the consequences of the injury on the player's life outside the sport tended to become the focus of conversation. The majority of the injuries that I recorded were acute in nature and, therefore, so was the pain. However, within the context of a professional rugby club, acute injuries often take on chronic traits since time away from the field of play is viewed as a possible loss of earnings for the club.[2] At VRFC, pain and injury experiences that were acknowledged were mostly associated with injuries that could be "played through." Injuries such as broken limbs were "obvious," whereas *playable* injuries could be used as an escape from a poor performance as well as a vehicle to elevate the player's kudos because it demonstrated desire to make physical sacrifice for the team. Therefore, I became concerned with how and why pain and injury varied from player to player and how this was associated with the treatment that was administered by the medical support team.

Commercialism in British rugby union has led to the recent professionalisation of the sport as well as to the transformation of the players into commodities (Howe 1999). Because of this transformation, the way that injuries are treated has also changed. Players at Valley appeared to be placed under more pressure to come to terms with pain and injury when their position within the squad lacked security. This is illustrated by the following comment made by a long-standing member of the club and former player:

---

[2] Acute pain and injury is experienced when the body is subjected to uncomfortable irregular action or force placed upon it whereas a chronic pain or injury is a state in which the body is impaired for an extended period of time.

> Since you have been around asking odd questions about my injuries
> and stuff I have really noticed how things have changed at the club.
> In the past, I would 'cry-off' due to pain and minor injury; now my
> livelihood is dependent on performing well every Saturday. You
> have to suck it up in the modern era — hide the pain and play on.

Furthermore, evidence suggests that players became more or less vocal about
their pain depending on to what advantage they thought it could be turned. For
example, I found that the mention of pain after a match could be used to save
face when a player's performance was below par as a result of carrying an injury.
Likewise, when a player sustained a minor injury in training and could easily
be replaced in a subsequent match, there was a tendency to conceal the pain and
injury (cf. Young *et al.* 1994: 183). On the other hand, a player who was a certain
starter for every match and much better than his understudies would do less to
cover up the pain that he might have been feeling. Such a player would not have
wanted to cope with a pain that hindered his performance and in the long term
impacted upon his chances of being the club's first choice starter.

Discussions among the players often focused around pain and playing hurt[3]
rather than injury because injury was seen as an indication of inferior biomechanics. The idea of injury detracts from a player's notion of perfection on the
pitch, in spite of the fact that every player at VRFC was injured while I was in
residence. There was a strong association between the type of injury, the pain
that was involved, and the way it was discussed. The club's star "Number 8" was
very aware of the problems that his third broken arm in two years had brought
to bear on him and his playing style: "It is not so much the pain of breaking this
thing [arm]. To have it happen so often really gets me down. Maybe the coach is
right. It is about time I try to change my tackling 'cause every time I start playing
good I get injured again." In other words, an injury may undermine a players'
self-confidence and as a result may lead to personal reassessment on a number
of levels. Therefore, with an injury of a serious nature there is little kudos to be
gained by talking about the pain. However, with injuries that are related to over-use
of particular parts of the body, most often aggravated by too much training, the
talk of pain increases. A "centre," approaching his mid-thirties and continually
struggling with sore abdominals, suggested: "Remember, when you play in the
centre it is important to have strong abs. [abdominal muscles], and at times I push
myself too hard . . . the pain gets, well, bad. You gotta remember that you gotta
push that barrier if you want to keep your place at my age." To this player, then,

---

[3] See Roderick *et al.* (2000) for a discussion of playing hurt in the context of professional soccer.

pain became a positive indicator of hard work. The same player commented that at times he was in pain and that he believed it was in his own best interest if the team did not know: "My abs are in constant pain and the trainer says that I have to be really careful with them. I try not to let any of the team selectors know that they bother me, or I may not get picked to play."

Such a scenario highlights the difficult position the sports medicine team occupies within the sporting community. When pain and injury are acute, the rugby club is aware that the injured player should not play, but when the situation becomes chronic there is scope for the player to conceal the problem. The player may say he is fit because he may be afraid of losing his place on the team or, with the advent of professionalism, may need the match fee which he will be paid. On the other hand, the coaching staff may try to manipulate the medical team into convincing the player that the pain does not exist and that therefore he should play. This is a clear example of how acute pain can manifest itself chronically within the environment of VRFC as a result of social pressures. Far from being unique to professional rugby union, other contact sports such as American football have been dealing with these types of dilemmas for some time (Huizenga 1994: 70).

Treating Pain Medically at Valley RFC

In the context of VRFC, the severity of each individual's pain was always relative. The lack of objectivity[4] in the measurement of pain has posed a serious problem for research into the social role of pain in various communities. As Bendelow & Williams (1995: 146) have suggested, this is a difficulty with investigations of pain throughout Western society:

> The elevation of sensation over emotion in traditional medical and psychological approaches results in the lack of attention to subjectivity, which in turn leads to a limited approach towards sufferers and a neglect of broader cultural and sociological components of pain.

In spite of these challenges associated with measuring pain, medical teams still have to deal with its consequences. When an athlete is injured, because of the

---

[4] It is possible to objectify pain using laboratory conditions and equipment to measure the physiological response of the nerves to pain (Good *et al.* 1992: 9). These conditions do not exist during competition or training and, therefore, the measurement of pain I am discussing in this chapter is captured in the subjective response of the athletes.

subjective nature of pain, a physiotherapist will often poke, pitch and twist in the region of the injury, in order to determine the extent of physical damage. Therefore, the treatment team increases the level of pain in the short-term in order to achieve a better understanding of the injury and thus speed up pain relief in the long-term.

The treatment of injury after the onset of pain can be a problematic process. From time to time it is possible for the medical practitioner to misdiagnose an injury because she/he is not taking into account all the relevant information. Ethnographic data related to rates of injury in rugby (Howe 2004) suggest that minor injuries become compounded when pain is inappropriately interpreted by medical staff leading to the wrong ailment being treated. This again provides justification for why diachronic research is beneficial in cataloguing the development of injuries. Although pain is the key marker for injuries, because there are no rigid rules about the elimination and/or severity of duration of pain (due in part to the subjective nature of the concept), it is therefore a problematic indicator of injury.

That pain can be misleading in the treatment of injury can be highlighted by the most significant injury case during my study. This involved the club's international "outside-half" who missed several games during the 1994/95 season with a supposed hamstring injury. The injury had been sustained during an important cup match, but the player had continued in the match despite feeling pain in the back of his leg. After playing in several more matches, the player succumbed to the crippling pain coming from the area of his hamstring which had been passed as healthy. Several weeks later the team osteopath diagnosed the injury correctly as a misalignment of the pelvis.

During the following season the medical team was unable to immediately detect a broken collarbone that the "outside-half" had sustained. A late diagnosis meant that the player was unable to take his place at outside-half for Wales for the first three matches of the 1996 Five Nations Championships,[5] all of which were lost. In this specific case, X-rays were taken but they did not appear to indicate a fracture. Therefore, if the player had been more vocal about the pain, the injury could have been properly treated. In the player's words: "You may think I'm thick but the pressure for me to play is unbelievable. When no fracture showed [on the X-ray] I thought, hell, it [the pain] must be in my mind . . . Now, with the

---

[5] This is an annual tournament involving the best teams from Europe (England, France, Ireland, Scotland and Wales). In its current format, the tournament, now with the inclusion of Italy, is known as the "Six Nations Championships."

injury like it is, I may lose my spot on the Welsh squad." In some cases, therefore, the pain of an injury may be a better indicator of an injury than the diagnostic equipment used by the sports medicine team. This in itself raises questions about how the level of pain tolerated by an individual on a daily basis affects the quality of service that he receives when he becomes injured.

Because of the subjective nature of pain, an understanding of how each player reacts to it may become important in determining the functioning of sports medicine clinics. Research on both male and female American collegiate athletes suggests that "they typically play while hurt to the extent possible and get help when their pain level reflects an injury that prevents them from performing" (Nixon 1996: 83). At VRFC, the habitus at the club allowed for open communication between the sports medicine team and the players. Therefore, the players would often seek medical treatment before an injury became serious.

Squad size has a lot to do with personal communication and availability of medical treatment. At the time of the study, VRFC only had a squad of 36 players and a treatment staff of four (including a doctor). An international "second row forward" commented: "One of the physios is always about . . . if I feel any real pain I go to them right away . . . I have missed several opportunities to play for Wales in the past because I was concealing an injury so I don't want to miss my next crack." In spite of such access to medical treatment and expertise, it is impossible to detail objectively and with complete accuracy the level of pain, regardless of how well the treatment staff know the player. The amount of pain a player is willing to tolerate will often depend on the demands at hand. For instance, at the start of a Six Nations campaign, pain tolerance would arguably be greater than that which would be considered acceptable for a regular club league fixture. Each competitive situation has a relative value to the player preparing to perform in it, and the more important it is for the player to play in a match, apparently, the more pain he will be willing to endure.

To many rugby club officials, the player's pain is no longer a prime concern. In the professional era, when a winning team is paramount to a healthy balance sheet, the elimination of injury is all-important. The reduction in the amount of time needed to treat injury leads to team management getting more value for their money in relation to player contracts. This shift in treatment patterns occurring in conjunction with wider professionalising trends had clearly left some long-serving members of the team concerned: "In the past when I was injured, I recovered at my own pace. Now, it seems that my feelings about my fitness are not as important . . . the club seems so concerned about getting their money's worth [that] they have little time for me." This statement illustrates how the bodies of players are becoming increasingly commodified.

Access to Medical Treatment at Valley RFC

The advent of professionalism in rugby union and the desire of both the club and the player to protect their investment in the sporting body have elevated accessibility to treatment to paramount importance. It appears from my research that accessibility to sports medicine clinics is key to the way an athlete deals with pain. If the player can easily access a physiotherapist when he has a minor complaint, it will clearly reduce the chances of further and more serious injury.

Some injury treatments may only work short-term; indeed, my data suggest that the selection of treatment method was not always successful. A player may return from injury only to find that he has failed to fully recover and is once again "sidelined." This is an indication of a number of possible problems. Firstly, the player may be unable to cope with the physical roughness of the game. Second, it may be an unlucky coincidence or, finally, it may be a flaw in the method of treatment administered for the injury. If pain and therefore injury start to become chronic (in the traditional sense), then a number of choices have to be made; do you retire from your sport or do you have an operation that may save and even prolong your playing career? A high profile player at VRFC provided a response to this question: "The fact that I am paid to play the game places great stress on me. I want to play well in every match and that means playing pain-free . . . It would be devastating when Wales comes calling if I am out with an injury." Such decisions about the health of a player in the professional era of rugby union not only affects the player's well-being but also the financial success of the whole club; as a result, greater emphasis is placed on the care and maintenance of the body. Therefore, one would think that effective treatment of injury should be paramount, but my data showed that this was not necessarily the case.

Treatment of injury at VRFC was observed to be very unsystematic, yet players were regularly seen leaving the treatment room "cured." Unless the injury was a common occurrence, such as a sprained ankle, the players appeared to be given different treatments until one of them began to relieve the pain. As players came into the treatment room they would be given the next available modality machine (such as ultrasound and/or interferential),[6] apparently regardless of the injury sustained. In spite of this unscientific approach to the treatment of injuries of various kinds, the players would return to fitness within reasonable time.

---

[6] Ultrasound is a machine/technique that uses sound waves to treat damaged tissue, whereas interferential treatment uses electrical pulses for the same purpose.

What is of importance is that the players believe and expect to be healed by the treatment staff. The acquisition of the services of a professional physiotherapist[7] brought scientific medicine to VRFC. Although this professional inevitably introduced a different personal approach, which altered the treatment environment, this was not inconsistent with the club's habitus, and therefore did not hinder the speed of recovery in the treatment room. As one of the players commented:

> Ever since the physio has arrived at the club, I have been happier in the treatment room, if you can be happy there! I don't know what is up with [the trainer] but we just don't get on. It gives me a feeling of security to know that the physio is looking after me.

This is not to say that all the players did not trust the trainer, but just to say that his personality was different to that of the physiotherapist. Players were therefore able to choose whom they wished to be treated by. Another option for pain and injury treatment at VRFC was an osteopath whose "alternative" form of medicine was more holistic than that provided by the physiotherapists. The treatment of injury provided by an osteopath was essentially done via manipulation of the skeletal system. This was often accompanied by heavy massage to loosen muscles around the various joints in the body before realignment could safely take place. Despite concerns on the part of the players that professionalism had had economic implications not necessarily in their interests, as noted earlier, the adoption of non-traditional medical practices is also a clear indication of the rugby club valuing its players, albeit as assets, in the professional era.

By increasingly giving the players a choice of treatment, the sports medicine team at VRFC had arguably enhanced the placebo effect and the speed of recovery from injury. A former Welsh international "flanker" at the club commented on the treatment using osteopathy:

> Ever since I have gone to see him [the osteopath] on a monthly basis for a physical, I have had no serious injury. I think it was great for the club to employ his services although I must confess to being sceptical of his techniques on my first few visits.

The introduction of an osteopath as well as qualified physiotherapists at the club may be seen as a shift in medical practice from a curative to preventative

---

[7] Before my time at VRFC, the club had used the services of a number of amateur trainers who typically adopted a bucket-and-magic-sponge "technology" toward the treatment of injury.

paradigm (Howe 2001). This is again in line with the value that has been added to the bodies of rugby players since the onset of professionalism. In the long-run, preventing injury is more cost-effective and better for the players than curing them once hurt. With the increased commercialisation of the sport of rugby (Howe 1999), the consumption of sports placebos such as sports drinks and other nutritional supplements has also been encouraged by the medical team at VRFC as well as regular flexibility exercises that can also help to limit the onset of injury. Ultimately, the nature of the game of rugby means that all injury cannot be prevented, but the habitus at Valley RFC has been transformed by the way in which pain and injury is treated in a changing club environment.

Conclusion

Exact measurement of the social significance of pain within the sporting world is problematic. By realising that pain is the signifier of injury, some explanations of the concept's cultural importance may be established. This chapter shows that as well as being a physical marker of injury, pain may be seen, in the environment of a rugby club, as a symbol of social distinction, the personal and social experience of which has been altered as the habitus of the club is transformed through professionalisation. No longer is the health and well-being of players considered, by management, above the desire to win games. In a sporting environment where "perfect" performance is the objective, acute pain often develops chronic traits as the desire for success is increased. As the need for success increases, so too does the risk of acquiring pain and injury. For better or worse, this is the legacy of professionalism in elite rugby in Wales.

The timing of the occurrence of pain and injury in the sporting context is ambiguous and manifests itself in an unstructured form. Ethnography is a research approach equipped to deal with this ambiguity. However, there is a paradox to the diachronic scope that the ethnographic method provides. On the one hand, the ethnographer is present when pain occurs, but she/he is also there to record the treatment and injury management regimes, which are in themselves very revealing of the social importance of pain and injury. Rugby players at Valley frequently discussed pain and its function in determining the time required by a player to return to activity after an acute injury, but such discourse was limited to the environment of the changing room. On the other hand, ethnography is clearly not appropriate in every research context as it is extremely time-consuming. It is suggested, therefore, that ethnographic research into pain and injury complements, but should not replace, the more established and less time-demanding methodologies of survey and interviews (Nixon 1993a; White *et al.* 1995; Young 1993). If used together, these techniques can enable the social science of sport to develop a more complete understanding of the sporting universals of pain and injury.

Acknowledgements

Thank you to Sage Publications Ltd. for allowing the reprint of part of a paper that first appeared as Howe (2001).

References

Armstrong, G. (1998). *Football hooligans: Knowing the score*. Oxford: Berg.

Bendelow, G., & Williams, S. (1995). Transcending the dualism: Towards a sociology of pain. *Sociology of Health and Illness, 17*(2), 139–165.

Bourdieu, P. (1977). *Outline of a theory of practice*. Cambridge: Cambridge University Press.

Bourdieu, P. (1990). *In other words: Essays towards a reflective sociology*. London: Polity Press.

Bourdieu, P. (1993). *Sociology in question*. London: Sage.

Dunning, E., & Sheard, K. (1979). *Barbarians, gentlemen and players: A sociological study of the development of rugby football*. Oxford: Martin Robinson.

Foley, D. (1990). *Learning capitalist culture*. Philadelphia: University of Pennsylvania Press.

Foucault, M. (1979). *Discipline and punish: The birth of the prison*. London: Hammonworth.

Good, M. J. D., Brodwin, P. E., Good, B. J., & Kleinman, A. (Eds) (1992). *Pain as human experience: An anthropological perspective*. Los Angeles: University of California Press.

Howe, P. D. (1999). Professionalism, commercialism and the rugby club: From embryo to infant at Pontypridd RFC. In: T. L. C. Chandler, & J. Nauright (Eds), *The rugby world: Race, gender, commerce and rugby union* (pp. 165–180). London: CASS.

Howe, P. D. (2001). An ethnography of pain and injury in professional rugby union: The case of Pontypridd RFC. *International Review for the Sociology of Sport, 36*(3), 289–303.

Howe, P. D. (2004). *Sport, professionalism and pain: Ethnographies of injury and risk*. London: Routledge.

Huizenga, R. (1994). *"You're okay, it's just a bruise": A doctor's sideline secrets about pro football's most outrageous team*. New York: St. Martin's Griffin.

Leder, D. (1990). *The absent body*. London: University of Chicago Press.

Nauright, J., & Chandler, T. J. L. (Eds) (1996). *Making men: Rugby and masculine identity*. London: Frank Cass.

Nixon, H. L. (1992). A social network analysis of influences on athletes to play with pain and injuries. *Journal of Sport and Social Issues, 16*(2), 127–135.

Nixon, H. L. (1993a). Accepting the risks of pain and injury in sport: Mediated cultural influences on playing hurt. *Sociology of Sport Journal, 10*(2), 183–196.

Nixon, H. L. (1993b). Social network analysis of sport: Emphasizing social structure in sport sociology. *Sociology of Sport Journal, 10*(3), 315–321.

Nixon, H. L. (1996). The relationship of friendship networks, sports experences, and gender to express pain thresholds. *Sociology of Sport Journal, 13*(1), 78–86.

Roderick, M., Waddington, I., & Parker, G. (2000). Playing hurt: Managing injuries in English professional football. *International Review for the Sociology of Sport, 35*(2), 165–180.

Smith, D., & Williams, G. (1980). *Fields of praise: Official history of the Welsh Rugby Union 1881–1981.* Cardiff: University of Wales Press.

Sugden, J. (1996). *Boxing and society: An international analysis.* Manchester: University of Manchester Press.

Wheaton, B. (1997). Covert ethnography and the ethics of research: Studying sport subcultures. In: A. Tomlinson, & S. Fleming (Eds), *Ethics, sport and leisure: Crises and critiques* (pp. 163–171). Aachen, Germany: Meyer and Meyer.

Wheaton, B. (2000). "Just do it": Consumption, commitment, and identity in windsurfing subculture. *Sociology of Sport Journal, 17*(3), 254–274.

White, P. G., Young, K., & McTeer, W. G. (1995). Sport, masculinity and the injured body. In: D. Sabo, & F. Gordon (Eds), *Men's health and illness: Gender, power, and the body* (pp. 158–182). London: Sage.

Williams, G. (1991). *1905 and all that: Essays on rugby football and Welsh society.* Llandysul, Wales: Gomer Press.

Young, K. (1993). Violence, risk, and liability in male sports culture. *Sociology of Sport Journal, 10*(4), 373–396.

Young, K., White, P., & McTeer, W. (1994). Body talk: Male athletes reflect on sport, injury, and pain. *Sociology of Sport Journal, 11*(2), 175–195.

Part III

Pain Parameters

Chapter 14

Athletic Trainers: Between Care and Social Control

Stephan R. Walk

The presence of medical professionals in sports facilities is an obvious testament to the unique health risks of sport and the normalisation of athletic injury. Athletic training in the United States, and similar professions around the world,[1] developed in response to the regularity of sports injuries and the need to provide on-site medical services for athletes. For those concerned with risk-taking, pain, and injury in sport, the existence of a profession singularly interested in treating sports injuries would seem a welcome development. However, like scholars who have studied institutionalised medicine (e.g. Foucault 1973; Goffman 1961), sociologists who have shown an interest in the study of risk, pain and injury in sport have been circumspect about the practice of sports medicine (e.g. Nixon 1998). While qualifications of sports medicine personnel, standards of medical care for athletes, and sports injury treatment facilities have all seemingly improved, sport is still characterised by health compromises, pain, and unreasonable risk taking.

Prompted by recent deaths of college and professional American football players, there is also increasing popular awareness and criticism of the medical

---

[1] "Athletic training" is a distinctively American term (also adopted in Japan and Taiwan) rooted in the idea that the athlete should be physiologically "trained" for athletic competition. This suggests that athletic training originally had a preventative focus. Like the medical profession in the U.S., however, there seems to have been a clear shift in the direction of a disease model, in that athletic trainers are principally prepared to treat injuries after they occur. Athletic trainers in the U.S. are analogous to sports physiotherapists in the U.K., athletic therapists in Canada, and biokineticists in South Africa.

Sporting Bodies, Damaged Selves
Research in the Sociology of Sport, Volume 2, 251–267
Copyright © 2004 by Elsevier Ltd.
All rights of reproduction in any form reserved
ISSN: 1476-2854/doi:10.1016/S1476-2854(04)02014-X

services athletes receive (e.g. Cowin 2001; Van Valkenberg 2001). The *Kansas City Star*, in an exposé on the National Collegiate Athletics Association (NCAA), suggested that health care services for college athletes are inconsistent across institutions and woefully inadequate in some cases (Rock 1997). The *Star* identified incidents of athlete deaths and long-term disabilities it claimed could have been prevented, pointing to a lack of medical safeguards across NCAA institutions, a lack of basic medical training among coaches, and insufficient resources for the acquisition of medical supplies and personnel. They suggested that the NCAA institute a requirement for a specific ratio of certified athletic trainers to athletes, require coaches to undergo CPR training, and include a review of health care services as part of NCAA institutional certification processes.

How might we understand the seeming paradox between the growth of the athletic training profession within sports medicine and the persistence of a health-compromising sports culture? This chapter will attempt to address this question by focusing on three primary topics. First, the historical development of athletic training into an allied health profession in the United States will be briefly summarised. Second, the social location of athletic training services within larger institutions, such as medical organisations and university sports programmes, will be discussed, noting in particular the conflicts of interest and gender dynamics they feature. Finally, the conflicting obligations of athletic trainers to establish and maintain trust with athletes while also attempting to win their compliance with an array of competitive, institutional, and social obligations will be summarised. The chapter will attempt to show the tensions in athletic training between providing effective medical services to athletes and performing social control functions.

Growing Pains: From Rubbers to Athletic Trainers

While sociology has an extensive history of scholarship on the institutionalisation of medicine and its allied professions (e.g. Freidson 1970; Starr 1982), athletic training has escaped all but brief mention in work by sport historians and sport sociologists. This is true of sport sociologists who have recently undertaken the study of risk, pain and injury among athletes. Hence, while athletic training has not been studied, it is a profession made possible by injured athletes. In the absence of such work, we might be guided by insights from early scholarship in the sociology of medicine on the way to tracing the historical development of athletic training.

In *Profession of Medicine*, Freidson (1970) studied the evolution of the medical profession in the United States. He observed how the term "medicine" was historically used to describe a wide range of *practices*, from individual self-healing techniques to the most scientifically sophisticated forms of medical services. He therefore looked at medicine first as an occupation — that is, as a set of practices for diagnosing and treating illnesses — and only secondarily as a body of scientific knowledge. Starr (1982) noted that the growth of the authority of medicine in the U.S. was made possible by mechanisms of both legitimation and dependency. The legitimations were the establishment by medicine of standardised education and legal licensing, which convinced the public to allow the medical establishment to essentially govern its own industry. Dependency upon the medical establishment was built by instituting controls over the dispensation of drugs, the formation of health insurance, and the founding of medical institutions, including hospitals and clinics. We might add to the latter that allied medical professions, such as nursing, were also ultimately dependent upon organised medicine for their legitimacy (Starr 1982).

The growth in the power of individual physicians was also permitted by these legitimations and dependencies — the physician gained public prestige as a result of services provided directly to the public, not necessarily as a result of the growth of scientific medical knowledge. Indeed, Freidson (1970) saw as radically different those activities associated with solving practical medical problems and those associated with the production of knowledge in the form of scientific journals and medical education. Thus, the distinction between the scientific knowledge created for the purposes of public licensure and the autonomy of a *profession*, and the "recipe knowledge" and sedimented traditions (Berger & Luckmann 1966) of the institutionalised practice of an *occupation* should be kept in mind. This suggests that any medical or paramedical occupation, like athletic training, should be analysed as much for its actual clinical practices as it is for its identification with a centralised professional organisation or body of scientific knowledge.

As was the case with medicine, some of the practices and techniques of athletic training predate its establishment both as an occupation and a profession, some having originated in antiquity (Fahey 1986; O'Shea 1980). These include the massage, taping and wrapping of the body historically associated with the paidotribes (*"boy rubber"*), *aleittes* (*"anointer"*), and *gymnastes* of Ancient Greece (Harris 1964). As we shall see, some of these practices continue in spite of limited scientific evidence demonstrating their usefulness. It was, however, the meteoric rise of a corrupt[2] and injurious college sports system in the early 20th century that set the stage for the emergence of the athletic training profession in the U.S.

---

[2] The founding of the National Collegiate Athletics Association in 1905 was a direct response to concerns over corruption, deaths, and serious injuries in college football expressed by President Theodore Roosevelt.

In 1916, S. E. Bilik, a "trainer" for the University of Illinois football team, published the seminal work, *The Trainer's Bible* (Bilik 1956). Prompted by an alarming number of catastrophic injuries and fatalities in college football, Bilik criticised those athletic programmes and coaches willing to garner money and prestige from the efforts of players, but who saw no need to adequately "train" athletes to participate in such a violent game. He chastised the "old-fashioned rubber," the drinking and swearing "know-it-all" ditch-digger masquerading as the team trainer (Bilik 1916: 8) and praised those trainers "thoroughly versed in conditioning, selection and care of protective equipment, bandaging, diet, psychology, physical therapy, [and] first aid of common athletic injuries" (p. 9). In doing so, Bilik foretold, almost formulaically, that athletic trainers would follow the actions of other successful occupational groups to establish themselves as a profession: namely, offering a service valued by the public; presenting the occupation as being motivated by public beneficence; identifying with and claiming a monopoly on a body of scientific knowledge; seeking licensure by claiming expertise on certain procedures; publishing research and professional journals; and calling attention to charlatans (Freidson 1970). While these efforts may have worked to the benefit of athletes, they, of course, also worked to preserve college football by implying that, with the right medical professionals, the game could be played safely.[3]

Accordingly, after failed efforts in the 1930s and 1940s, athletic trainers from nine U.S. regions met and founded the National Athletic Trainer's Association (NATA) in 1950 (O'Shea 1980). A few observations about this initial meeting will foreshadow issues that will come up later in this chapter. First, all but two of the 125 athletic trainers attending the 1950 meeting were white and all were male.[4] Indeed, it would be 16 years before a woman would become an NATA member, and 34 years before a woman would be elected to a board position in the NATA. Second, as in the case of S. E. Bilik, nearly all of these men had historical roots and strong alliances with university sports programmes. Indeed, all of the members of the first NATA Board of Directors had positions as athletic trainers at universities and most of them had been hired by coaches (O'Shea 1980). Third, the expenses for this meeting, and the five subsequent annual meetings, were underwritten entirely by the Cramer Chemical Company, a firm founded in 1918 by former track athlete Charles Cramer and his brother Frank, inventors of "Cramer Athletic

---

[3] Ominously, Bilik (1956) warned school authorities that they ought not allow "the alumni, the press, or the public" to run their athletic programmes, and suggested that when a coach "uses injured or fatigued youngsters; leaving them in the game too long, driving them in practice too hard, teaching them apparently unfair tactics — look for 'the power behind the throne' " (p. 13).

[4] Interestingly, the American Physical Therapy Association, founded as the American Women's Physical Therapeutic Association in 1921, did not admit its first male members until the late 1930s.

Liniment" and other products used by athletic trainers (Ebel 1999). Today, Cramer is one of the largest suppliers of products used by athletic trainers.

Despite these efforts, some 40 years passed before the profession of athletic training developed adequate curricular and clinical practices in university programmes to receive accreditation by the American Medical Association as an allied health field (Weithaus & Fauser 1991). A couple of factors may explain this gap. First, it was not until nine years after its founding that the NATA established what it termed a "model curriculum" by which to standardise the education of practitioners. That curriculum included a core of courses normally taken by physical education majors at universities, with the addition of a core of physical therapy and other courses. Unfortunately, not only did physical education have its own credibility problems within higher education, the inclusion of the physical therapy content of the curriculum created competitive tensions with physical therapy professionals. Second, a 1968 study by the NATA concluded that not a single university programme had instituted the then nine-year-old model curriculum (Ebel 1999). For at least 20 years, and perhaps many more, it was evidently quite possible, and socially acceptable, to practise athletic training as an occupation without the credentials and competencies suggested by the field's own professional organisation.

Starting in the mid-1970s, NATA reacted by instituting curricular changes that would distinguish it from physical therapy, establishing competencies, delineated roles and a certification examination, accrediting university programmes, and lobbying school administrators and state officials for recognition and licensure of the profession. These efforts persist today. By 2004, only students from programmes offering curriculum-based, as opposed to internship-based, programmes will be permitted to sit for the NATA certification examination, and only the former will be eligible for accreditation. As of 2002, the field was licensed in 38 States, although the most populous state, California, was still considering such legislation as of this writing.[5]

Freidson's (1970) distinctions between the knowledge required for licensure and that which informs actual clinical practices remains relevant to athletic training. Indeed, although many of the practices of athletic trainers are grounded in medical literature, some of the most common and well-known procedures are done with little scientific evidence to support their efficacy. These include procedures done with the ostensible objective of preventing injuries. Indeed, although athletic trainers develop considerable expertise in taping, the taping of body parts, insofar as it is

---

[5] In these and other efforts, athletic training struggles to distinguish itself from the physical therapy profession, which indeed has its own section called "sports physical therapy." The California Physical Therapy Association appears to be opposed to the licensure effort in California.

used to support or limit the range of motion of injured joint segments, has, at best, mixed scientific support in the research literature (e.g. Callaghan 1997). Moreover, although some American football programmes may require players to wear them, there is little scientific evidence to support the use of knee braces to prevent injury (Mueller *et al.* 1996; Paluska & McKeag 2000). In the case of both procedures, it would seem that the effect is to orient athletes toward re/entering participation with the, perhaps false, hope of being protected. Tellingly, Parkkari *et al.* (2001) reported that only 16 randomised trials on the prevention of sports injuries have been done. This seems to strongly suggest that clinical sports medicine is overwhelmingly focused on treating injuries, as opposed to preventing their occurrence.

Nevertheless, despite very little research on the efficacy of a number of products in sports medicine, NATA has an elaborate marketing programme for manu-facturers of such products entitled "NATA: First aid in health care marketing," and offers opportunities for corporate sponsorship of the organisation. Indeed, the website lists the companies supporting the organisation and states, "Please support companies that support the profession" (http://www.nata.org/downloads/marketing/2002MarketGuide.pdf).

The Sport of Medicine: Athletic Training on the Field

How is athletic training currently practised and how does its social position affect the health care athletes receive? We will attempt to answer these questions by examining three themes noted above. First, as we have seen, athletic training is a medical "para-profession" (Freidson 1970) both subordinate to and dependent upon institutionalised medicine. By the mandates of its own "Role Delineation Study" (NATA 1991), athletic trainers work under the authority of a licensed physician, the latter of whom are exclusively permitted to diagnose sport-related illnesses and injuries. Second, despite this fact, athletic training is a profession that grew not out of medicine, but instead out of a male-dominated and distinctively violent sports culture. Most athletic trainers in universities work closely with coaches and are hired and paid out of the budgets of athletic departments, as opposed to those of the school's student health services or hospital. Men dominate the positions of leadership in the field, and earn on average nearly $10,000 more per year than their women counterparts.[6] Not surprisingly, as we shall see, the

---

[6] See http://www.nata.org/downloads/2000SurveyResults.pdf. It should be noted that in 2000, NATA elected its first woman as President of the association. She was re-elected in 2002 for another two-year term. In the interest of full disclosure, she is a colleague and friend of this author at California State University, Fullerton.

social atmospheres of athletic training rooms share much in common with locker rooms in their being historically masculine spaces. Finally, the professional preparation of athletic trainers within universities also places the field under the political and economic structures of academic departments, whose students must prepare to sit for the NATA certification examination by being given clinical experiences in treating athletes.

Because there are no national or state mandates, the organisation of health care for athletes in the United States, particularly in school and university programmes, is determined locally.[7] In college and university settings, with which most of the remainder of this chapter will be concerned, the sports medicine programme is supervised by one or more team physicians, although it is rare that such physicians oversee the daily athletic training services provided. The links of these physicians to their institutions vary widely from informal, consultative arrangements to full-time employment (Stockard 1997), and are commonly an addition to private practice. Team physicians also come from a variety of medical subspecialties, including pediatrics, orthopedics, cardiology, gynecology, and dermatology, and thus the standards of care that apply to those subspecialties, not those of sports medicine, legally govern their care of athletes (Mitten 2001).

In fact, sports medicine, as an area of specialty for physicians, is itself not recognised by the American Board of Medical Specialties (Mitten 2001). Only the American Osteopathic Medical Association has a certification board for sports medicine. Due to the wide variety of specialties, team physicians at universities may not be fully versed in the varieties of sports injuries with which they may be presented, some researchers suggesting that this may lead to substandard care (Strickland 1995). As an example of the undeveloped nature of clinical sports medicine, a study of the elective sports medicine component of pediatric residency programmes involved an average of fewer than six hours of lecture, and less than five hours of clinical exposure (Stirling & Landry 1996). Indeed, the chief residents surveyed in the latter study reported that they referred the majority of pediatric sports injuries they encountered to other physicians.

Despite the considerable variation in the employment arrangements and medical specialities among team physicians, athletic trainers and athletic training rooms are by contrast nearly universal at such institutions. Moreover, athletic trainers and, as we shall see, their students, often operate quite autonomously

---

[7] Primary and secondary schools in the U.S. have been utterly dependent on local physicians to volunteer their services for athlete health care. In these settings, many physicians perform pre-participation examinations on athletes and agree to be "on call" at competitions in case of emergencies. To this day, most on-site athlete medical care in these settings is in the hands of coaches. Increasing numbers of schools, however, are hiring certified athletic trainers, some in response to state mandates.

from physicians and academic administrators. Generally, the athletic training programme in university sports is under the direction of a head athletic trainer, a full-time, paid position which, depending upon the size and resources of the institution, may also have paid assistant athletic trainers. These head athletic trainers may have one or a combination of clinical, administrative, and educational responsibilities, reflecting the fact that they ultimately work under the supervision of physicians, athletic directors, and/or heads of academic departments. The latter responsibility also obviously entails the supervision of students whom, as we shall see, constitute a significant portion of the clinical labour force for the delivery of health care services to intercollegiate athletes in the U.S. Perhaps as important, those head athletic trainers with principally clinical duties, along with their interning students, work closely with, and in many cases, at the pleasure of, powerful and politically influential coaches.

Divided Loyalties and the Context of Care

Given the organisational structures in which athletic trainers work, we should not be surprised that Kotarba (1983), in his book on chronic pain, found athletic trainers functioning as "bridges" among athletes, coaches, physicians, administrators, and others. This suggests that health care professionals in sport often find themselves in the middle of conflicts of interest. Athletic trainers in Kotarba's study had to resist pressures from coaches to clear injured athletes for play but were also frustrated by athletes who hid serious injuries from them. Reflecting the fact that most athletic trainers had insufficient time to attend to all athletes, they tended to prefer athletes they considered "gamers." Gamers were those athletes who were tolerant of injury, who seldom complained about pain, and who evidenced a strong commitment to achievement within their sports. "Nongamers," on the other hand, constantly complained about pain and frequently sought the trainer's services.

Such research brings up two important issues. First, do athletic trainers and other sports medicine personnel, in some cases, identify more closely with the dominant values and interests of coaches and others in sport than they do with the values and interests of their medical colleagues? Second, might these tendencies be especially the case if athletic trainers work in an organisation that does not provide them sufficient resources and personnel? Clearly, the term "gamer" is not among the medical categories developed to manage patients and their conditions, and is instead an example of the clear adoption of the language and ideologies of coaches, fans, sports media, and others (Nixon 1993). Moreover, "gamers" are those athletes who display the values historically associated with an androcentric sports environment, an indication that the gender ideologies of sport have found their way into athletic training spaces.

To what degree do athletic trainers appear to adopt the values and language of masculininst sports culture? A few studies have explored these issues, although somewhat tangentially. Nixon (1996) conducted surveys of college athletes focusing on the degree to which they have experienced and normalised pain and injury. Nearly 70% of the athletes in the study had been seriously injured; almost all of them reported playing while hurt; nearly half said that they received pressure from coaches to play while hurt; and, significantly, over 40% reported being pressured by athletic trainers to play while hurt. On the other hand, Nixon (1994) conducted a study on the interactions of college athletes with coaches, teammates, and athletic trainers. He found that the receptivity of athletic trainers to the health problems of athletes played a key role in whether athletes decided to hide their injuries and pain. Studies in the professional athletic training literature have also found that the receptivity of athletic trainers to athlete concerns plays an important role in maintaining their contact with health care personnel (e.g. Fisher & Hoisington 1993; Fisher, Mullins & Frye 1993). These results suggest that athletic trainers have the potential to insulate themselves and their athletes from an otherwise health-compromising atmosphere but may not do so for reasons related to their organisational and culture environments.

The View from the Bottom

Other studies on these issues have focused on the social situations, acquired practices and belief systems of athletic trainers during their career socialisation. My own research (Walk 1997) has shown that, for a number of reasons, *student* athletic trainers in university sport programmes provide a significant portion of health care services to college athletes. The ostensible reasons for this are manifold, but most appear to be rooted in the educational and economic considerations of universities and their athletic programmes. As interns requiring a minimum number of clinical hours in order to be able to take the NATA examination, these students are assigned by head athletic trainers to work with the university's intercollegiate athletes. In most programmes, students are assigned to teams, first under the supervision of certified athletic trainers or more advanced student athletic trainers, and eventually serve as the sole athletic trainers for the teams to which they are assigned. These assignments represent "opportunities" for student athletic trainers to witness the comprehensive process of athlete health care, including caring for actual sports injuries, experiences that will also develop their clinical competencies. Perhaps as important, however, student athletic trainers allow athletic departments and universities to save considerable sums of money that might otherwise have to be spent on supplying paid athletic trainers for every practice and event in which athletes are active.[8] Considering that some athletic departments offer more than 25 sports, the savings are considerable. Thus, the dependency of the students on the credential-granting programme comes with a counter-dependence of the programme on unpaid student labour to deliver the majority of its services.

As such, student athletic trainers are at the very bottom of a "support system" for athletes. They are uncompensated assistants in a paramedical profession; interns who work for athletes who are also their peers; and students requiring credentials for graduation and for professional certification. In their clinical work, they appear as overburdened and share many of the same frustrations as their supervising staff trainers in their inability to care for all of the athletes who require it. Athletes sometimes treat them poorly, calling them "water boys" or "water girls," given their responsibility to provide water to athletes. Finally, similar to their professional counterparts, they are pressured by coaches to return players to action when it is medically inadvisable and feel unable to exert influence on coaches who do not show concern for the health and well-being of athletes (Walk 1997).

Student athletic trainers in my research (Walk 1994) have also reported disputes among their superiors about rehabilitative modalities and their medical indications. They described disagreements about the appropriate sequences of modalities and preventative measures, including taping techniques, indicating differences in athletic training philosophies. Of course, as we have seen, these differences appear more closely related to institutional traditions than to practices validated by research. Once students acquired the skills associated with these procedures, their applications to actual cases of injury were complicated by the competing agendas of coaches, athletes and staff athletic trainers, lending a political significance to the decisions the student trainers made. Because the programme and its medical staff in this study seemed to be under the hegemony of a few powerful male coaches — who apparently were granted managerial carte blanche in the programme — student athletic trainers often felt powerless to act counter to their wishes.

My research has also shown that women student athletic trainers are subject to sexual harassment and sexualisation in their work contexts (Walk 1999). Women

---

[8] Note that most epidemiologies of sports injuries have found that more injuries occur in practices than in games reflecting, of course, that there are vastly more practice sessions than games in a typical athletic season. Many university sports programmes assign student athletic trainers to these practice sessions, depending on them primarily to provide first aid and emergency care until a more qualified person is available.

working with male athletes and coaches are often subject to both overt and subtle forms of harassment that bear similarities to the experiences of women physicians (Phillips & Schneider 1993). In the course of attempting to provide medical information and services, women health care workers are often seen as nurturing figures, as vulnerable and in need of protection, and as potential sexual interests of men. In my study (Walk 1999), the women's attempts to establish the trusting relationships that they believed led to better care, in addition to the contact required in medical procedures, was sometimes construed as sexual invitation by male athletes. The specific consequences of these dynamics are not entirely clear as they relate to athlete health and well-being. Nevertheless, this important and often hidden feature of the practice of sports medicine should not only be identified and condemned, but also further explored as a potentially health-compromising characteristic of the social milieu of clinical sports medicine.

Given these social circumstances, what does the limited research on the career socialisation of student athletic trainers reveal about the degree to which they adopt the injury-legitimising ethos of elite sports? Again, my own studies of student athletic trainers paralleled the results of Kotarba (1983) in a number of ways. Student athletic trainers in my study (Walk 1997) reported that athletes often hid their injuries and pain from them because they feared losing playing time and status on their teams. Being immersed in lengthy interactions with them, some student athletic trainers also adopted the pain and injury ideologies and language of athletes and coaches. Although they were self conscious about doing so, they also stereotyped athletes, using terms such as "headcases" and "babies," in addition to "egos" and "dedicated" athletes. Headcases were athletes the student athletic trainers alleged were faking injuries, presumably, to avoid difficult practice sessions or to "explain" poor performances. Babies were described as athletes who reported very minor health problems or who had very low pain tolerance. Student athletic trainers would often validate these assessments of athletes with staff athletic trainers, coaches, and even other athletes. Note that both the "egos" and "dedicated" stereotypes are consistent with the notion of a "gamer," in that they validate stoicism, ostracise those unwilling to tolerate pain, psychological or otherwise, and are solely focused on returning the athlete to play.

More generally, these stereotypes are responses to the management problems involved in athletic training, and suggest that athletic trainers engage in activities that are essentially social control mechanisms. Athletes who fail to report injuries, as well as those whose complaints are seen as false or unworthy of medical attention, represent problems for institutionalised sports medicine and are met with responses often found in other areas of medical practice. As we shall see, the health problems of athletes may originate outside the scope of institutional surveillance, and thus athletic trainers are often faced with a vexing set of problems.

Compliance and Social Control

As noted earlier, athletic trainers able to gain the trust of athletes are sometimes in a better position to detect medical problems and render care than those who are not. Predictably, athletes are less apt to hide injuries from those they trust. Student athletic trainers, in particular, may form close relationships with athletes with whom they work, particularly given their status as peers and students, although these associations may extend beyond that which is considered "professional" and include intimate friendships and romantic relationships. As such, student athletic trainers may help athletes they consider friends to circumvent procedures and violate policies, and generally provide some sanctuary for athletes who wish to rest, avoid competition, or simply escape the strictures of the institution (Walk 1997).

Indeed, athletes in university sports programmes are often immersed in systems of regimented practices they often consider invasive, humiliating, and, in some cases, without foundation, and may work to resist such efforts. These include various forms of academic monitoring, team rules on appearance and "off the field" conduct, drug use surveillance, as well as income and other "benefit" restrictions instituted by organisations like the NCAA. However, in some cases, athletic trainers and student athletic trainers are part of these regimented practices for athletes, and may have obligations to monitor and report violations in one or all of these areas. Athletes may therefore see athletic trainers as duplicitous, in that they foster trust in what is outwardly a support system, while actually working on behalf of invasive and manipulative coaches, sports governing bodies, and educational institutions.

Of course, athletes may also show disparate forms of opposition or indifference to the medical services rendered by athletic trainers. As noted earlier, athletes may sustain injuries they do not report and report maladies that do not exist, or they may refuse treatment for injuries requiring it and request treatment for injuries they seemingly should handle themselves. As other research has reported, athletes who are anxious or frustrated by their injuries may report for treatments and not comply with instructions (Ford & Gordon 1997). They may stay in rehabilitation with false claims about pain or exit rehabilitation with false claims about comfort. In addition, athletes sometimes visit "outside" physicians to obtain second opinions based on beliefs that the medical staff at their universities is incompetent, even though they do not fully utilise of all the services the university offers.

Further complicating such issues are problems that appear to exist outside the areas over which athletic trainers, and the institutions for which they work, have control. Two studies in the medical literature have shown that college athletes demonstrate less healthy lifestyles and engage in more health risk behaviour than their non-athlete counterparts (Nattiv & Puffer 1991; Nattiv *et al.* 1997). An early study showed that college athletes, versus their non-athlete counterparts, tended to consume more alcohol, drive while intoxicated, ride with an intoxicated driver, fail to use seatbelts and motorcycle helmets, and engage in high risk sexual behaviour resulting in sexually transmitted diseases (Nattiv & Puffer 1991). A later study found identical results, in addition to finding that athletes engaged in more physical fights than non-athletes (Nattiv *et al.* 1997). Additionally, the latter study found that male athletes engaged in more risk-taking behaviours than female athletes and that athletes involved in contact sports were higher risk-takers than those in non-contact sports. Finally, the Nattiv *et al.* (1997) study found that those athletes who demonstrated one risk-taking behaviour were more likely to engage in a number of other risk-taking behaviours.

These considerations point to a number of potentially health-compromising behaviours by athletes that seem to extend beyond competitive pressures or challenges to sport-related masculinity, and which follow similar patterns of patient behaviours in non-sport contexts. We would also anticipate that such actions would be followed by institutionalised responses. Indeed, patient compliance, including adherence to appointments, medication regimens, rehabilitation regimes, and home therapies is among the most pervasive issues in the medical literature. Burgoon *et al.* (1991) reported that, as long ago as 1979, there had been over 1,400 published articles on various forms of patient noncompliance (Haynes *et al.* 1979, in Burgoon *et al.* 1991). Additionally, some authors have cited noncompliance as the single most important issue in health care (Eraker *et al.* 1984, in Burgoon *et al.* 1991).

Burgoon *et al.* (1991) have noted two principles among others that underlie the definition and study of medical noncompliance by patients. The first is that "[patients] enter into the transaction voluntarily and are free to choose whether or not to comply with the suggestions and directives of the [physician]" (p. 178). The second states that "[c]ompliance can almost always be viewed as benefiting the patient or significant others and is rarely viewed as a benefit to the [physician]" (p. 179). These principles also seem to inform the practices of athletic trainers. That is, athletes are seen as autonomous individuals whose health-related decision-making is viewed in an "informed consumer" framework — athletes are expected to become competent users of the services available to them. Moreover, noncompliance is conceptualised on the basis of benefits to the athletes, not in terms of the management benefits to sports medicine personnel or the universities for which they play.

Considering the benefits for sports medicine personnel (i.e. rather than the assumed benefits to athletes) suggests a rethinking of compliance issues in terms of social control (Kotarba & Seidel 1984). In such a model, athlete noncompliance is viewed as a form of deviance that hinders the ability of institutionalised medicine to render athletes as serviceable entities. Athletic trainers may attempt to win athlete compliance by reporting noncompliance to staff trainers or coaches, or threatening to do so. As such, they use the same social capital as coaches in order to win athlete cooperation. Moreover, the athlete's failure to comply with medical instructions and institutionalised policies, as we have seen, may also be met by various forms of stigmatisation and marginalisation. As Kotarba & Seidel (1984) summarised, these stigmas may include the labeling of athletes as malingerers, substance abusers, hypochondriacs, counfounders, lazy or undedicated, or simply "pains in the ass." A social control framework recognises that sports medicine rarely involves dyadic relationships between athlete and athletic trainer. Indeed, sports medicine is sometimes not effective, involves parties other than the autonomous athlete (i.e. including coaches, teammates, parents, peers, and others), and may involve intense conflict between athletes and medical personnel (Kotarba & Seidel 1984).

An athlete whose identity has been spoiled by various failures to measure up to the expectations of medical staff might be particularly hesitant to seek treatment and counsel. For example, an athlete who fakes an injury in order to avoid a difficult practice session may thereafter be labeled as undedicated, a "headcase" or as someone who "cries wolf." Athletes who become aware of their own stigmatisation will likely lose trust in the medical staff, under-report health problems, and fail to comply with medical instructions and advice, although they will likely remain athletes. These would appear to be the most problematic cases, in that they are often hidden from view and athletes in such circumstances may feel they have no place to turn for help.

Given its pervasiveness in the medical literature, however, it is untenable to assume that the non-compliance, risk-taking and unhealthy actions of athletes stem exclusively from pressures within sports, let alone stigmatising by sports medicine staff, coaches, and others. But, not all athletes take unreasonable health risks and indeed some appear to have elevated concerns for health in ways similar to their non-athlete counterparts to the extent that they develop a dependency on the medical staffs at their institutions. Perhaps most importantly, the larger social context in which college athletes are a part, including those of college students in general, appears to be quite accepting of pain (Nixon 1996), tolerant of health risks, and non-compliant with medical advice. If it is our goal to understand the distinctive ways in which sport fosters pain acceptance, risk-taking, and the neglect of health and well-being, we must also understand these processes outside of sport contexts. While it is true that athletes are involved in intensely competitive, often health-compromising, and sometimes abusive environments, these facts, unfortunately, are also true of the larger society.

Summary

Our knowledge of the role of sports medicine personnel in studies of athlete risk, pain, and injury is obviously in its infancy and there are many questions to be answered. While it is clear that athletic trainers often act on behalf of athletes over and against an injurious sports culture, they may also accept the values of that culture as well as the pitfalls of their medical colleagues when facing the difficulties of managing difficult patients in trying circumstances. Among the looming issues is the licensure of athletic trainers in the United States, which may affect the health care of athletes in unforeseen ways. Indeed, some athletic trainers, rather than receiving a salary for their services, may now bill the health insurance providers of their athletes, as do physicians and other medical professionals. As a result, in addition to their immersion in health-compromising sports cultures, there may be new pressures on athletic trainers to treat as many athletes as possible and in ways dictated by insurance companies (McKinlay *et al.* 1996). New studies will require a focus not only on the practices and beliefs in institutionalised sports medicine, but also on the changing nature of the relationships among health care personnel and athletes. Finally, research must focus on the relative amounts of power over decision-making among all those involved in athlete health care, including coaches, athletic trainers, physicians, parents and, alas, the athletes themselves.

References

Berger, P. L., & Luckmann, T. (1966). *The social construction of reality: A treatise on the sociology of knowledge.* New York: Anchor Books.

Bilik, S. E. (1956). *The trainer's bible* (Ninth Revised Edition). New York: T. J. Reed.

Burgoon, M., Birk, T. S., & Hall, J. R. (1991). Compliance and satisfaction with physician-patient communication: An expectancy theory interpretation of gender differences. *Human Communication Research, 18*(2), 177–208.

Callaghan, M. J. (1997). Role of ankle taping and bracing in the athlete. *British Journal of Sports Medicine, 31*(2), 102–108.

Cowin, J. (2001, March 15). Is there a trainer in the house? Greater participation in athletics has led to more sports injuries – and a greater need for medical care inside area schools. *The Boston Globe*, 12.

Ebel, R. G. (1999). *Far beyond the shoebox: Fifty years of the national athletic trainer's association.* New York: Forbes Custom Publishing.

Fahey, T. D. (1986). *Athletic training: Principles and practice.* Palo Alto, CA: Mayfield.

Fisher, A. C., & Hoisington, L. L. (1993). Injured athletes' attitudes and judgments toward rehabilitation adherence. *Journal of Athletic Training, 28*(1), 48–54.

Fisher, A. C., Mullins, S. A., & Frye, P. A. (1993). Athletic trainers' attitudes and judgments of injured athletes' rehabilitation adherence. *Journal of Athletic Training, 28*(1), 43–47.

Foucault, M. (1973). *The birth of the clinic: An archaeology of medical perception.* New York: Pantheon.

Ford, I. W., & Gordon, S. (1997). Perspectives of sports physiotherapists on the frequency and significance of psychological factors in professional practice: Implications for curriculum design in professional training. *Australian Journal of Science and Medicine in Sports, 29*(2), 34–40.

Freidson, E. (1970). *Profession of medicine: A study of the sociology of applied knowledge.* New York: Dodd, Mead.

Goffman, E. (1961). *Asylums: Essays on the social situations of mental patients and other inmates.* New York: Doubleday.

Harris, H. A. (1964). *Greek athletes and athletics.* London: Hutchinson of London.

Kotarba, J. A. (1983). *Chronic pain: Its social dimensions.* Newbury Park, CA: Sage.

Kotarba, J. A., & Seidel, J. V. (1984). Managing the problem pain patient: Compliance or social control? *Social Science and Medicine, 19*(12), 1393–1400.

McKinlay, J. B., Potter, D. A., & Feldman, H. A. (1996). Non-medical influences on medical decision-making. *Social Science and Medicine, 42*, 769–776.

Mitten, M. J. (2001). The law and sports medicine. In: W. E. Garret, D. T. Kirkendall, & D. L. Squire (Eds), *Principles and practice of primary care sports medicine* (pp. 47–56). Philadelphia: Lippincott, Williams, & Wilkins.

Mueller, F., Zemper, E. D., & Peters, A. (1996). American football. In: D. J. Caine, C. G. Caine, & K. J. Lindner (Eds), *Epidemiology of sports injuries* (pp. 41–62). Champaign, IL: Human Kinetics.

NATA Board of Certification, Inc. (1991). *Role delineation study: Certification examination.* Raleigh, NC: Columbia Assessment Services.

Nattiv, A., & Puffer (1991). Lifestyles and health risks of collegiate athletes. *Journal of Family Practice, 33*, 585–590.

Nattiv, A., Puffer, J. C., & Green, G. A. (1997). Lifestyles and health risks of collegiate athletes: A multi-center study. *Clinical Journal of Sports Medicine, 7*, 262–272.

Nixon, H. L. (1993). Accepting the risks of pain and injury in sport: Mediated cultural influences on playing hurt. *Sociology of Sport Journal, 10*(2), 183–196.

Nixon, H. L., II (1994). Coaches' views of risk, pain, and injury in sport, with special reference to gender differences. *Sociology of Sport Journal, 11*, 79–87.

Nixon, H. L., II (1996). Explaining pain and injury attitudes and experiences in sport in terms of gender, race, and sports status factors. *Journal of Sport and Social Issues, 20*, 33–44.

Nixon, H. L., II (1998). Response to Martin Roderick's comment on the work of Howard L. Nixon, II. *Sociology of Sport Journal, 15*, 80–85.

O'Shea, M. E. (1980). *A history of the national athletic trainer's association.* National Athletic Trainer's Association.

Paluska, S. A., & McKeag, D. B. (2000). Knee braces: Current evidence and clinical recommendations for their use. *American Family Physician, 15, 61*(2), 411–418, 423–424.

Parkkari, J., Kujala, U. M., & Kannus, P. (2001). Is it possible to prevent sports injuries? Review of controlled clinical trials and recommendations for future work. *Sports Medicine, 31*(14), 985–995.

Phillips, S. P., & Schneider, M. S. (1993). Sexual harassment of female doctors by patients. *New England Journal of Medicine, 329,* 1933–1939.

Rock, S. (1997, October 8). Risking players' safety: NCAA does not require medical supervision. *The Kansas City Star,* A1.

Stirling, J. M., & Landry, G. L. (1996). Sports medicine training during pediatric residency. *Archives of Pediatric Medicine, 150*(2), 211–215.

Starr, P. (1982). *The social transformation of American medicine.* New York: Basic Books.

Stockard, A. R. (1997). Team physician preferences at National Collegiate Athletic Association Division I universities. *Journal of the American Osteopathic Association, 97*(2), 89–95.

Strickland, J. W. (1995). Philosophy of the treatment of athletes. *Clinical Sports Medicine, 14*(2), 285–288.

Van Valkenberg, K. (2001, January, 30). Getting low grades for safety in high schools: Many area schools don't provide for trainers to be athletic events, and some coaches are saying the situation is a disaster waiting to happen. *The Baltimore Sun,* D1.

Walk, S. R. (1994). *Information and injury: The experiences of student athletic trainers.* Unpublished doctoral dissertation, Michigan State University.

Walk, S. R. (1997). Peers in pain: The experiences of student athletic trainers. *Sociology of Sport Journal, 14,* 22–56.

Walk, S. R. (1999). Moms, sisters, and ladies: Women student trainers in men's intercollegiate sports. *Men and Masculinites, 1,* 33.

Weithaus, B., & Fauser, J. J. (1991). Committee on accreditation: Assessing educational outcomes and assuring quality. *Journal of the American Medical Association, 266*(7), 968–969.

Chapter 15

Negotiating with Risk: Exploring the Role of the Sport Medicine Clinician

Parissa Safai

In a rare television moment, a former team doctor admits that during his tenure with the Toronto Argonauts of the Canadian Football League, he allowed players to play even though he "should have failed them on their physicals" (McIlvride 1994). With "swollen and arthritic knees," he allowed athletes who were at "the last stages [of their careers]" to play because they were "smart, team leaders, and [because] the coaches wanted them" (McIlvride 1994). For the athletes in question, playing with decimated bodies was an unspoken requirement of their sport. However, for this physician, supporting patients in doing further harm to themselves was a violation of his professional code of conduct. The clinician acknowledges, on tape, that he acted inappropriately (in violating the Hippocratic Oath that he took as a physician) on *behalf* of the organisation he worked for, and at the *behest* of the players and coaches. He accepted the conflicting responsibilities of being a team clinician — the professional duty to treat patients to improve their health and the contractual obligation to support these same athletes as they risked their health. In many ways, he failed to provide duty of care in safeguarding the health and well-being of his patients and yet did so without professional or legal repercussions because of the context in which he worked — sport.

While this anecdote is a point of departure for numerous questions and debates about the broader culture of pain for many men *and* women in competitive sport, the dangerous demands of professional sport, as well as medico-legal issues surrounding duty of care, it points sharply to the role of the sport medicine clinician and to the dynamics of the clinician-patient relationship. We must

Sporting Bodies, Damaged Selves
Research in the Sociology of Sport, Volume 2, 269–286
Copyright © 2004 by Elsevier Ltd.
All rights of reproduction in any form reserved
ISSN: 1476-2854/doi:10.1016/S1476-2854(04)02015-1

continually raise questions about the lived contradictions for athletes regarding the supposed healthfulness of competitive sport and the real experiences of pain and injury. However, we must also critically examine the roles of medical clinicians (physicians, therapists and trainers), and how they negotiate with patient-athletes regarding the maintenance of over-conformity to the sport ethic (Hughes & Coakley's (1991) notion of "positive deviance") that is widely believed to involve what has been termed a "culture of risk" (Nixon 1992).

Research is limited in this field, but this chapter focuses on three studies that examine the nature of the relationship between the "culture of risk" and the negotiation of treatment in sport medicine. Studies by Walk (1997), the Centre for Research into Sport and Society at Leicester University, U.K. (e.g. Roderick & Waddington 2000; Waddington 1999, 2000), and Safai (2001) all examine and problematise the role of the sport medicine clinician in different sport settings — U.S. intercollegiate sport (NCAA), professional English soccer and Canadian intercollegiate sport, respectively. Given that the existing literature and anecdotal evidence predict that a "culture of risk" is promoted in clinician-athlete negotiations, the studies investigate how clinicians interact with athletes beyond the level of clinical diagnoses, and attempt to determine whether they implicitly contribute to and reinforce overconformity to the sport ethic (Hughes & Coakley 1991). Drawing on these studies, the chapter then focuses on the clinicians themselves. Their work is bound by the ethical and legal requirements of their profession, their personal experiences and by their positions in the competitive sport hierarchy and administrative structures of sport. In particular, this chapter focuses on the way in which their work takes place in a policy vacuum. This vacuum creates a situation in which student and professional athletes are, at times, stranded between competing demands for health and the drive to participate. I argue that the situation is the outcome of limitations imposed on sport medicine clinicians in a competitive sport system.

Exploring the Clinician-Patient Relationship in Health Care and Sport Medicine

While this chapter cannot do full justice to the complex subject of the clinician-patient relationship (see Chapters 7, 10, 13, 14 & 16), we can briefly explore some of the ways in which the dynamics of this relationship are understood (Williams & Calnan 1996). Although the literature mostly deals with the physician-patient relationship, much of it relates to all types of clinician-patient interactions.

According to Freidson (1970: 206), physicians [read clinicians] embody dominant values in society and create the social possibilities for acting sick because they are deemed society's authority on what "illness really is." They are "gatekeepers" (Freidson 1970: 206) to most mainstream health resources (e.g. prescription drugs, surgery, physiotherapy, hospitals, etc.) since these cannot be used without their permission. There are three main ways that a patient may respond to a clinician. She/he may: (i) do everything a clinician recommends (Parsons 1951); (ii) ignore everything a clinician recommends; or (iii) discuss and negotiate the form of treatment that the clinician recommends (Hayes-Bautista 1976a, b).

In cases where the interests of the patient and clinician may conflict, as can potentially be the case in sport where an injured athlete may want to train and compete when the clinician would like the patient to rest and heal, the final two options are most often used. The third option, however, lends itself best to sociological analysis. This option views clinician-patient interaction as *a process of negotiation*, rather than the physician simply giving orders and the patient following or ignoring them in an automatic, unquestioning manner.[1] This trend in participation is arguably a recent phenomenon with a shift towards the questioning of authority, including medical authority, and seen most recently in the increased use of the internet in accessing medical information (Shorter 1991). Numerous individuals with access to the internet "do" medical research of some sort before approaching and interacting with clinicians (Lupton 1994: 113–117).

While these processes also apply to sport medicine, in contrast to general practitioners or other specialists, there are other competing demands unique to sport medicine clinicians. Sport medicine clinicians parallel other clinicians who negotiate with patients engaged in risky behaviours such as smoking, alcohol, and/or substance abuse, and/or in high-risk occupational settings/professions such as mining, construction, oil and gas exploration, and the military (Young 1993). With the exception of a few occupations, there are no other activities in social life where people assume risk in the same ways as they do in competitive sport, resulting in an almost blasé acceptance of pain and injury, and an unquestioned tolerance of the "culture of risk." Thus, clinicians interact with patients who may not co-operate with their treatment plans because of their involvement in a "macho" (and evidently increasingly "macha") "culture of risk" that fosters pain tolerance, and may hold negative consequences of those who fail to play with pain (Curry 1993; Sabo & Panepinto 1990; Theberge 1997; Young *et al.* 1994; Young & White 1995). All of this occurs within a context of (otherwise) excellent health, resulting in a perception of bodily betrayal on the part of athletes. In combination, the

---

[1] Interestingly, Rier's (2000) personal account of dealing with an acute and traumatic illness highlights and incorporates elements of both models. For more in-depth discussions of the changing views of the clinician-patient relationship in the sociology of health and medicine, see Gerhardt (1989), Lupton (1994) and Annandale (1998).

culture and experience prompts some athletes to return to action as soon as they possibly can — sometimes at the cost of their overall health and well-being (cf. Klein 1995; Messner 1989).

Three Case Studies

How does this apply to the study of pain and injury in sport? Are clinicians helping injured athletes by offering specialised treatment, or are they reinforcing the "culture of risk?" Is it simply an "either/or" situation? As Walk notes, through survey research and theory, Nixon argues that there is also a network in place in the NCAA, specifically Division I, that reinforces risk-taking — a "conspiratorial alliance of coaches, athletic administrators, sport medicine personnel, and others whose activities perpetuate the acceptance by athletes of risk, pain, and injury in sport" (Walk 1997: 23). Nixon (1992) terms these alliances "sportsnets," and argues that the insulation and immersion of medical systems within the larger framework of producing winning teams and athletes is detrimental to the health and safety of athletes. He proposes the establishment of independent systems of medical personnel who are not intimately connected to the sportsnets, and urges athletes to seek second opinions from independent medical personnel in the assessment of persistent injury. Other ethnographic studies (e.g. Walk 1997; Young *et al.* 1994; Young & White 1995) show that the "culture of risk" is far more complex than Nixon implies. While all recognise that there is widespread acceptance of injury in competitive sport, they also recognise the intricate ways in which athletes and others produce and respond to this culture.

Walk's Study of Student Athletic Trainers

Walk (1997) examines the experiences of student athletic trainers (SATs) in a study that questions and subjects Nixon's theory to empirical "test" (see Chapters 3 & 14). Walk writes of the experiences of SATs in a large, NCAA Division I institution via group and individual semi-structured interviews. He contends that Nixon's notion of a sportsnet is questionable in that "even a sportsnet may be characterised by flaws in its systems of control, related negotiation and conflict, and some measures of freedom for its members, even those with the least amount of power — in the present case, student athletes and SATs" (p. 50).

Documented in the study were the often contradictory views held by the clinicians towards the "culture of risk" — concern for the welfare of the student-athlete and the reproduction of injury-legitimating norms. Walk (1997) argues that the sportsnet was not as all-encompassing as Nixon suggests, particularly in the relationships between clinicians and student-athletes that "worked to undermine some of the totalizing and exploitative tendencies the [institutional] sportsnet may have had" (p. 50). SATs, often exploited student workers themselves, were often seen occupying the paradoxical "middle" position between athletes and others, such as coaches, administrators, and health professionals, where they form close bonds with athletes and occasionally reinforce the "culture of risk," and yet also guard the athlete against external pressures to compete. However, as one of his key points, Walk (1997) stresses that while student-athletes often have the least amount of power in the sportsnet, they should not be viewed as " 'dupes' by minimising the roles and responsibilities they may play in exercising sovereignty over the treatment of their own bodies" (p. 54). This reinforces the importance of individual choice and action, not just of athletes, but for all individuals involved in the negotiation process.

CRSS Studies in Professional Soccer in the U.K.

Researchers from the Centre for Research into Sport and Society at the University of Leicester, U.K. have also contributed to our knowledge of the medical clinician in sport (Roderick *et al.* 1999; Roderick & Waddington 2000; Waddington 1999, 2000 — see Chapter 16). In critically examining the management of injuries in professional English football (soccer), interestingly on behalf of the Professional Footballers Association, they highlight not only the assimilation of participants into the "culture of risk," but also the highly problematic and antithetical situations in which medical clinicians are often immersed. Their investigation, including surveys of and interviews with club physicians, physiotherapists and current and former players, supports existing research on the ways in which athletes, particularly professional athletes, tolerate injury as part of their sport careers. However, also documented are the ways in which clinicians are, at times, swayed by athletes and management to support and reinforce injury tolerance. As one clinician they interviewed noted, "In private practice, my *modus operandi* is to cure the injury. In professional football, my *modus operandi* is to get the player on the pitch as quickly as possible" (Roderick & Waddington 2000: 172).

The evidence shows that not only do clinicians work without a uniform code of ethics, there are often conflicts of interest between the responsibilities clinicians have to their patients and the responsibilities clinicians have to their employers (the managers and the owners of the professional teams). The subject of patient confidentiality is a particularly strong example of this since, as one clinician noted, "the problem is that I'm employed by the football club. I'm employed by the manager and I'm supposed to be working with him and if I withhold information which he thinks he should have, then he would say that I wasn't working for the club or for him, so it puts me in a difficult position . . ." (Waddington 2000b: 52). This is of great concern to therapists who have a particular ethical responsibility because they, as Waddington (2000b) notes, ". . . perhaps more so than doctors . . . often get to know a great deal about players' private lives" (p. 51). According to the Leicester researchers, there is a tremendous amount of ambiguity around the responsibilities of the clinician, the rights of the patient-athlete, and the power and scope of both coach and the club — ambiguity that is potentially devastating for athletes.

Safai's Study of Clinician-Athlete Negotiations

Safai's (2001) study of the process of negotiation between clinicians and injured intercollegiate athletes in a Canadian university offers another angle from which to examine the tripartite relationship between clinicians, patients and coaches.[2] The case study used a combination of interviews with sport medicine clinicians (physicians, physiotherapists and athletic therapists) and student-athletes, as well as focus groups with athletes and coaches, to investigate whether clinicians reinforce the "culture of risk" evident in elite sport. In contrast to the other studies, it is important to note the distinct nature of competitive sport at the university under study. The intercollegiate program and sport medicine clinic for the university were both administered by an academic Faculty which had an *explicit* emphasis on both physical education *and* health. The institution had internalised the critiques of injury tolerance in sport and had created policy in attempts to counter it. For example, each year, a handbook had been created for intercollegiate athletes as a resource and guide. The handbook contained information on a variety of subjects, including personal and academic development, and stated that "[This university] is committed to *whole person development*. Students are at a crucial stage of their intellectual, physical and social development. Athletic skill development should be encouraged alongside: *health and well-being, including self-knowledge about*

---

[2] Canadian intercollegiate sport provides a relatively distinct setting in which to examine the interactions between sport medicine clinicians and athletes. Unlike other levels of elite sport, including the highest levels of U.S. intercollegiate sport, Canadian Interuniversity Sport (CIS, formerly CIAU) athletes are subject to strict academic guidelines, generally do not receive significant athletic scholarships, playing seasons are relatively short, and the pressures regarding revenue generation are less pronounced. Furthermore, sport medicine staff are often required to attend to numerous athletes from various teams throughout the year, and are thus not affiliated with a specific team as much as with the entire institution.

health and well-being..." (Student-athlete Handbook 2001–2002: 6; emphasis added). Any evidence of a "culture of risk" here, given the explicit emphasis on positive and healthy sport participation, suggests that such a "culture of risk" may exist to a greater extent at other institutions with less emphasis on health and well-being in their guiding principles.

In some ways, the focus on health and well-being has filtered down to the participants as can be seen in a dialectical relationship between the "culture of risk" and the "culture of precaution" (Safai 2001). A "culture of risk" *does* exist here, and it "frames the medical practices" of the clinicians (Walk 1997: 33). However, it is not all encompassing. There also exists a "culture of precaution" that resists injury and pain tolerance (Safai 2001). Head injuries highlight the "culture of precaution," since such injuries are negotiated in a significantly different manner than other types of injury. Where the limits of playing or not playing with injury can be shifted and blurred if the injury is musculo-skeletal, there is zero-tolerance for, and for the most part, non-negotiation of playing with head/brain injuries (Safai 2001).

Safai's case is somewhat distinct from the other two. Her focus is on an institution, a sport medicine clinic, and sport medicine clinicians attempting to resolve the policy vacuum surrounding the treatment of pain and injury in sport. However, while these clinicians are taking a step in the direction in safeguarding the health of their athletes, they are not sheltered from the broader systemic attitudes and norms that legitimate injury and pain in sport *or* the ambiguity and contradiction surrounding their roles in the competitive sport system.

An Absence of Policy

While this institution has adopted a zero-tolerance policy towards head injuries, such policy (regarding head injuries or otherwise) is not uniform among Canadian post-secondary institutions, and points our discussion to the general lack of uniform policy or code of ethics in sport medicine. This absence constrains sport medicine clinicians in that there is a great deal of ambiguity around their roles and responsibilities, which in turn has significant consequences for patients that fall under clinician care (cf. Waddington 2000b).

Much of the limited work in sport medico-legal circles centres on issues of drug use and abuse, as well as incidents of violence in sport at the professional or elite amateur level (see Young 1993; Grayson 1999). Little attention is paid to the daily ethical and legal obligations of the sport medicine practitioner in competitive sports systems, such as Canadian Interuniversity Sport (CIS). One possible explanation of this is that criminal and civil law is rarely seen to cross the boundaries of the playing field, the arena, or the locker room. Furthermore, much attention is paid to the role of the physician, while the roles and responsibilities of paramedical clinicians are largely overlooked. Thus, we need to extend our discussion to the ethical and legal responsibilities of all sport medicine clinicians.

As mentioned, many sport medicine clinicians shoulder contradictory responsibilities — while those involved in sport have a duty to provide competent medical services, they are also participants within competitive sport systems. While Grayson (1990, 1999), Macleod (1990) and Payne (1990) discuss the general responsibilities of the sport medicine clinician, Pipe (1998) recognises the conflicting role of the team clinician in intercollegiate sport:

> Our primary responsibility is to protect athletes' health and well-being as defined most broadly. Superficially, this role may seem perfectly compatible with the interest of the sports organization with which we and the athlete are associated. However, what's best for an athlete's long-term health may conflict with the organization's short-term interest in winning. As a result, we may have a problem of divided loyalty, which raises significant questions about the ethical practice of our profession (p. 40).

In the context of professional English football, Waddington (2000b: 49) acknowledges that the assumptions that normally underpin the clinician-patient relationship: "may not apply in the same way, or to the same degree, in the work situation of the club doctor or physiotherapist in professional sport; as . . . the 'team [clinician] . . . is acting as an agent of that club.'" He questions the conflict of loyalties between clinicians and patient-athletes, and points out that there are no commonly held codes of ethics governing such matters as the amount and kind of information medical practitioners pass on to team management (see also Roderick & Waddington 2000).

This points to the need for "an agreed code of ethics for dealing with issues involving player/patient confidentiality and, more generally, for defining the obligations of . . . doctors and physiotherapists towards the [club, team or organisation] and towards the individual player-as-patient" (Waddington, 2000b: 53).[3] Grayson (1999) recommends the World Medical Association's (WMA)

---

[3] In the U.K., based on the work done by the Centre for Research into Sport and Society, the General Medical Council urged the National Sports Medicine Institute to examine and address the problems they highlighted. Since then, the British Olympic Association, the Football Association and the British Medical Association have all published guidelines regarding clinician-patient confidentiality, and argue that patient confidentiality outweighs contractual obligations (Waddington, 2000b).

"Principles of Health Care for Sports Medicine" as one such global code of ethics. He suggests that the WMA's guidelines for the ethical conduct of physicians should be used by all sport medicine practitioners to protect the patient-athletes and to outline the clinician's ethical and legal responsibilities. Grayson argues the importance of each guideline, and relates each to the Declaration of Geneva — the international code of medical ethics.

While the WMA guidelines and Declaration of Geneva represent international policy relating to medico-legal issues in sport medicine, what is available in Canada and in Canadian universities? While other organisations exist that outline the role and responsibilities of athletic therapists, physiotherapists, massage therapists and the like, the Canadian Academy of Sport Medicine (CASM) is the umbrella organisation that develops policies and guidelines for the conduct of physicians in sport medicine contexts. According to Safai (2001), the CASM does not offer a set of guidelines or specific policies for the clinician-patient relationship. Rather, it directs attention to position statements by CASM members on various committees (none of which address intercollegiate or elite level sport), as well as to the Canadian Medical Association (CMA). The CMA, of which the CASM is an affiliate society, does offer a code of ethics for physicians, but this is generalised and not specific to the particularities of sport medicine.

In the CIS system, there is a similar absence of policy relating to the nature and conduct of sport medicine in varsity programs. The CIS handbook (2001–2002) has a section devoted to its doping policy, but largely ignores sport medicine. Since, within the CIS, there is no policy relating to the nature and conduct of sport medicine in varsity programs, the sport medicine policies and codes of conduct tend to be specific to individual universities (e.g. the university's Student-Athlete Handbook). Within the institution, the increased focus on health policy is a function of the Faculty in which the teams, the athletes, the coaches, the clinic and the clinicians are located. The significance of this lies in the fact that it is not only an athletic centre, but an academic one as well. The sport medicine clinic is located within an educational space, follows such a mandate, and has its own services geared towards health education (Safai 2001).

This discussion points to the reality that since there is no broad policy or code of ethics, clinicians rely heavily upon their own sense of professional ethics and their own personal experiences during the negotiation of treatment. As one clinician in Safai's (2001: 87) study acknowledged, "All this stuff is so grey. And so I, as a medical professional, find myself relying on my belief system and my value system to determine what is a potential catastrophic situation versus what is a nuisance situation." There are no clear cut answers to how clinicians negotiate the "culture of risk" with their patient-athletes, just continuous weighing of the perceived risks and benefits of playing and/or not playing with pain. For another clinician in the same university, the negotiation process was continually filled with bargaining and weighing:

> The bargaining begins in my head before they say anything. As soon as I hear the story and they say 'I got this injury and I have a meet in three weeks', I'm already wondering what strategy I'm going to use to bargain with them — how forceful I'm going to be in my opinion? And I'm already calculating the risk in my head that if I let them hedge — what's the chance that they'll do some damage? And there's two sides to that, there's the one side that's the primary concern which is, how much damage are they going to do to themselves? And the second is, if they do some damage to themselves, what's the chance that I'm going to get repercussions for that? (Safai 2001: 164).

While there are protocols and guidelines in place for clinicians to deal with particular injuries and/or to help ascertain relevant information, much of what occurs between clinicians and patient-athletes occurs in a space of ambiguity. Having a code of ethics in place for clinicians may not necessarily change the way in which the negotiation of treatment proceeds, but it may help to guide clinicians in their interactions with athletes. Furthermore, and perhaps more importantly, such policy may help back-up clinicians when their recommendations counter the interests and desires of other individuals involved in the sportsnet.

This is particularly poignant when considering that clinicians are *only* able to offer their recommendations. As one clinician in Safai's (2001: 190) study explains:

> It's up to the athlete to make up her mind about what she wants to do. Because we can only give advice if they're competent — we can't say 'You can't play'. If the coach says 'I'm not gonna put you on', then the athlete doesn't go on. But if the coach says 'I'm gonna put you on', and the athlete doesn't want to go on, then there's nothing you can do either. So, if you had a difficult coach, you'd have to emphasize to the athlete that they can't play.
>
> Interviewer: You can't order athletes, for lack of a better word?
>
> Clinician: No, you can't order. The only time that we can actually insist on any type of care is with psychiatric cases or if we feel the person is not competent to make decisions, which we can't say, so we can only advise.

Patients tend to follow clinicians' recommendations based on their belief in the authority and knowledge of clinicians — a function of the social, historical and political power gained by medicine (see Coburn & Willis 2000; Freidson 1970; Johnson 1972; Navarro 1986; Turner 1995). However, if clinicians can only recommend (other than unique situations where the patient is at risk or places others at risk), and if there is no policy to back their positions when those recommendations go against the interests of the others, then problems may arise.

What the evidence from Safai's study shows is that even while there is an accountability structure in place within the institution, there are still moments when the clinician is rendered powerless within the sport hierarchy. As mentioned earlier, clinicians are immersed in the dialectical relationship between risk and precaution and, at times, are complicit in reinforcing the tolerance of pain and injury. However, the following anecdote highlights a problematic situation when the clinician's recommendations go against the desires of the coaches and athletes. While covering a collision sport game, with a team that was en route to the national championships, a clinician recounted a situation that resulted in him garnering a negative reputation and a great deal of criticism:

> One of the athletes had a mild concussion, and I got into a fairly heated argument . . . about whether this [player] should play or not. And I didn't think he should, and everyone else, including the player, thought he should play, so I lost the argument. And he got hurt again, and I really started screaming. And so he did wind up sitting out a few games, and that's when I acquired the nickname Dr. Death from the team. And got called that for the next couple of years, until all those people who were on that team graduated.

> Interviewer: Was that athlete . . . a key player?

> Clinician: Yes, starting offensive star.

> Interviewer: Do you think there would have been such a stink if he wasn't?

> Clinician: No, it was that I was trying to gut the offense by making this [player] sit . . . and this was a team that was undefeated. A championship calibre team, and they were on a roll and I was rocking the boat (Safai 2001: 130).

This example shows how some situations render the clinician powerless, and also hints at some of the potential consequences for athletes. In this case, the athlete resisted the recommendation of the clinician voluntarily. However, as we shall see below, other examples show how athletes can become dangerously stranded between the recommendations of the clinician and the pressure from peers, coaches and their own overconformity to the sport ethic.

Stranding the Athlete

This evidence from Safai's study highlights the fact that the primary objective of clinicians is to inform the patient-athlete of the perceived risks and benefits of playing with the injury, and to place the decision-making responsibility in the hands of the athlete (cf. Roderick & Waddington 2000; Walk 1997). As one clinician noted, "I put the burden on [the athlete], so they realize they're making the decision for themselves 'cause I can't force a cast on them' " (Safai 2001: 183). Another clinician reiterated: "I always put the onus on the patient [so] mainly, if it doesn't work out, I [can] say, 'Hey, you didn't do your work. It's not my fault. I told you what you needed to do, and you didn't do it' " (Safai 2001: 184).

Informing the patient is part of the clinician's duty. However, what is interesting here is that in the Canadian intercollegiate context, the power to "order" an athlete to participate or not participate rests in the hands of the coach. Although the clinicians do point out that both the coach and the player have "the ultimate say," the ability to make that decision does not rest equally in the hands of the athlete and the coach. Whereas a clinician cannot "bench" a patient-athlete because of injury, a coach can. As a clinician noted:

> Physicians do not make decisions about return to play. We give advice. The advice is given to athletes and to coaches, and the athletes and coaches make the decision. The American courts would think that the athletes make the decision, but in fact, there are very few cases where the athlete challenges the coach's right to decide who plays. So in fact it's the coach who makes the decision. 'Cause if the doc says to the coach, 'So and so shouldn't play', even if so and so says 'I refuse to follow the advice and I'm putting my uniform on', if the coach says 'Park it on the bench', the athlete parks it on the bench. So, it's kinda interesting that physicians do not have the authority or the right to tell someone they may not play, but coaches do. However coaches do not have the knowledge they should have to make those decisions based

on injury, so they rely on advice from the doctor. So, there's a triangle there between the athlete, the team official and the physician (Safai 2001: 185).

What this clinician acknowledges deals directly with the amount of real "power" held by clinicians in comparison to that of coaches and the perceived "power" of the clinicians based on their expertise and knowledge. His mention of case law touches squarely on a central theme in the negotiation process — liability.

Liability is a key issue for both clinicians and coaches (see Chapter 18). One could argue that fear of liability is a function of the setting — a large academic institution that has a particular hierarchical structure. Every level of this structure is accountable to the other levels above and below it. Thus as one clinician suggests: "To be in such a big university, with so many administrative levels, you have to cover your ass and have protocols set out" (Safai 2001: 185). For this clinician, the sense of being overprotective and "covering your ass" was a function of the clinic's location within an educational institution.

The sense of accountability is echoed in conversation with coaches, although for them the first level of accountability is perceived to be the physicians. In fact, the amount of power held by the clinicians, as *perceived* by the coaches, has a tremendous impact on the decisions they make about playing or not playing injured athletes. Since the focus here is clinicians, suffice it to say that based on the evidence, one could argue that for some coaches, their decisions have more to do with fear of being held liable than with safeguarding their athletes' health. It is not unrealistic for coaches, or even clinicians, to be concerned about liability, particularly in a North American culture that Grayson (1999) calls "litigation hungry." But, it does influence the ways in which decisions are made about the health and safety of the athlete.

While the clinician has the advantage of a high level of perceived power, the patient-athlete also wields a certain degree of power in that s/he can accept, modify, or refuse the advice. However, the evidence shows that athletes negotiate their health from a position that is entrenched in a "culture of risk." The amount of decision-making responsibility placed into the hands of the athlete can be problematic as one athlete acknowledges: " . . . it's really pushed at [this university], that [the decision to play with pain or not to is] up to the maturity of the athlete. Where it gets scary is when they assume that, but the athlete doesn't really see the need to take care of themselves" (Safai 2001: 189). This is not to suggest that athletes should be treated like children. But we need to question whether placing the burden of responsibility on the shoulders of athletes is fair considering that athletes may be immersed in a "culture of risk," and often make their choices under the influence of their coaches, teammates, and injury-legitimating attitudes.

This concern is exemplified by an athlete involved in a high-risk contact sport recounting the experiences of her teammate who was concussed during playoffs and needed to continue competing in order to help the team maintain their playoff status:

> Interviewer: So, if it was the beginning of the season, and she had a concussion, would she have competed?
>
> Athlete: She wouldn't have [competed]. She's alright now, but she's still getting treatment.
>
> Interviewer: She's getting treatment now for the head injury [from last season]?
>
> Athlete: Yes.
>
> Interviewer: When that happened, did the therapist step in?
>
> Athlete: He told her, this is a possible concussion, but . . . [pause] it was left up to her.
>
> Interviewer: And what did your coach say?
>
> Athlete: He really didn't give much of an option (Safai 2001: 191).

The last sentence sums up the situation that some student-athletes are placed in with their coaches — they have no option but to compete with injury. Even though clinicians claim to place the onus of responsibility on the patient-athlete, and the coaches claim that they follow the advice of the clinicians out of fear of being held legally liable for endangering the athletes, the reality in some situations is radically different and potentially devastating for the athlete. If a coach is heavily assimilated into a "culture of risk," influences his or her athletes to accept and tolerate injuries, or does not recognise the seriousness of head injuries, then the athlete is "stranded" between going against his/her clinician's recommendation or going against her/his coach and team. Having said that, while the majority the situations outlined in Safai's study did not have such negative results, this is an area where we need to know more and where there is a need for more research.

Conclusion

This chapter focuses on and attempts to further problematise the role of the sport medicine clinician in various sport settings. Based on studies by Walk (1997), the Leicester University Centre for Research into Sport and Society (e.g. Roderick & Waddington 2000; Waddington 2000) and Safai (2001), we see that clinicians negotiate injury issues in sport involving risk and *with* risk, not only in the sense that their medical practices are situated in and framed by the "culture of risk," but also in the sense that the ambiguity and contradiction surrounding their responsibilities and authority renders their recommendations and actions precarious.

While a main emphasis in this chapter was to highlight the policy vacuum in which most sport medicine clinicians work, we cannot overlook Safai's (2001) study of a Canadian institution that attempts to rectify this absence. We see that some of the measures taken have resulted in a "culture of precaution" that works to counteract injury-legitimating norms — itself an extension of the institution's emphasis on healthy and positive *life-long* sport participation. However, while this dialectical relationship exists and while clinicians and administrators are attempting to address the pervasiveness of the "culture of risk," the evidence still reveals the *reproduction* of injury-tolerant attitudes, the absence of *uniform* policy or code of ethics, and the *consequence* of this absence on the clinician-athlete relationship. The lack of policy renders the negotiation of treatment problematic at times, because where there is conflict of interests in the competitive sport hierarchy, the clinician is effectively powerless in the face of the coach's authority, and the immersion of the patient-athlete in the "culture of risk." The clinicians resort to "ending" their professional responsibilities by informing participants of the risks. However, such a solution offers only an escape hatch from the trap they feel they are in, not a proper resolution to the ambiguity surrounding them.

In general, these studies represent sociology *in* sport medicine and not *of* sport medicine. Future research must continue to examine the ways in which policy articulates with sport medicine in all types of sport settings. However, it must also examine the ways in which clinicians are complicit in the construction of injury and injury tolerance. The paradox of competitive sport implicates the role of the clinician in that as athletes work on and wear down their bodies, there is an ever-increasing need for the specialised knowledge and abilities of these practitioners. This fosters a supply-demand scenario, where the commodity being exchanged is the health of the human beings. We cannot ignore the fact that sport medicine professions are intensely involved in asserting themselves as *the* medical and paramedical disciplines of the athletic body (see Coburn & Willis 2000; Hoberman 1990; Johnson 1972; Navarro 1986; Turner 1995; see also Harvey 1983 for parallels to other bodily professions). Thus, we have a field that is carving out a niche for itself within both the healthcare and sport markets, that is rhetorically committed to health, but which also sustains itself using voluntarily injured bodies. Thus, one could suggest that the fact that sport medicine clinicians are not and have not been vocal in creating a code of ethics is indicative of their complicity in reproducing injury tolerance. This is certainly a provocative statement, and is meant to spark further research, policy development and education in this area.

Acknowledgements

I would like to thank Peter Donnelly for his guidance with this project and Bruce Kidd for feedback on an earlier draft.

References

Annandale, E. (1998). *The sociology of health and medicine: A critical introduction.* Cambridge: Polity Press.

Canadian Interuniversity Sport (CIS) (2001–2002). *Operating and policy manual.* Ottawa: Author.

Coburn, D., & Willis, E. (2000). The medical profession: Knowledge, power, and autonomy. In: G. Albrecht, R. Fitzpatrick, & S. Scrimshaw (Eds), *Handbook of social studies in health and medicine* (pp. 379–393). Newbury Park: Sage.

Curry, T. J. (1993). A little pain never hurt anyone: Athletic career socialization and the normalization of sports injury. *Symbolic Interaction, 16,* 273–290.

Freidson, E. (1970). *Profession of Medicine.* New York: Dodd, Mead.

Gerhardt, U. (1989). *Ideas about illness: An intellectual and political history of medical sociology.* London: Macmillan.

Grayson, E. (1990). Sports medicine and the law. In: S. Payne (Ed.), *Medicine, sport and the law* (pp. 3–49). Oxford: Blackwell Scientific Publications.

Grayson, E. (1999). *Ethics, injuries and the law in sports medicine.* Oxford: Butterworth Heinemann, Reed Educational and Professional Publishing Ltd.

Harvey, J. (1983). *Le corps programmé ou la rhetoriqué de Kino-Québec.* Montréal: Albert Saint-Martin.

Hayes-Bautista, D. (1976a). Modifying the treatment: Patient compliance, patient control and medical care. *Social Science and Medicine, 10,* 233–238.

Hayes-Bautista, D. (1976b). Termination of the patient-practitioner relationship: Divorce, patient style. *Journal of Health and Social Behaviour, 17,* 12–21.

Hoberman, J. (1990). *Mortal engines: The science of performance and the dehumanization of sport.* New York: Free Press.

Hughes, R., & Coakley, J. (1991). Positive deviance among athletes: The implications of the sport ethic. *Sociology of Sport Journal, 8*, 307–325.

Johnson, T. (1972). *Professions and power.* London: Macmillan.

Klein, A. (1995). Life's too short to die small: Steroid use among male bodybuilders. In: D. Sabo, & D. F. Gordon (Eds), *Men's health and illness: Gender, power, and the body* (pp. 105–120). London: Sage.

Lupton, D. (1994). *Medicine as culture: Illness, disease and the body in western societies.* London: Sage.

Macleod, D. (1990). The doctor's contribution towards safety in sport – an exercise in preventive medicine. In: S. Payne (Ed.), *Medicine, sport and the law* (pp. 61–69). Oxford: Blackwell Scientific Publications.

McIlvride, D. (1994). Playing hurt (D. McIlvride, Director). In: A. Scherberger (Producer), *For the love of the game.* Toronto: The Sports Network.

Messner, M. (1989). When bodies are weapons. In: D. Sabo, & M. Messner (Eds), *Sex, violence & power in sports* (pp. 89–98). California: Crossing Press.

Navarro, V. (1986). *Crisis, health and medicine.* New York: Tavistock.

Nixon, H. (1992). A social network analysis of influences on athletes to play with pain and injuries. *Journal of Sport and Social Issues, 16*(2), 127–135.

Parsons, T. (1951). *The social system.* Glencoe: Free Press.

Payne, S. (1990). *Medicine, sport and the law.* Oxford: Blackwell Scientific Publications.

Pipe, A. (1998). Reviving ethics in sport: Time for physicians to act. *The Physician and Sports Medicine, 26*(9), 39–41.

Rier, D. (2000). The missing voice of the critically ill: A medical sociologist's first-person account. *Sociology of Health and Illness, 22*, 68–93.

Roderick, M., & Waddington, I. (2000). Playing hurt: Managing injuries in English professional football. *International Review for the Sociology of Sport, 35*(2), 165–180.

Roderick, M., Waddington, I., & Parker, G. (1999). Playing hurt: Professional footballers and their injuries. In: P. Murphy (Ed.), *Singer & Friedlander Review* (pp. 3–7). London: Singer & Friedlander.

Sabo, D., & Panepinto, J. (1990). Football ritual and the social reproduction of masculinity. In: M. Messner, & D. Sabo (Eds), *Sport, men, and the gender order: Critical feminist perspectives* (pp. 115–126). Champaign: Human Kinetics.

Safai, P. (2001). *Healing the body in the 'culture of risk', pain and injury: Negotiations between clinicians and injured athletes in Canadian competitive intercollegiate sport.* Unpublished master's thesis, University of Toronto.

Shorter, E. (1991). *Doctors and their patients: A social history.* New Brunswick, NJ: Transaction.

Student-athlete handbook (2001–2002). Faculty of _____: Large Canadian University (CU).

Theberge, N. (1997). It's part of the game: Physicality and production of gender in women's hockey. *Gender and Society, 11*(1), 69–87.

Turner, B. (1995). *Medical power and social knowledge* (2nd ed.). London: Sage.

Waddington, I. (1999). On medical grounds: The club doctor in professional football. In: P. Murphy (Ed.), *Singer & Friedlander review* (pp. 53–56). London: Singer & Friedlander.

Waddington, I. (2000). In confidence? Aspects of the medical relationships in professional football clubs. In: P. Murphy (Ed.), *Singer & Friedlander review* (pp. 49–54). London: Singer & Friedlander.

Walk, S. R. (1997). Peers in pain: The experience of student athletic trainers. *Sociology of Sport Journal, 14*, 22–56.

Williams, S., & Calnan, M. (1996). *Modern medicine: Lay perspectives and experiences.* London: UCL Press.

Young, K. (1993). Violence, risk, and liability in male sports culture. *Sociology of Sport Journal, 10*(4), 373–396.

Young, K., & White, P. (1995). Sport, physical danger and injury: The experience of elite women athletes. *Journal of Sport and Social Issues, 19*(1), 45–61.

Young, K., White, P., & McTeer, W. G. (1994). Body talk: Male athletes reflect on sport, injury, and pain. *Sociology of Sport Journal, 11*, 175–194.

Chapter 16

Sport, Health and Public Policy

Ivan Waddington

In many countries — and not just in the developed world — governments are involved, either directly or indirectly, in promoting sport, both inside and outside of the educational context. The central goals of this paper are to examine: (i) the assumptions underlying what is one of the central objectives of many government sport programmes, namely to improve the nation's health; and (ii) *via* the use of policy case studies from Britain and the United States, some of the complexities involved in the relationships between sport, health and public policy.

Sport, Exercise and the Healthy Body Ethos

There are probably few ideas which are as widely and uncritically accepted as that linking sport and exercise with good health. What is particularly striking about this ideology is its near universal acceptance across a range of societies for, in developing and developed societies, there is a broad consensus that "sport is good for you."

The ideology linking sport and health has a long history. In 19th century Britain, the birthplace of many modern sports, an ideology of athleticism which linked sport with health, both physical and "moral," was developed in the Victorian public schools (Mangan 1981), while the promotion and maintenance of the health of schoolchildren has long been an area of concern to physical educators (Colquhoun & Kirk 1987: 100). The idea that sport and exercise are associated with health is widely known and accepted by British schoolchildren today; one study for the Sports Council (1995: 128) noted that "the health and fitness message seems to be well known by children. Virtually all of them, 92% agreed that it was important to

Sporting Bodies, Damaged Selves
Research in the Sociology of Sport, Volume 2, 287–307
Copyright © 2004 by Elsevier Ltd.
All rights of reproduction in any form reserved
ISSN: 1476-2854/doi:10.1016/S1476-2854(04)02016-3

keep fit... In addition... 82% agreed that they felt fit and healthy when they did sport and exercise." Not surprisingly, the idea that sport is health-promoting is one which is frequently stressed by those involved in sport; to quote the British runner and former Olympic gold medalist Sebastian Coe: "Sport is an integral part of a healthy lifestyle in today's society" (foreword to Mottram 1988).

Such views have been endorsed over many years in a variety of official and semi-official health publications in Britain. The *Allied Dunbar National Fitness Survey* (Sports Council and Health Education Authority 1992) and the Department of Health in its *Health of the Nation* (1992) both noted a number of health benefits associated with regular physical activity. The Health Education Authority (1997: 2–4) has suggested that "the health benefits of an active lifestyle for adults are well established," while the same organisation, in its *Young and Active?* policy framework (1998), similarly drew attention to the health benefits of physical activity for young people. In similar fashion, the English Sports Council, in its strategy document *England, the Sporting Nation* (1997: 3), pointed to what it called the "well rehearsed" health benefits of sport.

In the United States, an authoritative report from the American College of Sports Medicine and the Center for Disease Control recommended that adults should take 30 minutes of moderate activity on most days of the week (Wimbush 1994), while the Surgeon General's report, *Physical Activity and Health* (U.S. Department of Health and Human Services 1996: 10), argued that "significant health benefits can be obtained by including a moderate amount of physical activity on most, if not all, days of the week." In Canada, a discussion paper prepared for Health Canada and Active Living Canada (Donnelly & Harvey 1996) noted that a comprehensive examination of Canadian data had similarly identified several significant health benefits of physical activity.

Nor are such views confined to countries in the developed world. Riordan (1986: 291), for example, has pointed out that governments in developing societies frequently place considerable stress on the development of sport, not only for the consequences which sport can have for nation-building and national integration but also for the effects it can have on hygiene and health.

It is clear that the ideology linking sport and health is widely accepted across a range of societies. But to what extent does this ideology stand up to critical examination?

Exercise, Sport and Health

There is a substantial body of data which indicates that moderate, rhythmic and regular exercise has a significant and beneficial impact on health. In Britain, the Royal College of Physicians of London (1991: 28) concluded that:

There is substantial evidence that regular aerobic exercise such as walking, jogging, dancing or swimming is beneficial to general physical and psychological health. Regular exercise appears to be particularly effective in prevention of coronary disease and osteoporosis and of some value in the management of obesity and diabetes.

More recently, the Department of Health (2001: 1) has stated that there "is now compelling evidence that physical activity is important for health and has great potential for health gains." More specifically, the Department of Health stated that regular physical activity:

- decreases the risk of cardiovascular disease mortality in general and coronary heart disease mortality in particular;
- prevents or delays the development of high blood pressure and reduces blood pressure in people with hypertension;
- helps to control body weight and diabetes;
- can help reduce the risk of falls and accidents by improving bone health and maintaining strength, co-ordination, cognitive functioning and balance;
- reduces the risk of colon cancer and possibly other forms of cancer;
- reduces the risk of depression, reduces anxiety and enhances mood and self-esteem;
- can help prevent non-specific chronic low back pain (Department of Health 2001: 1).

Studies in North America point to similar conclusions, and suggest that regular exercise is associated with reduced mortality from all causes, from cardiovascular disease and from cancer of combined sites (Blair *et al.* 1989; Paffenbarger *et al.* 1986), while a review of four population surveys (two carried out in Canada and two in the United States), suggests a positive association between physical activity and lower levels of anxiety and depression (Stephens 1988). The report of the U.S. Surgeon General (U.S. Department of Health and Human Services 1996) brought together, for the first time, what has been learned about physical activity and health from decades of American research, and produced a list of health benefits very similar to those identified above by the Department of Health in Britain.

At first glance, studies like those cited above might seem to indicate that the health-based arguments in favour of sport and exercise are overwhelming. Donnelly and Harvey (1996: 5) have noted, tongue-in-cheek, that the "numerous, almost miraculous claims for the benefits of physical activity lead one to wonder why it has not been patented by an innovative company" but, more seriously, they go on to point out that the widespread nature of these claims should serve as a warning against a too easy and uncritical acceptance of these claims, and that the context of the claims needs to be examined carefully. There are indeed some important provisos to be borne in mind when considering studies on the relationship between exercise and health. In particular, it is important to note that almost all of those studies which are cited to support the idea that sport is good for health refer *not* to sport, but to physical activity or exercise. But physical activity and sport are *not* the same thing. Physical activity or exercise might involve walking or cycling to work, dancing, working in the garden, or walking upstairs instead of taking the elevator. None of these are sport. There are several important differences between physical activity and exercise, on the one hand, and sport on the other. Perhaps the most important of these is that, whereas the competitive element is not central to most forms of physical activity, sport, in contrast, is inherently competitive. Moreover, it is becoming increasingly competitive not just at the elite level (Waddington 2000), but at local levels too. The increased competitiveness of modern sport — one aspect of which is the increased emphasis which has come to be placed on winning — means that, unlike most people who take part in non-competitive physical activities, those who play sport are, particularly at the higher levels, frequently subject to strong constraints to "play hurt"; that is, to continue playing while injured, or to play with painkilling injections "for the good of the team," with all the associated health risks these behaviours entail (Roderick *et al.* 2000; Young *et al.* 1994).

It is also important to remember that many sports — and not just the obvious combat sports — are mock battles in which aggression and the use of physical violence are, to a greater or lesser degree, central characteristics (Dunning 1986: 270). In this context, we might note that many sports have, in present-day societies, become enclaves for the expression of physical violence, not in the form of unlicensed or uncontrolled violence, but in the form of socially sanctioned violence as expressed in violently aggressive "body contact"; indeed, in the relatively highly pacified societies of the modern West, sport is probably the main — for many people the only — activity in which they are regularly involved in aggressive physical contact with others. Moreover, as Messner (1990: 203) has noted, in the more violent contact sports, "the human body is routinely turned into a weapon to be used against other bodies, resulting in pain, serious injury, and even death."

The link between sport, aggression and violence also provides an important key to understanding why sport is a major context for the inculcation and expression of gender differences and identities and, in particular, for the expression of traditional forms of aggressive masculinity. As Young *et al.* (1994) have pointed out, these traditional concepts of masculinity involve, as a central proposition, the idea that "real" men play sport in an intensely confrontational manner and, in this context, players are expected to give and to take hard knocks, to hurt and to be hurt and, when injured, to "take it like a man" and not show pain; injury thus becomes what Guttmann (1978: 121) has called a "certificate of virility, a badge of courage" and, for many players and fans alike, relatively violent sports such as American football and rugby are, precisely because of their violent character, arenas *par excellence* for young men to demonstrate their masculinity.

Writing of professional sport, Young (1993: 373) has noted:

> By any measure, professional sport is a violent and hazardous work-place, replete with its own unique forms of 'industrial disease'. No other single milieu, including the risky and labor-intensive settings of miners, oil drillers, or construction site workers, can compare with the routine injuries of team sports such as football, ice-hockey, soccer, rugby and the like.

In this context, it is instructive to note that one recent study of injuries in English professional football found that the overall risk of injury to professional foot-ballers is 1000 times greater than the risk of injury in other occupations normally considered high risk such as construction and mining (Hawkins & Fuller 1999). But it is not just elite level sport which involves health risks. The increasingly competitive nature of sport, even at the local level, means that there is a cost to be paid for participation in sport. Part of that cost is paid in the form of sports injuries.

The Epidemiology of Sports Injuries

Sports injuries are extremely common and, clearly, they have to be taken into account in any attempt to assess the "health costs" and "benefits" of sport and exercise. One large-scale study (Sports Council 1991) estimated that in England and Wales there are 19.3 million new injuries each year and a further 10.4 million recurrent injuries, making a total of 29.7 million injuries a year. The direct treatment costs of injuries were estimated at £422 million, with costs of lost production (11.5 million working days a year are lost due to sports injuries) estimated at £575 million, giving a total annual cost of sporting injuries of £997 million (1991: 25, 31). In the light of these data, one can understand why one American text on sports injuries (Vinger & Hoerner 1982) is subtitled "The Unthwarted Epidemic."

Three years after the Sports Council study, a team from Sheffield University Medical School (Nicholl *et al.* 1994) sought to ascertain the direct economic costs and benefits of exercise to the healthcare system. The health benefits of exercise (e.g. avoidance of costs associated with the management of chronic illnesses such as cardiovascular disease) were weighed against the costs of treatment of exercise-related injuries and it was found that, while there were clear economic benefits associated with exercise for adults aged 45 and over, for younger adults (15–44 years old), the costs avoided by the disease-prevention effects of exercise (less than £5 per person per year) were more than offset by the medical costs resulting from participation in sport and exercise (approximately £30 per person per year). Put another way, for every 15–44 year old adult who regularly participates in sport, there is a net cost to the British taxpayer of £25 per year. The authors conclude "there are strong economic arguments in favour of exercise in adults aged 45 and over, but *not* in younger adults" (1994: 109, emphasis added). A Dutch study which produced similar results to those of Nicholl *et al.* noted that "this is an amazing result, and it contrasts heavily with statements of people who use the supposed health effect of sport as an economic argument to promote sport" (Reijnen & Velthuijsen 1989, cited in Nicholl *et al.* 1994).

Injury risks vary markedly from one sport to another; not surprisingly, the highest risks are associated with contact sports. The Sports Council study (1991: 33) found that rugby was by far the most dangerous sport, in terms of risk of injury, with an injury rate of 59.3 per 100 participants per four weeks. The second most dangerous sport was soccer (39.3) followed by martial arts (36.3), hockey (24.8) and cricket (20.2). A study in New Zealand (Hume & Marshall 1994) similarly found that rugby union had the highest injury rate, while other high-risk sports included horse riding, soccer, cricket, netball, rugby league, basketball and snow skiing. That there is a close association between physical contact and injury risk is clear; Lynch and Carcasona (1994: 170–171) cite a study of youth outdoor and indoor soccer in the United States which found that 66% of injuries in the outdoor league and 70% of injuries in the indoor league resulted from physical contact. Perhaps not surprisingly, and very much in line with the analysis presented earlier, the Sports Council study found that the activities with the lowest risks of injury were the non-contact, rhythmic (and largely non-competitive) activities involved in "keep fit" (6.5 incidents per 100 participants per 4 weeks) and swimming and diving (2.9).

Studies of this kind suggest that, if a major goal of sport development policies is to improve people's health, then we should give rather more thought to the kinds of physical activities we wish to encourage. It is clear that gentle or moderate and regular physical activity has a beneficial impact on health. However, as we move: (i) from non-competitive activity to competitive sport; and (ii) from non-contact to contact sports, so the health costs, in the form of injuries, begin to mount. Similarly, as we move from mass sport to elite sport, the constraints to train longer and more intensively and to continue competing through pain and injury also increase, with a concomitant increase in the health risks. The health-related arguments in favour of regular and moderate physical activity may be clear, but such arguments are considerably less persuasive in relation to competitive, and especially contact, sport and very much less persuasive in relation to elite, or professional sport. What are the implications of this analysis for public policy in the areas of physical activity, exercise, sport and health?

Sport, Health and Public Policy

In order to examine this problem it is useful to differentiate between two broad kinds of public policy. The first of these is policy of the kind which has been associated with the work of the Health Education Authority (HEA) in the United Kingdom, and the Surgeon General in the United States. Such policies are firmly embedded within a public health framework and have relatively clearly stated goals which are concerned with improving the health of the community; in this context, encouraging people to adopt more active lifestyles is seen, not as a desirable end in itself, but as a means of improving public health.

In contrast to policies which are oriented primarily towards public health concerns are policies like those which have emanated from the Sports Councils in the U.K., or from government departments which have an interest in promoting sport; a good example of the latter, to be examined later, is the *Sport: Raising the Game* policy which was produced by the Department of National Heritage (DNH) in July 1995. Such policies, it is important to note, have their origins not within the public health policy community, but within the sports policy community, and those who are responsible for developing and implementing such policies are not oriented primarily towards public health issues, but towards the promotion of sport *per se*. In relation to the latter, there is, of course, no doubt that many (though not all) people find participation in sport intrinsically enjoyable and rewarding. However, in the battle for public funding, in which sport has to compete with many other services which might generally be thought to have a more pressing claim on public funds — for example health, education, or pensions — the fact that many people enjoy sport might be thought to constitute a relatively poor basis for a claim for public expenditure. Within this context, the widely accepted view that "sport is good for health" might be seen to provide a more persuasive justification for public funding for sport; perhaps not surprisingly, many people within the sporting policy community have, by uncritically conflating the concepts of physical activity, exercise and sport, been able to claim for sport health benefits which are certainly associated with many forms of physical activity but whose relationship to competitive sport is, as we saw earlier, much more problematic. Moreover, those within the sporting community have also been able to call upon a number of other ideologies — for example, that the provision of sporting facilities fosters community development, reduces crime, helps to break down barriers of race/ethnicity and enhances the country's international prestige — to advance their claims for public expenditure on sport. My primary concern here is with the health-related issues, though it should be noted that, as the recent review by Long and Sanderson (2001) makes clear, the evidence to support most of these claims is, at best, very skimpy. Of more immediate significance within the present context, however, is the fact that, largely because of the way in which sport has become linked with a variety of pro-sport ideologies, the goals of public policy in relation to sport have — much more so than in the case of the policy goals deriving from the public health policy community — become diffuse and unclear. More specifically, health-related concerns have often been subordinated to other goals of sporting policy, and have sometimes resulted in the development of policies whose impact on health may actually be a *negative* one. These issues are best explored *via* an examination of the two rather different forms of public policy identified earlier: public health policy and policy for sport. It is recognised, of course, that there is some overlap between the activities of the public health and the sports policy communities — for example, the Allied Dunbar National Fitness Survey (Sports Council and Health Education Authority 1992) was funded by the HEA, the Department of Health and the Sports Council — but nevertheless the central thrusts of public health policy and sports development policy are sufficiently different to justify this distinction.

Public Health Policy and Physical Activity

Although the health benefits of physical activity have long been extolled, it has only been in recent years that bodies concerned with public health have begun to formulate clear guidelines about what was considered, in terms of health benefits, an appropriate amount of physical activity. The early recommendations — most notably, the "position stand" of the American College of Sports Medicine (1990) — focused on cardio-respiratory endurance and specified sustained periods of *vigorous* physical activity involving large muscle groups. However, in more recent years, the recommended level of physical activity has been scaled down, largely as a result of two developments. Firstly, more recent research has indicated that it is not necessary to engage in very vigorous activity to derive substantial health benefits, for there are major health gains to be obtained from exercise of *moderate* intensity. Secondly, there was a growing realisation that programmes involving vigorous physical activity were, for many people, simply unrealistic, and that programmes involving more moderate levels of activity were associated with improved adherence; in these respects the latter were, in terms of public health policy, more effective.

In line with these developments, the executive summary of the U.S. Surgeon General's report, *Physical Activity and Health* (U.S. Department of Health and Public Services 1996: 1) lists its key finding as follows:

> people of all ages can improve the quality of their lives through a lifelong practice of moderate physical activity. You don't have to be training for the Boston Marathon to derive real health benefits from physical activity. A regular, preferably daily regimen of at least 30–45 minutes of brisk walking, bicycling, or even working around the house or yard will reduce your risks of developing coronary heart disease, hypertension, colon cancer, and diabetes.

It is worth emphasising that the primary concern of the report is with physical activity rather than sport; indeed it is striking that almost all of the examples of moderate physical activity recommended in the report are either lifestyle activities such as washing and waxing a car, washing windows or floors, gardening, dancing, pushing a stroller, raking leaves or shovelling snow, or non-contact, rhythmic exercises such as water aerobics, swimming laps, bicycling gently, jumping rope, stairwalking, walking and shooting baskets. The only competitive sports which figure in the list of recommended examples of moderate activity are playing basketball for 15–20 minutes and playing volleyball for 45 minutes; significantly, the major competitive sports in the United States — notably grid-iron football, baseball and ice-hockey — are conspicuous by their absence from this list of recommended activities! The emphasis on lifestyle activities, rather than competitive sport, is further reinforced by the observation that, in the United States, the "most popular leisure-time activities among adults are walking and gardening or yard work" (1996: 14).

This emphasis on lifestyle activities rather than sport also comes out very clearly in the "Physical Activity. It's Everywhere You Go!" campaign which was launched by the Centers for Disease Control and Prevention (CDC) in 1997 and which is on-going at the time of writing (May 2002). The CDC website currently promoting the campaign emphasises the role of physical activity, not in the context of competitive sport, but as a part of everyday lifestyle: physical activity, it says, is "in the house. It's in the yard. It's at the office. It's even at the mall! It's everywhere you go!"

(CDC 2001). The campaign explicitly acknowledges that the central campaign theme — "It's Everywhere You Go" — "raises awareness that the physical activity needed for a healthier life can be included in many everyday activities" and, in launching the campaign, the CDC Director emphasised that: "You do not have to be a star athlete or join an expensive gym to receive health benefits from physical activity —- taking the stairs instead of the elevator or taking a walk with the family instead of watching television — you can fit physical activity in everywhere you go" (CDC 1997).

The Children's Lifetime Physical Activity Model (Corbin *et al.* 1994) reflects a similar emphasis on lifestyle activities of moderate intensity, rather than competitive sports. The model suggests that children should, as an optimum, participate three or more times a week in a volume of activity involving the expenditure of at least 6–8 kcal/kg/day. This level of activity is, as Harris & Cale (1997: 59) have pointed out, "one that inactive children can achieve with a modest commitment to childhood games and activities, or lifestyle activities such as walking or riding a bicycle to school or performing physical tasks around the home."

Within Britain, the evolution of public health policy in relation to physical activity has followed a broadly similar pattern to that in the United States. In September 1993, the Government established a Task Force to develop a national strategy for promoting physical activity and, in the following year, the HEA convened an international symposium charged with the task of identifying the most effective health education messages for promoting physical activity. The symposium report (*Moving On*, HEA 1995) suggested that, in relation to physical activity, public health policy should, firstly, seek to reduce the proportion of the population who are sedentary and, secondly, to increase the proportion of the population engaging in regular physical activity of a moderate intensity. The report did recommend that policy should also be oriented towards increasing the proportion of the population engaging in regular vigorous intensity physical activity, though particular stress was laid on the first two objectives; the third objective, it was pointed out, represented the more traditional goal of exercise programmes, while the first two objectives "represent a shift in thinking towards the promotion of physical activity of a more moderate intensity" (HEA 1995: 4). This led to the main physical activity recommendation: that adults should take 30 minutes of moderate intensity physical activity, such as a sustained brisk walk, on at least five days of the week.

Particular concern was expressed about the large number of people — nearly a third of all adults, and 55% of those aged 65 or older — who take part in no physical activity on a regular basis, and who have at least a two-fold increase in mortality risk. In this context, the HEA (1995: 8) noted that:

The greatest public health benefits are likely to be gained from encouraging an increase in moderate activity. Therefore, sedentary individuals and those who are active on an irregular basis are the priority audiences to be reached.

The HEA later produced a series of policy documents about physical activity and health; these included *Promoting Physical Activity in Primary Health Care* (1996), which was targeted at primary healthcare teams, the three year campaign, *Active for Life*, which was launched in 1996, and *Young and Active?* (1998), a policy framework for young people. The HEA ceased to exist in 2000, since when its functions have been taken over by a number of other organisations, including the Health Development Agency and the Department of Health. The Department recently issued a major policy statement on exercise referral systems, designed to encourage primary care practitioners to refer patients who are physically inactive and/or who have other identifiable health needs for supervised exercise sessions, which take place mainly in public leisure facilities (Department of Health 2001). In all of these policy documents the emphasis has consistently been placed on encouraging people to engage in physical activity of *moderate* intensity. For example, the publicity material for Phase Three of the *Active for Life* campaign, which ran from April 1998 to March 1999, pointed out that "Being active doesn't have to be hard work; everyday activities like dancing, cycling, walking and swimming can improve health."

Moreover — and like the report of the Surgeon General in the United States — HEA policy revolved centrally around the concept of *physical activity* and, within that policy, competitive sport hardly figured at all. The *Young and Active?* policy statement (p. 2), for example, provided definitions of key concepts underlying the policy; these key concepts include physical activity, exercise, physical fitness, physical education and health-related exercise but, significantly, *not* sport. It might also be noted that, in that same policy document, the HEA, in pointing to the health benefits of physical activity, noted that some of these benefits, for example in terms of enhanced self-esteem, "can be limited by an over-emphasis on competitive performance" (HEA 1998: 2). In its earlier *Moving On* policy statement, the HEA also recognised that negative perceptions of what it called "sporty image" constitute one of the barriers to more widespread participation in health-enhancing physical activity.

In considering these policy statements, two points are clear. The first is that these policies are unambiguously and very firmly embedded in a public health framework and express public health concerns. This is clearly illustrated by the nature of the groups which were targeted by the HEA campaigns. Thus while the three year *Active for Life* campaign was aimed at the whole population of England aged 16–74 years, it echoed the thrust of the public health priorities of the earlier *Moving On* policy in that it particularly targeted more sedentary population groups, which it identified as:

- young women aged 16–24 years;
- middle aged men and women aged 44–55 years;
- older people aged over 50 years.

The earlier *Moving On* policy also suggested that people with disabilities and those from low-income groups were also particularly likely to be sedentary. These target groups, it hardly needs saying, were identified on the basis of their health needs, rather than on the basis of any likely contribution they might be able to make to the nation's sporting achievements.

The second, equally clear, point is that competitive sport is, at best, marginal to policies like those developed by the HEA. What is important is physical activity; in terms of their impact on health, physical activities such as heavy DIY, gardening, heavy housework or dancing are just as valuable as are, for example, gentle swimming or doubles tennis. In this context, it might be suggested that what policies like those developed by the HEA *are* about — that is, public health — is thrown into sharper relief by what they are *not* about — namely competitive sport. HEA policy as it developed in the 1990s, for example, was emphatically *not* about improving levels of sporting performance; there is nothing in the HEA documents which corresponds in any way with the English Sports Council's "sports development continuum" described as a "framework for helping individuals to achieve their personal best [which] is expressed as a continuum moving from foundation, through participation and performance, to [sporting] excellence" (English Sports Council 1997: 5). Policies such as those developed by the HEA, in contrast, are *not* about achieving personal bests. They are *not* about identifying talented young athletes. They are *not* about producing future Olympic champions. And they are *not* about enhancing Britain's international reputation through sporting performance. They are about improving health and saving lives, and it is this which accounts for the fact that two of the three major target groups identified by the HEA — middle aged and elderly people — involve people who, in sporting terms, will generally be some way past their personal bests.

Sports Development Policy

Within Britain the Government, both directly through the Ministry of Sport and indirectly through government-funded organisations such as the Sports Councils, takes an active part in promoting the development of sport. That such policies are valuable, and that they effectively promote a number of desirable objectives, seems to be generally taken for granted. But are the goals of such policies clear? And if these policies have several goals, are those goals mutually compatible, or might the achievement of one goal undermine the achievement of other goals? And, in particular, what is the relationship between sports development policies and health promotion?

In order to try to resolve some of these problems, it may be useful to look at some examples of sports policy, and the claims which are made in those policy statements on behalf of sport. The English Sports Council (1997: 3), in its *England, the Sporting Nation* strategy document, claimed that the "benefits of sport are well rehearsed — national identity and prestige, community development, personal challenge, as well as economic and health benefits. Sport is a central element in the English way of life..."

Two years previously, the then Prime Minister, John Major, wrote in the preface to the Government's *Sport: Raising the Game* policy document (DNH 1995) that sport:

> enriches the lives of the thousands of millions of people of all ages around the world who know and enjoy it. Sport is a central part of Britain's National Heritage.
>
> ... Sport is a binding force between generations and across borders. But, by a miraculous paradox, it is at the same time one of the defining characteristics of nationhood and of local pride. We should cherish it for both those reasons.
>
> ... Competitive sport teaches valuable lessons which last for life. Every game delivers both a winner and a loser. Sports men (sic) must learn to be both. Sport only thrives if both parties play by the rules, and accept the results with good grace. It is one of the best means of learning how to live alongside others and make a contribution as part of a team. It improves health and it opens the door to new friendships (p.2).

In the light of such sweeping claims, it is appropriate to ask a number of questions about the goals of public policy for sport (Waddington & Murphy 1998). Are such policies, like those of the HEA, oriented primarily towards public health goals? In other words, is the primary goal to encourage mass participation in sport with a view to improving the health of the nation? Or is the primary goal to encourage participation in sport in order to have a broader base from which future world or Olympic champions can be selected and trained? Or is the goal to encourage people to participate in sport because this is felt to be a useful means of teaching what may be held to be desirable values — for example the values of fair play, of respect for one's opponent, and of sporting behaviour? Or is the goal to develop local communities? Or is it to encourage young people, in particular, to play sport as a means of diverting them away from drugs or crime?

It is important to clarify these questions, not least because the way in which these questions are answered determines what other questions we need to ask. For example, if sports development policies derive primarily from health considerations, then we need to locate such policies within the context of the kind of issues examined earlier. If, on the other hand, the primary concern is to provide a wider base for the production of elite athletes whose sporting achievements in international competition will reflect favourably upon Britain's international standing, then we need to ask questions about the relationship between sport, politics and international relations. And if the primary goal is to provide non-criminal outlets for the energies of disaffected youth, then we need to ask questions about sport as a means of social control. The way in which we answer these questions may also indicate which government department (or departments) should have major responsibility for sports development policies. Should it be the Ministry for Sport? Or the Department of Health? Or Education? Or even the Home Office?

It is not possible to examine all these questions here; my primary concern is with health-related issues and it is upon these that I will focus. More specifically, I want to examine the policies pursued from the mid-1990s by successive British Governments, Conservative and Labour, in relation to sport for children and young people. As we noted earlier, there may be several reasons why governments adopt particular policies in relation to sport — for example, to produce future Olympic champions — but the question I wish to address here is as follows: does recent government policy for sport and PE make sense on *health* grounds?

Sport, Physical Education and Public Policy in the U.K.

The most striking characteristic of government policy in relation to sport and PE for school-age children from the mid-1990s has been the way in which successive governments have sought not only, in their view, to re-establish the centrality of sport in schools, but also to prioritise certain kinds of physical activities whilst marginalising others.

National Curriculum Physical Education (NCPE) has been taught in British schools since 1992 and features six activity areas: competitive games, athletics, swimming, gymnastics, dance and outdoor and adventurous activities. Within a couple of years of the introduction of the NCPE, however, powerful voices within the then Conservative government, most notably those of the Prime Minister, John Major, and his Minister for Sport, began to make clear their unhappiness at what they perceived as a lack of sufficient emphasis on competitive sport (and especially team games) in the NCPE and they sought to re-prioritise sport and, in particular, "traditional" team games, within NCPE (Penney & Evans 1997). This resulted in two major initiatives: the revised NCPE (implemented in August 1995) and the government's 1995 policy statement *Sport: Raising the Game*. As the latter document pointed out, "in the revised National Curriculum the government has greatly increased the importance of competitive sport," while "the focus of this Policy Statement [*Sport: Raising the Game*] is deliberately on sport rather than physical education" (p. 7). The central thrust of government policy was thus quite clear; in the Prime Minister's words, it was "to put sport [by which the Government meant competitive sport, rather than physical activities in general] back at the heart of weekly life in school" (DNH 1995: 2).

As Penney & Evans (1997) have pointed out, the policy of the Conservative Government thus effectively privileged defined "activity areas" — specifically competitive sports and, in particular, traditional team games — over broader, permeating themes such as "health-related exercise." The broad thrust of these policies has been taken over by the Labour Government which has been in office since 1997; there was a minor modification to NCPE in 2000[1] but in all other respects the emphasis on competitive sport has been continued and, indeed, further accentuated.

The continued — indeed enhanced — emphasis on competitive sport runs like a central thread throughout the recent government policy statements *A Sporting Policy for All* (Department for Culture, Media and Sport [DCMS] 2000) and *The Government's Plan for Sport* (DCMS 2001). The former, for example, identifies in its Introduction the two key goals of government policy: "more people of all ages and all social groups taking part in sport; and more success for our top competitors and teams in international competition." Moreover, levels of participation and competitive sporting success are inextricably intertwined in government policy. For example, in the Introduction the document identifies "the key issues which

---

[1] The only change to NCPE was introduced in September 2000. Since that date, competitive games have remained compulsory in Key Stages 1–3 (five to 14 year olds), but are now no longer compulsory in Key Stage 4 (14–16 year olds); instead, 14–16 year olds are allowed to choose any two from six activities: games, gymnastics, athletics, dance, swimming and water safety, or outdoor and adventurous activities. This was a small step by the Labour Government away from the prioritisation of games within the PE policy which it had inherited from John Major's Conservative Government. However, all the key aspects of the previous government's *Sport: Raising the Game* policy, including the emphasis on team sports, remain intact.

must be tackled if we are to improve our performance in sport"; one of these is that "people lose interest as they get older, reducing participation and diminishing the pool of talent" (DCMS 2000: 5). The document makes no reference to the likely consequences of this emphasis on competitive sport for the health of young people, though there is an explicit attempt to use sport as an instrument to tackle other social problems. In the chapter on "Sport in the Community," for example, there is a discussion of how sport may be used to tackle problems of social exclusion. Even here, however, the emphasis on success in competitive sport reappears; the document points out that not all groups have equal access to sporting facilities, and says that not only is this unfair, "it also wastes the talents of too many young people. We cannot expect to compete at international level, if we don't draw from the widest possible pool of talent" (p. 11). There is a chapter on "Sporting Excellence," the focus of which is self-explanatory, while the chapter on "Modernisation" begins: "Getting England winning again — and putting in place the strong base of participation to make that possible — means getting things right, off the pitch as well as on." It continues that "Cups are not won in committee rooms, but we know . . . that professional organisation and modern administration . . . can increase the likelihood of international success" (DCMS 2000: 19). The focus on competitive sport, rather than — as in the case of public health campaigns — physical activity as an aspect of everyday life, could not be more clear.

However, this increased emphasis on competitive sport for young people, both inside and outside of school, has potentially significant consequences for their health. Put most simply, the question is: does government policy in relation to sport and physical education make sense in terms of its likely health consequences for young people? It is to this issue that I now turn.

Sport, Physical Education and Health

The taken-for-granted relationship between sport, physical education and health is clearly illustrated in the comment of Alderson and Crutchley that "the essential focus for physical education in schools should be sport," to which they add that the role of physical educationalists "should be to prepare children for sport culture within our society so that they may make best use of it in relation to their personal development, their effective use of leisure time and their *physical and psychological well-being*" (1990: 54; emphasis added).

However, as we have seen, the health "costs" associated with contact sports such as rugby, football and hockey are considerably greater than those associated with non-contact sports or with non-competitive exercise. In this context, it is important to note that those activities which successive governments have sought to prioritise are precisely those competitive sports, and often contact sports, in which the health "costs" are greatest while those activities which are increasingly being marginalised within the physical education curriculum — most notably dance and outdoor and adventurous activities (Penney & Evans 1994; Waddington, Malcolm & Cobb 1998; Waddington, Malcolm & Green 1997) — are those which offer substantial health benefits but with far fewer health "costs." Such a policy might make sense if the central objective is to produce successful sportspeople capable of boosting Britain's international sporting prestige, but it would not seem to be the most appropriate policy if the priority is to improve the health of young people.

In this regard, it should be noted that many of the injuries typically associated with sports in the physical education curriculum have potentially serious ramifications for physically developing children. Helm (cited in Pool & Carnall 1997: 10) has pointed out that at the age of about 12 (girls) and 14 (boys) "the skeleton is at its most vulnerable to fracture. During these years the bones are growing rapidly and muscle cannot keep up, so there is a danger of dislocation and fracture." In this context, Pool and Carnall have identified a number of injuries which are commonly associated with sports on the physical education curriculum. These include fractured cheekbones, often sustained in sports such as hockey and lacrosse; torn cartilages and damaged hamstrings, tendons and ligaments which are common in athletics, many team sports and indeed all contact sports involving extensive twisting, turning and rapid explosive movements; and spinal injuries, most common in games like rugby, particularly where opponents are mismatched in terms of size, strength and fitness, which is often the case in age-grouped school sport and representative teams. It is not perhaps unreasonable to suggest that, in many respects, the structure of school sport *appears routinely to court the risk of injury for growing youngsters.*

Moreover, the renewed prioritising of sport in the physical education curriculum, together with concern about the low level of activity of some children, has led some teachers to adopt what Harris and Cale (1997: 61) call a "hard line approach" which involves "increasingly forcing pupils into 'hard' exercise, such as arduous cross-country running or fitness testing." If we are genuinely concerned about the health of young people, such an approach should be questioned. It is important to note that while physical education teachers may be aware and generally accepting of the role they are encouraged to play in promoting physical activity for health they also appear to be largely unaware of recent exercise recommendations and may not appreciate the implications for health-related physical activity (Harris & Cale 1997). While the Children's Lifetime Physical Activity Model (Corbin *et al.* 1994) highlights the fact that exercise does not have to be strenuous to be beneficial to health and that "moderate activity is associated with improved adherence in children . . . and a lower risk of injury" (Harris & Cale 1997: 61), it appears that teachers may be reluctant to recognise and incorporate moderate rather than vigorous forms of activity into health-related exercise lessons and frequently promote vigorous physical activity "at the expense of less strenuous forms of exercise" (Harris & Cale 1997: 61). Given this situation, it is not altogether surprising that children's and young people's perceptions of fitness and health are such that "fitness tends to be associated with high levels of performance and uncomfortable physical exertion" and that fitness is often viewed "in relation to sporting achievement rather than relative to everyday life activities" (Harris 1994: 146). This, it might be noted, is almost the exact opposite of the view of health-promoting physical activity which organisations concerned with public health are seeking to promote. As we noted earlier, public health organisations in Britain and the United States have repeatedly stressed that being active does *not* have to be hard work, and that everyday lifestyle activities such as dancing or walking can improve health; the view that being active involves high levels of performance and uncomfortable physical exertion is likely, for many people — and perhaps particularly for girls — to generate negative perceptions of what more active lifestyles involve.

Conclusion

The concepts of physical activity, exercise and health have often been conflated, particularly by people within the sports lobby, who frequently claim for sport the health benefits associated with non-competitive physical activity or exercise. It is time to reject such sleight-of-hand, for it is intellectually dishonest and it provides a misleading basis for public policy. Whereas the public health case in favour of regular, moderate-intensity physical activity has been made very clearly, the public health arguments in favour of competitive sport — and, in particular, team sports like those which have been at the centre of recent British government policy — are hardly persuasive.

References

Alderson, J., & Crutchley, D. (1990). Physical education and the National Curriculum. In: N. Armstrong (Ed.), *New directions in physical education* (Vol. 1, pp. 37–62). Champaign, IL: Human Kinetics.
American College of Sports Medicine (1990). Position stand: The recommended quantity and quality of exercise for developing and maintaining cardiorespiratory and

muscular fitness in healthy adults. *Medicine and Exercise in Sports and Exercise, 22,* 265–74.

Blair, S. N., Paffenbarger, R. S., Clark, D. G., Cooper, K. H., & Gibbons, L. W. (1989). Physical fitness and all-cause mortality. *Journal of the American Medical Association, 262*(17), 2395–2401.

Centers for Disease Control and Prevention (1997). CDC launches new campaign to increase physical activity among adults, http:/www.cdc.gov/nccdphp/dnpa/readyset/press.htm accessed 07/05/2002.

Centers for Disease Control and Prevention (2001). Physical activity. Ready. Set. It's everywhere you go! http:www.cdc.gov/nccdphp/dnpa/readyset/ accessed 08/05/2002.

Colquhoun, D., & Kirk, D. (1987). Investigating the problematic relationship between health and physical education: An Australian study. *Physical Education Review, 10*(2), 100–109.

Corbin, C. B., Pangrazi, R. P., & Welk, G. J. (1994). Towards an understanding of appropriate physical activity levels for youth. *Physical Activity and Research Digest Series, 1*(8), President's Council on Fitness and Sport, USA, 1–8.

Department for Culture, Media and Sport (2000). *A Sporting Future for All.* London: DCMS.

Department for Culture, Media and Sport and Department for Education and Employment (2001). *The Government's Plan for Sport.* London: DCMS and DFEE.

Department of Health (1992). *The health of the nation: A strategy for health in England.* London: HMSO.

Department of Health (2001). *Exercise referral systems: A national quality assurance framework.* London.

Department of National Heritage (DNH) (1995). *Sport:Raising the game.* London: DNH.

Donnelly, P., & Harvey, J. (1996). *Overcoming systematic barriers to active living.* Discussion paper prepared for Fitness Branch, Health Canada and Active Living Canada.

Dunning, E. (1986). Sport as a male preserve: Notes on the social sources of masculine identity and its transformation. In: N. Elias, & E. Dunning (Eds), *Op. cit* (pp. 267–283).

English Sports Council (1997). *England, the sporting nation.* London: English Sports Council.

Guttmann, A. (1978). *From ritual to record.* New York: Columbia University Press.

Harris, J. (1994). Young people's perceptions of health, fitness and exercise: Implications for the teaching of health related exercise. *Physical Education Review, 17*(2), 143–151.

Harris, J., & Cale, L. (1997). Activity promotion in physical education. *European Physical Education Review, 3*(1), 58–67.

Hawkins, R. D., & Fuller, C. W. (1999). A prospective epidemiological study of injuries in four English professional football clubs. *British Journal of Sports Medicine, 33,* 196–203.

Health Education Authority (HEA) (1995). *Moving on: A summary.* London: HEA.

Health Education Authority (1996). *Promoting physical activity in primary health care: Guidance for the primary healthcare team.* London: HEA.

Health Education Authority (1997). *Young people and physical activity: Promoting better practice.* London: HEA.

Health Education Authority (1998). *Young and active?* London: HEA.

Hume, P. A., & Marshall, S. W. (1994). Sports injuries in New Zealand: Exploratory analyses. *New Zealand Journal of Sports Medicine, 22,* 18–22.

Long, J., & Sanderson, I. (2001). The social benefits of sport: Where's the proof?' In: C. Gratton, & I. P. Henry (Eds), *Sport in the city* (pp. 187–203). London and New York: E & F N Spon.

Lynch, J. M., & Carcasona, C. B. (1994). The team physician. In: B. Ekblom (Ed.), *Handbook of sports medicine and science: Football (Soccer)* (pp. 166–174). Oxford: Blackwell Scientific Publications.

Mangan, J. A. (1981). *Athleticism in the Victorian and Edwardian public school.* Cambridge: Cambridge University Press.

Messner, M. (1990). When bodies are weapons: Masculinity and violence in sport. *International Review for the Sociology of Sport, 25*(3), 203–218.

Mottram, D. R. (Ed.) (1988). *Drugs in Sport.* London: E. & F. N. Spon.

Nicholl, J. P., Coleman, P., & Brazier, J. E. (1994). Health and healthcare costs and benefits of exercise. *PharmacoEconomics, 5*(2), 109–122.

Paffenbarger, R. S., Hyde, R. T., Wing, A. L., & Hsieh, C.-C. (1986). Physical activity, all-cause mortality, and longevity of college alumni. *New England Journal of Medicine, 314*(10), 605–613.

Penney, D., & Evans, J. (1994). It's just not (and not just) cricket. *The British Journal of Physical Education, 25*(3), 9–12.

Penney, D., & Evans, J. (1997). Naming the game. Discourse and domination in physical education and sport development in England and Wales. *European Physical Education Review, 3*(1), 21–32.

Pool, H., & Carnall, D. (1997, February 18). Sport is war minus the shooting! *Guardian Education,* 10–11.

Reijnen, J., & Velthuijsen, J.-W. (1989, November 20–22). *Economic aspects of health through sport.* Proceedings of an international conference: Sport – an economic force in Europe, 76–90. Lilleshall, UK.

Riordan, J. (1986). State and sport in developing societies. *International Review for the Sociology of Sport, 21*(4), 287–303.

Roderick, M., Waddington, I., & Parker, G. (2000). Playing hurt: Managing injuries in English professional football. *International Review for the Sociology of Sport, 35*(2), 165–180.

Royal College of Physicians of London (1991). *Medical aspects of exercise.* London: Royal College of Physicians.

Sports Council (1991). *Injuries in sport and exercise.* London: Sports Council.

Sports Council (1995). *Young people and sport in England 1994.* London: Sports Council.

Sports Council and Health Education Authority (1992). *Allied Dunbar national fitness survey.* London.

Stephens, T. (1988). Physical activity and mental health in the United States and Canada: Evidence from four population surveys. *Preventive Medicine, 17,* 35–47.

U.S. Department of Health and Human Services (1996). *Physical activity and health: A report of the surgeon general, executive summary.* Department of Health and Human Services.

Vinger, P. F., & Hoerner, E. F. (Eds) (1982). *Sports injuries: The unthwarted epidemic.* Littleton, MA: PSG Publishing.

Waddington, I. (2000). *Sport, health and drugs.* London and New York: E & F N Spon.

Waddington, I., Malcolm, D., & Cobb, J. (1998). Gender stereotyping and physical education. *European Physical Education Review, 4*(1), 34–46.

Waddington, I., Malcolm, D., & Green, K. (1997). Sport, health and physical education: A reconsideration. *European Physical Education Review, 3*(2), 165–182.

Waddington, I., & Murphy, P. (1998). Sport for all: Some public health policy issues and problems. *Critical Public Health, 8*(3), 193–205.

Wimbush, E. (1994). A moderate approach to promoting physical activity: The evidence and implications. *Health Education Journal, 53,* 322–336.

Young, K. (1993). Violence, risk and liability in male sports culture. *Sociology of Sport Journal, 10,* 373–396.

Young, K., White, P., & McTeer, W. (1994). Body talk: Male athletes reflect on sport, injury, and pain. *Sociology of Sport Journal, 11*(2), 175–194.

Chapter 17

The Costs of Injury from Sport, Exercise and Physical Activity: A Review of the Evidence

Philip White

Perhaps the best way to begin this chapter is to start with what will be my conclusion: the available epidemiological information on the costs of sport, physical activity and exercise (variously conceptualised and measured) is inconsistent, far from complete, and merits further attention. Initiatives needed to redress various gaps in the extant research literature will be discussed much later in the chapter (see De Loes 1997; Finch & Owen 2001; Janda 1997; Koplan *et al.* 1985; Van Mechelen 1997 for further discussion on the need for better injury data). In the meantime, I will embark on a review of the research which is available, although I must emphasise at the outset that a *precise assessment of costs* is not possible given the available data. Further, although it is possible to make assessments of the absolute extent of injury resulting from sport, exercise and physical activity and the attendant costs of those injuries in various countries and regions of countries, relative comparisons are problematic because of variability in measurement protocols (not to mention different currencies and variable inflation rates within various currencies over time). This is not to say, however, that an overview of existing studies cannot offer an interesting, if sometimes alarming, assessment of the downside of participation in sport, physical activity and exercise. For public health planning purposes, it is also useful to have an understanding of the benefits and costs of involvement in various types of participation for particular sub-groups of the population.

Sporting Bodies, Damaged Selves
Research in the Sociology of Sport, Volume 2, 309–331
© 2004 Published by Elsevier Ltd.
ISSN: 1476-2854/doi:10.1016/S1476-2854(04)02017-5

Participation in physical activity (a term I will use henceforth to encompass exercise, sport, physical recreation and physical activity) results in a number of well-documented health benefits (Curtis & Russell 1997; U.S. Department of Health and Human Services 2000). It also involves the risk of injury. As we will see, the rates of incidence of such injuries are higher than many would suspect and risks of injury increase with greater frequency and duration of participation. As Jones *et al.* (1994: 202–203) have argued, "the strongest and most consistent association exists between total amounts of exercise and higher risks of injury." Despite such concerns, and based seemingly on the relatively untested assumption that the benefits of participation in physical activity outweigh the costs, we have seen in the last few decades the launching of public health initiatives aimed at increasing the proportion of populations engaging in physical activity (Koplan *et al.* 1985). This chapter interrogates that assumption by reviewing the evidence that is currently available.

Conventional Wisdoms on the Physical Benefits of Sport and Physical Activity

It has become by now a commonplace that greater participation in sport and physical activity in the population leads to positive health benefits on a range of dimensions (Royal College of Physicians 1991; Siscovick *et al.* 1985). As Anterno Kesaniemi *et al.* (2001: S351) suggest: "Regular physical activity is widely accepted as a behaviour to reduce all-cause mortality rates and to improve a number of health outcomes." The many positive outcomes have been shown to be physical and psychological (see Bouchard *et al.* 1990; Quinney *et al.* 1994 for reviews of various types of benefits). As Nicholl *et al.* (1994: 111) have suggested:

> Compared with a sedentary lifestyle, regular participation in exercise improves body functioning — for example, circulation, strength, stamina, and joint mobility. More specifically, exercise is associated with reduced risk of certain chronic illnesses, such as cardiovascular diseases and osteoporosis, and it is effective in treating diabetes, mild stress and anxiety.

In terms of broad outcomes, in a study of a large cohort of U.S. college graduates aged 45 or older, the death rate of moderate exercisers was between 23 and 29% lower than non-exercisers (Paffenbarger *et al.* 1993). The findings also indicated that those in the sample who took up moderately vigorous sports added, on average, nine months to their lives.

There is also a body of research that points to estimated savings to the health care system and to increased economic productivity resulting from increased physical activity in the population (see Wood 1993 for a detailed review). Other quantified estimates are summarised in a number of publications (cf. Nicholl *et al.* 1991). In Canada, a report prepared for the Canadian Fitness and Lifestyle Institute in 1996 reported that the annual reduction of direct treatment costs from a 1% increase in the number of people who are physically active to be $10,233,000 for ischemic heart disease, $407,000 for colon cancer, and $877,000 for diabetes mellitus (type II) (Conference Board of Canada 1996). In the U.K. the Royal College of Physicians (1991: 28) has made similar conclusions from accumulated evidence: "There is substantial evidence that regular aerobic exercise such as walking, jogging, dancing or swimming is beneficial to general physical and psychological health" (see Chapter 16).

At first glance, the evidence seems to indicate that as a public heath policy issue, physical activity should indeed be promoted. As indicated above, there are a large number of studies indicating that substantial health benefits and significant saving to the health care system would accrue from only small increments of increased rates of physical activity. There is also reason, however, to be cautious when making prognostications about the public health benefits of exercise promotion. First, as Nicholl *et al.* (1994) point out, the relationship between physical fitness and physical exercise might be at least partially accounted for by the possibility that healthy people exercise more than unhealthy people. Second, not all exercise is beneficial. While prescriptions for the types and amounts of exercise have varied considerably in recent years, there is broad consensus that adequate amounts of activity for benefit are "by no means extreme" (Morris *et al.* 1980). This is to say, then, that activity that is more intense or of longer duration might potentially invoke costs associated with injury that exceed the benefits (see McCutcheon *et al.* 1997). As Waddington (2000) has suggested:

> In short, to suggest that a thirty minute gentle swim three times a week is good for one's health does not mean that running 70 miles a week as a means of preparing for running marathons is good for one's health in an equally simple or unproblematic way. Indeed it might be noted that one of the American studies, which found that death rates generally went down as levels of physical activity increased, also found a reversed trend at the highest levels of physical activity.

Third, there has been relatively little research attention paid to the costs attached to injury (for example, direct medical costs incurred through attendance at emergency departments at hospitals, costs associated with rehabilitation from injury with professionals such as physiotherapists, or time lost from work) associated with participation in physical activity. Clearly, for informed public health policy initiatives around physical activity promotion both the benefits and the costs have to be assessed.

It is to the incidence and cost of such physical activity-related injuries that we now turn. Before doing so, it is important to make the proviso that this area of research remains in its formative stages. There are many competing, sometimes contradictory, patterns of findings in the literature. For example, there are some, such as McCutcheon *et al.* (1997), who have concluded from a secondary analysis of Canadian national survey data that "employee absenteeism due to sport-related injuries are quite inconsequential." In other reports, though (see, for example, Nicholl *et al.* 1991: foreword) it has been suggested that "sports injuries are not uncommon, affect a large number of people and make considerable demands on the nation's health services." Elsewhere, professionals working "in the field" have reported on their personal experiences. As a pair of emergency room physicians at a hospital adjacent to a Canadian ski resort concluded:

> If the number of injuries seen on the ski hills occurred on a section of highway, that section of highway would be closed down (Dr. Harry O'Halloran).

> If ski injuries were caused by a virus, they would be viewed as a major public health issue (Dr. John McCall) (Taylor 2000: D1).

In order to make sense of this area of research, I will first examine evidence on the incidence of injury. Subsequently, the economic costs of injury will be evaluated.

The Injury Toll

Sport injuries are perhaps more common than popularly believed. In what follows below, I will substantiate this view by reviewing the existing research on injury incidence. This is not a simple task given a conclusion offered by Koplan *et al.* (1985) that data enabling the calculation of exercise-related morbidity and attendant costs are essentially non-existent. As might be expected from this statement, the bulk of the studies available have been published relatively recently.

In order to make sense of the previous research on incidence of sport injuries, I will first attend to findings from large sample surveys. These sources of data will give us some sense of the extent of sport injury in broad populations and an understanding of the significance of sport injury as a public health issue. Following this I will turn to more specific issues such as the injury rates among particular groups of people or in different types on activities.

Since the mid-1980s, data from large-scale surveys have become available on rates of sport injuries for Canada, the U.S., Australia and the U.K. For Canada, there are four main sets of findings. The first findings, published by McCutcheon *et al.* (1997), were taken from the 1988 Campbell's Survey of Well-Being in Canada. From a nationally representative sample of Canadians age 18 and over it was found that 10.1% of respondents had experienced a sport injury in the previous 12 months. Slightly more than 13% of males had been injured, whereas 7.4% of women had experienced a sport-related injury. These estimates for the general Canadian population were somewhat higher than estimates from a 1987 Gallup Survey in the U.S. which was designed to examine the incidence of sports injuries among individuals who participated in recreational sporting activity. The rates from the U.S. survey for the previous two years were similar to the one year Canadian rate. The 2-year rates for the U.S. survey for adults were 14% for men and 6% for women. McCutcheon *et al.* (1997) suggested that the higher rates for Canadians might have been attributable to the greater popularity of the sports of ice hockey and downhill skiing in Canada. These sports yield relatively high levels of injuries among participants.

The second Canadian survey of injury rates was conducted for the province of Quebec (Impact Recherché 1993). The study examined the participation patterns of Quebec residents aged six years and older and the patterns of injuries requiring treatment by a health professional. The overall prevalence injury rate recorded in the study was 4.8% (400 injuries from a sample of 8,365 respondents). It was further estimated that 286,000 injuries were sustained in Quebec in 1991.

The third set of findings, a replication of the Quebec study, came from a large sample survey for the province of Ontario (McClaren 1996). The findings indicated that 7.4% of the total population over the age of five years in 1995 had been injured in the previous 12 months. The rates for males and females were 9.4 and 5.4% respectively. The prevalence rates for individuals who had participated in sport and physical recreation was 9.6%. An estimated 750,000 injuries (471,000 to males and 279,000 for females) were sustained by the Ontario population in 1995.

The final, and fourth set of injury findings for Canada comes from analyses of Statistics Canada's 1987 General Social Survey (Ministry of Culture, Tourism and Recreation Communiqué, April 1993). The patterns of findings indicated that for Canadians aged 15 and older, sport/recreation injuries were the most common type of injury, accounting for 29% of all injuries (42% for Canadians aged 15–24). Almost two-thirds (65%) of an estimated 430,000 injuries suffered during participation in sport/recreation activities were sustained by males.

In the U.S., Burt and Overpeck (2001) sought to estimate the proportion and characteristics of sport- and nonsport-related injury presented to hospital emergency rooms. Data from 16,997 emergency department encounters were analysed from the 1997 and 1998 National Hospital Ambulatory Medical Care Survey. After sample weights were applied to provide national estimates it was projected that there were an average of 2.6 million emergency visits by persons between the ages of five and 24 years, and 3.7 million visits for persons of all ages. As a proportion of total visits, sport-related injuries accounted for almost one quarter of the visits by persons five to 24 years old. The visit rate was twice as high for males as females.

According to another U.S. study, there are approximately 4.4 million sport injuries among Americans aged from five to 17 each year, 1.4 million of them serious. Over one third of all accidents happen in sport and recreational activities. Boys experienced nearly twice as many injuries as girls (Bijur *et al*. 1995). Elsewhere, Rutherford and Miles (1981), in their report to the U.S. Consumer Products Safety Commission, reported five million medically-treated injuries in the 15 most popular sports over a 12 month period. Injury estimates for winter sports alone extended to 800,661 injuries requiring medical care in 1999. Snow skiing accounted for the largest proportion of those injuries with 276,00, followed by ice hockey with 149,074 (Orthopaedics Update 2000).

It should also be noted that an American study, which found that death rates generally went down as levels of physical activity increased, also found a reversed trend at the highest levels of physical activity (Paffenbarger *et al*. 1986). The authors cautioned that this finding may have been a manifestion of their research method, although they also posited that it might have indicated factors that become hazardous with high levels of vigorous activity.

A study of the cost effectiveness of a safety intervention into the sport of softball gives a powerful indication of the preventability of many types of sport injuries (see Janda 1997). In the mid-1980s, Janda *et al*. (1986) determined that among 40 million recreational players in the U.S., 70% of all softball injuries were due to players sliding into base. Following further surveillance and a review of preventive techniques (Janda *et al*. 1988a) a study of the effectiveness of break-away bases was initiated. Subsequent findings (Janda *et al*. 1988b) found a 96% reduction in sliding-related injuries and a 99% reduction in associated health care costs. Subsequent calculations made in combination with the U.S. Centre for Disease Control estimated that if all bases in the U.S. were converted from stationary to break-away models there would be a reduction of 1.7 million injuries per year.

An interesting demographic dimension in recent years in the U.S. has been the growth of injuries to people of the "baby boomer" generation (aged 35–54).

An estimated 1 million boomers suffered medically-treated sport injuries in 1998. Those treated in emergency rooms rose by 33% from 276,000 to 365,000 from 1991 to 1998 (Consumer Products Safety Review 2000). It has also been reported that from 1987 to 1995 there was a 17% increase in patients seeing orthopedic surgeons for knee complaints, an increase largely attributed to baby boomers taking up active lifestyles (*Globe and Mail*, Nov. 8, 1995). While the growth in "boomer injuries" was attributed partly to greater number of people in that cohort, recent data for Americans aged 65 and over suggest that sport injury rates have increased over and above the growth in that section of the population (Rutherford & Schroeder 1998). Over a seven-year period from 1990 to 1997 sport-related injuries in this group rose from 34,000 to 53,000; an increase of 54%.

In Australia, although sport injury-related costs have been identified as a public health problem (Commonwealth Department of Human Services and Health 1994; Finch & McGrath 1997), systematic data collection on a national scale are currently not available (Finch & Owen 2001). Among the few published sources, Egger (1991) has estimated sport injuries at one million per year, with 200,000 regarded as serious and 40,000 requiring hospitalisation or surgical intervention (see also Centre for Health Promotion and Research 1990). Most of the remaining available data offer regional estimates. In New South Wales there are 10,000 hospitalisations due to sport injuries each year among young people with 54% of young people experiencing an injury in a six month period (Northern Sydney Area Health Service 1997). Based on a formula developed by the Monash University Accident Research Centre, these 10,000 hospitalisations were projected to indicate that over 2 million sport injury accidents occur among young people in the state each year. A recent study published by Finch *et al.* (1999) found that 27% of people injured during sport and physical activity in the Latrobe Valley required treatment, with 35% experiencing some negative effect from the injury on the quality of their life and 36% reporting that their injury had inhibited further participation. Hockey and Knowles (2000) of the Queensland Injury Research Unit indicate from data gathered from emergency departments at 9031 hospitals that 10% of all patients arriving for treatment were sport-related. Of these, 60% resulted from playing different forms of football (e.g. Australian Rules, Rugby Union, Rugby League, Soccer), 80% were sustained playing traditional organised sport forms, and males outnumbered females by a ratio of three to one.

The most comprehensive study of sport injuries to date was conducted in the U.K. by Nicholl *et al.* (1991; see also Nicholl *et al.* 1994, 1995). One of the few studies to attempt to quantify both the incidence and the costs of sport injuries, the project was commissioned by and carried out for the Research Unit of the Sports Council in the U.K. The purpose of the study was to:

> Make national estimates of the incidence and patterns of exercise
> related morbidity (on both a per capita and an exposure to risk
> basis) and to estimate the injury risk in different sub-groups of the
> population and for different activities (Nicholl *et al.* 1991: 4).

Their objective was also to suggest where research strategies for injury prevention might best be directed, so as to maximise the health benefits of exercise.

Data were collected for a large representative random sample of the population of England and Wales between the ages of 16 and 45 years. The survey itself involved a postal questionnaire which was sent to 28,857 respondents who were selected at random from lists of family physicians. 7,829 respondents from the 17,564 usable responses had participated in vigorous exercise or sport. Of these, 1,429 or 18% had been injured in the previous four weeks and they reported a total of 1,803 separate injuries in 1,705 incidents. Three-quarters of all injury incidents occurred in men.

Soccer accounted for 28.9% of all injury incidents. No other activity contributed more than 10% of all injury incidents. When combined, three activities associated with "fitness" (running, weight training and keep fit) were responsible for about the same number of injury incidents as soccer. In terms of risk per occasion of participation the higher risks were associated with contact/collision sports. Rugby was the "most dangerous" sport with an injury rate of 59.3 injuries per 100 participants per four weeks; a finding consistent with Hume & Marshall's (1994) study of sport injury in New Zealand. Soccer was the second most dangerous sport followed by martial arts, field hockey and cricket. Just over half of injuries (56%) were categorised as "extrinsic," meaning that they had resulted from being struck with objects (like balls), falls, or collisions with other people or equipment. The remainder of the injuries were "intrinsic" and were caused by factors such as over-exertion or over-use.

To arrive at an estimate of the annual incidence of sport injury in England and Wales the number of injury incidents in the sample were weighted and multiplied. The resulting estimate indicated 19.3 million new injury incidents during the year as a consequence of participation in vigorous activities. Approximately one half of these incidents (9.8 million) were potentially serious involving things like fractures, dislocations, or head injuries, or required medical attention or restriction of normal activity for those injured. With an additional estimated 10.4 million recurrent injury incidents (the reinjuring of a previous injury) per year, there was a calculated total of 29.7 million injury incidents during the year.

A portion of the research literature on sport injury deals with the tragic issue of injury with catastrophic outcomes. As Mueller *et al.* (1996: 1) have suggested:

Catastrophic athletic injuries, although accounting for a small percentage of all catastrophic injuries, are tragic events affecting the lives of mostly young healthy individuals. For example, of the 2,500 new cases of paraplegia and the 1,050 new cases of quadriplegia in the United States each year, about 7% (174 paraplegia and 74 quadriplegia) are related to sports injury. Of the 410,000 people who sustain brain injury each year, 17,600 are left with some kind of permanent disability. About 10% of brain injuries are the result of sport or recreational activity.

Canadian data collected for a 12 month period spanning 1991 and 1992 for the province of Ontario (Sport and Recreation Research Communiqué, July 1993) reported on serious and catastrophic (fatal or permanently disabling) sport/recreational injuries. A total of 561 cases were reported over the 12 month period from eleven regional trauma centres and from the office of the Chief Coroners of the Province of Ontario. 220 of these cases were fatalities. Four activities — snowmobiling, bicycling, boating (including fishing from a boat) and swimming — accounted for 52% of all cases and 73% of the fatalities. Approximately 85% of the cases recorded involved males.

In the U.K., statistics for fatal accidents during sport and leisure activities were calculated by Nicholl *et al.* (1991) from data made available by the Office of Population Censuses and Surveys. For the eight year period from 1982 to 1989, there were an average of 100 fatal accidents that occurred during sport activities (799 total). Air sports (such as hang-gliding and sky-diving), motor sports, horse riding and water sports accounted for the bulk of these fatalities. In terms of risk of fatality, however, even in a high risk sport like climbing the rate of death is very low at one death per 100,000 occasions of participation.

Athletes who participate at the highest levels of amateur and professional sport have a different relationship to the costs of injury. To this end, I will now review evidence from elite sport. To professionals, injury can mean lost income and to team owners and sport promoters injury means lost production. The expression "I went to a boxing match and a hockey game broke out" is a humourous "take" on the culture of professional ice hockey in North America. Behind the humour lie some grim statistics which are testament to the toll that hockey plays on the bodies its players. As Smith (1987: 15–16) indicated from his collation of injury data, "4,723 NHL man-games were lost in the 1984–1985 season owing to injury. The estimated injury bill for a single NHL team is between $500,000 and $1 million per season."

As Waddington (2000) has suggested, for elite performers to succeed in modern sport they have to train more intensely, for more extended periods of time, and start at an early age. The results of training may be extraordinary performance either in amateur or professional sport, but athletes may also pay a price for such intense training. One way in which their bodies may respond is to break down from overuse. They may also attempt to perform despite injury and/or develop injuries that become chronic. As Donohoe and Johnson (1986: 93) have noted, the "long-term effects of overuse injuries are not known, but some concerned doctors have asked whether today's gold medallists could be crippled by arthritis by the age of 30." Further statistics for injuries come from Canadian professional football. Smith (1987) reported 462 man-games lost in the 1981 Canadian Football League season owing to injury. On a broader level, no sport workplace creates injury with such regularity and severity in the U.S. as professional football (Adams *et al.* 1987). The evidence is striking, as Guttmann (1978: 161–162) has reported:

> The percentage of players incurring injuries severe enough to cause them to miss at least one game a season is over 100%; this means not that every NFL player is injured at least once every season, but that those who are not injured are more than offset by those who are injured several times. The average length of a playing career has dropped to 3.2 years, which is not long enough to qualify a player for inclusion into the league's pension plan.

In another study of National Football League injuries, Underwood (1979) reported that almost every player was injured at some point during a four-month span. The toll effected on the bodies of these athletes has been summarised as follows by Young (1993):

> No workplace matches football for either the regularity or severity of injury . . . football injuries may include arthritis, concussion, fracture, and, most catastrophically, blindness, paralysis, even death . . . a review of heat stresses such as cramp, exhaustion, and stroke related to amateur and professional football . . . reported 29 player deaths between 1968 and 1978 . . . the 1990 season represented the first in over 60 years without a player death (p. 377).

Comparisons across professional sport show that some sports are more dangerous than others. In an Australian comparison of rates of injury (the percentage of players missing through injury at any given time), professional cricket was shown to have a lower rate of injury at 7% (Orchard & James 2001) as compared to Australian Rules Football (15%), Rugby League (16%) and Rugby Union (13%) (Seward *et al.* 1995).

A similar sport-specific analysis in the U.K. examined soccer injuries among professional players. This analysis was carried out by the sport's organising body, The Football Association, from July 1997 to May 2000. Data from 91 of the 92 clubs revealed 6,030 injuries among 2,376 professional players. Furthermore, at any one time 10% of all the players in the study were unable to practice and each player missed, on average, four games a season (Chaudhary 2001).

The literature cited above has had much to offer in moving toward a better understanding of the relationship between physical activity (whether it be sport, exercise or physical recreation) and injury. With a few notable exceptions (Nicholl *et al.* 1994; Reijnen & Velthuijsen 1989; Van Puffelen *et al.* 1989), however, cost/benefit analyses assessing the public health consequences of injuries suffered from physical activity have not been factored in to the formulation of initiatives designed to promote physical activity in the population.

The Costs of Injury

This section will report on findings gleaned from a disparate body of research assessing the costs of injury suffered during physical activity. The emphasis here will be mainly on economic costs. As Tolpin and Bentkover (1986: 38) suggest:

> Economic costs of injuries are of two types: direct and indirect. Direct costs are those expenditures paid for by the patient, the patient's family, and third party reimbursement agencies. In particular, these expenditures result from the explicit outlay of resources necessary to diagnose and treat the injury under consideration. Direct costs of sports injuries thus include the costs of injury room and/or hospital treatment, physicians, dentists and other professional services, drugs, medical supplies, physical therapy, rehabilitation services, and follow-up care... Indirect costs are not directly associated with the care of the injury but are incurred as a result of the injury. The costs result primarily from reduced productivity and increased morbidity and mortality.

The main focus here will be a discussion of the aggregate costs of sport- and exercise-related injury. In looking at costs to nation-states or to regions of countries, very little attention will be paid to various social costs that might be accrued as a consequence of sport injury. For example, disruptions of a psycho-social nature either to injury victims or to families and friends will not be evaluated mostly because there has been insufficient research to date to warrant a review.

Other short- and long-term effects of a sport injury can cause a victim to lose a job, suffer family dislocation, enter into economic dependence, lose educational opportunities, incur legal expenses and so on. These are important issues with real and severe ramifications. Again, however, broad-based research on these issues is not extensive enough for a review to be conducted.

In discussing costs, the measures themselves found in the research to date are multitudinous. Existing reports have included: (a) aggregate costs of injury to health care systems in various countries or regions of countries; (b) the economic cost to a community of foregone productivity resulting when people are unable to work; (c) costs of injury as incurred by individuals in terms of the financial burden associated with treatment and rehabilitation, and with income foregone resulting from time away from work; (d) costs as measured by time away from training and physical activity; and (e) costs for professional sport organisations and individual athletes resulting from inability to compete through injury.

In Canada, there have been a number of studies undertaken to assess the economic impact of sports injuries. In 1986, the Environics Research Group (1987) conducted a study on behalf of the Ontario Sports Medicine and Safety Advisory Board. Based on a sample of 700 Ontario residents, this study projected that 1.3 million people are injured in Ontario each year at a total cost of between C$1.8 and 3.2 billion. This estimate far exceeded those arrived at by a series of studies on the economic costs of injury that have been conducted under the auspices of the Ontario Ministry of Culture, Tourism and Recreation (later the Ministry of Citizenship, Culture and Recreation).

The first of these studies estimating the economic cost of sport/recreation-related injury was reported for the period October 1988 to September 1989 and was based on data from three different sources (Ministry of Culture, Tourism and Recreation, April 1993). First, data made available by the Ontario Office of the Chief Coroner indicated that 213 accidental fatalities were recorded. The costs associated with these fatalities were calculated to include C$584,060 in direct medical costs and C$184,741,936 in value of lost time/productivity. Second, data taken from a survey of catastrophic and serious sport/recreational injuries in Ontario identified 34 permanently disabling injuries (in which the individual is left permanently disabled and requires lifetime care). The combined costs of the two categories exceeded C$21 million. The remaining "other" injuries (an estimated 70% of which were thought to require medical attention) were compiled from Canada's 1987 General Social Survey (Statistics Canada 1987) and resulted in associated costs in excess of C$67 million. All told, the 12-month cost of sport injuries for 1998/1999 was estimated to be over C$428 million, of which C$155 million was taken up in direct medical costs to the taxpayer.

The second study was conducted by SportSmart Canada in order to gather information of serious and catastrophic sport/recreation injury in Ontario (Sport and Recreation Research Communiqué 1993). Over a twelve month period beginning July 1, 1991 a total of 561 injuries were reported (220 of them being fatal). Based on an economic cost model developed by the Ministry the costs associated with the 541 cases that had complete data were calculated. Costs were reported for the following categories: fatal injuries ($N = 219$); permanently disabling injuries ($N = 19$); and, serious non-disabling injuries. The costs (in 1988 Canadian dollars) were as follows. For fatal injuries, the direct medical costs were C$372,300, the related expenses were C$231,045 and the value of lost time/productivity was C$183,799,866. The permanently disabling injuries generated C$17,788,932 in direct medical costs and C$12,252,277 in lost time/productivity. Serious non-disabling injuries cost Ontario taxpayers C$10,086,425 in direct medical expenses and C$414,900 in lost time/productivity. Summed across categories of injury the total costs of injury in 1991/1992 were estimated at C$224,945,745.

A third study, conducted in 1995 by the Institute of Social Research at York University and funded by the Ontario Ministry of Citizenship, Culture and Recreation yielded further estimates of cost associated with sport-related injuries (Sport and Recreation Research Communiqué, April 1996). The telephone survey of 8,367 individuals aged six years and over provided information on 604 individuals who in the previous 12 months had sustained a sport/recreation injury serious enough to require treatment by a health professional. Extrapolations from the sample to the population of Ontario suggested that 750,000 injuries occur each year. The components of costs associated with these injuries were as follows: visits to health care professional; hospitalisations; time off work/school; and, out-of-pocket expenses. Of the reported injuries, 70% were treated initially by a family doctor or emergency room doctor and 45% of those needed at least a second appointment with a health professional. There was an average of four visits to health professionals for each injury. Four percent of those injured were hospitalised, for an average of 4.4 nights. Over half (55%) said they had to take time off work or school as a result of their injuries. An average of 10.7 days were taken off work or school. Just under half (43%) of the injured respondents reported they had incurred out-of-pocket medical expenses, with an average expenditure of $188 per person.

Following the application of a model designed to quantify the costs (adjusted to 1995 Canadian dollars) associated with these injuries (see Thomson 1990; Thomson & Richardson 1989), the projected 750,800 injuries sustained in 1995 were estimated to have had an economic cost of over C$637 million dollars. About 46% of that amount was made up by the value of lost productivity and/or foregone earnings. About 12% of the total was estimated to have been borne directly by the individual or the family of the injured. Over 42% was taken up by the costs of visits to health care professionals or hospitalisations. In addition to the estimated economic cost of over C$637 million, McClaren (1996) pointed out that if the costs of some 200 individuals who are killed every year during participation in sport and recreation and over 20 who are permanently disabled (estimated at C$245 million) the annual costs of sport- and recreation-related injuries in Ontario may be about C$900 million.

In the U.S. one of the most staggering estimates of the cost of sport injury comes from a recent report that sport injuries occurring in the Spring are the most common reason for a visit to a physician's office (www.nbc.columbus.com/health/1357842.html). Further, it was reported that sport injuries cost the US $215 billion and 147 million work days lost each year. This is an increase from the statistics tabulated by the American Orthopaedic Society for Sports Medicine for the period from 1946 to 1964 when the total cost of all medically-treated sports injuries was estimated to have been US$18 billion (based on 309 million emergency room-treated injuries) (www.aaos.org/wordhtml/press/boomer/sports.htm). The U.S. Consumer Product Safety Division reports that in 2000 there were 176,904 fractures, dislocations and strains/sprains related only to the sport of football among children age 5–18. The cost of the consequent medical treatment was US$8.1 billion (www.aos.org). The cost of winter sports in 1999 have been estimated at US$14.9 billion in medical, legal, work loss and other expenses. Downhill skiing alone cost US$5.57 billion (Orthopaedics Update 2000).

Other data for the U.S. estimate that, even among baby boomers only (aged 35–54), the cost of medically treating all sport-related injuries was US$18.7 billion in 1998 (Consumer Products Safety Review 2000). This represented a 33% increase in emergency room visits in this age group from 276,000 to 365,000 annually. For Americans aged 65 years or over the costs of emergency room treatment for sport injuries increased from US$364 million to US$516 million. Expressed in 1996 dollars this was an increase of 42% (Rutherford & Schroeder 1998).

On another research tangent, Janda et al. (1988b) conducted a study on the economic savings associated with modification to bases used in softball. Their assessment of the benefits of replacing stationary softball bases with break-away bases estimated a projected reduction of 1.7 million injuries with an attendant saving of $2 billion in health care costs annually in the U.S.

In Australia, despite recognition of the impact of physical activity for health, information about the costs of injuries has been scarce (Finch & Owen 2001). The only available published study specific to the area was by Egger (1991) who estimated that approximately one million Australians experience a sport injury each year at a cost to the Australian health budget and to the economy in general in excess of A$1 billion. In other research, Watson and Ozanne-Smith (1998) reported that, for the state of Victoria, lifetime costs of injuries (sport-related or otherwise) accounted for an estimated A$556 million. Sport injuries accounted for 21% of these costs, second only to injuries caused by transportation. A Report to the Centre for Health Promotion and Research (1990) calculated that in 1987/1988 the total direct medical costs of sport injuries in Australia were between A$333 million and A$400 million with a further A$400 million lost through work absenteeism (a combined total of about A$1 billion in 1990 prices). As a consequence of its report, the Centre for Health Promotion and Research (1990) projected that since between 30 and 50% of sport injuries are preventable, an expenditure of A$0.5 million on preventative strategies could potentially save up to A$200 million. Mathers *et al.* (1999) reported that in 1996 sport injuries accounted for almost one quarter of "disability adjusted life years" lost due to non-traffic related unintentional injury in Australia. Elsewhere, sport-related eye injuries have been estimated to cost approximately A$28 million per annum (Fong 1994).

   In New Zealand, it has been suggested that "sporting injuries are costing New Zealand a fortune" (*New Zealand Sport Monthly*, 1993: 48–50). The Accident Compensation Commission (ACC) paid out nearly NZ$100 million in 1992 in new claims. Players in four popular sports — netball, rugby union, rugby league and cricket — cost the ACC NZ$13.5 million in new claims. Total sport-related claims were similar in 1996 at NZ$97 million. Nearly one in five of the compensated injuries resulted in permanent loss or impairment of bodily function (www.hrc.govt.nz/download/pdf/I&Rcomplete2001.pdf).

   In the sport of rugby, ACC payments increased between 1990 and 2001 from NZ$9.5 million to NZ$22.9 million. The extent of this cost has been controversial because the ACC Injury Prevention Manager for Rugby Union, Margaret Youmans, has argued that ACC payments have allowed some players to rest during the week only to play rugby on the weekend. Moreover, a recent ACC-funded study conducted by the Otago Injury Prevention Research unit reported that 39% of rugby players have played against medical advice (www.nzdoctor.co.nz/nov25rugby.html).

   The largest and most comprehensive study of the cost and benefits of sports injuries in Britain (Nicholl *et al.* 1991) reported that the direct treatment costs of new and recurrent injuries were estimated at £422 million. The costs of lost production (due to days off work) were estimated at £575 million, giving a total annual cost of sporting injuries of £997million (1991: 25, 31). This figure can be compared to some extent with an estimation by the National Sports Medicine Institute that the cost of sports injuries in the U.K. each year is in excess of £500 million (Cole 1995: 32). Figures released concurrently by the Association of British

Insurers indicated that 20 million sport injuries were recorded in 1994, nearly 15 million of which were bad enough to cause the victims to miss at least one day at work. In total, there were eight million working days lost to sport injury in 1994 at a cost of £405 million to the economy (Goodbody 1995: 7).

Three years after this major study, a team from Sheffield University Medical School (Nicholl *et al.* 1994) undertook to calculate the direct healthcare costs and benefits associated with exercise. The health benefits of exercise (e.g. avoidance of certain chronic illnesses such as cardiovascular disease and osteoporosis) were weighed against the costs of treatment of exercise-related injuries. Findings showed that, while there were clear economic benefits associated with exercise for adults aged 45 and over, for younger adults (aged 15–44), the costs avoided by the disease-prevention effects of exercise (less than £5 per person per year) were more than offset by the medical costs resulting from participation in sport and exercise (approximately £30 per person per year). In other words, for every 15–44 year old who regularly participates in exercise, there is a net cost to the British taxpayer of £25 per year. The authors (1994: 109) concluded that "there are strong economic arguments in favour of exercise in adults aged 45 or over, but *not* in younger adults."

At the professional level it has been suggested that: "sport is a more violent and dangerous occupation than mining, oil drilling or deep-sea fishing and, even at lower levels, injuries are commonplace" (cited in an editorial of *Ludus*, Leicester Centre for Research into Sport and Society 1998). The physical toll that the game takes on the bodies of professional athletes is perhaps most strikingly illustrated by NHL records from 1998 showing that by mid-March of that year (i.e. not even at the end of the regular season and preceding the play-offs) 64 players had suffered some form of brain trauma, resulting in 238 man-games lost to injury (McKenzie 1998). Two years previously, there had only been 60 concussions reported for the whole season with 190 man-games lost (Shoalts 1996). In 1997, 19 players had missed at least one game through injuries suffered in fights alone by mid-February (217 man-games lost in total) (Dryden 1997). Commenting on the costs of injuries to professional hockey teams, Glen Sather, then the General Manager of the Edmonton Oilers, suggested that "The average cost of an injured player is C$10,000 a game. It's costing us C$10 million a year. A lot of these injuries can be prevented" (quoted in Strachan 1994: C6). A 1998 study of players in the Canadian Football League showed that concussion is endemic in professional football. Scott Delaney, the team physician of the Montreal Alouettes who conducted the study (cited in Brooks 1999) found that 44.8% of the 300 players questioned had suffered at least one concussion during the previous season. Injuries are also rife in professional Australian rugby. Gibbs (1993) found that

27.7% of injuries in professional rugby league are major, resulting in five or more missed games.

The long term injury effects for former professional athletes also appear to often be debilitating. Meir *et al.* (1997) reported that 4–6% of retired professional rugby players experience long-term job limitations, medical costs and loss of income as a result of injuries sustained during their career. In professional soccer, the preliminary results from a study conducted at Coventry University (Hicks 1998) show that of 284 former professional football (soccer) players, 49% had been diagnosed with osteoarthritis, a rate of incidence five times higher than that in similarly aged males in the general population. Fifteen percent of all respondents were registered disabled while a third of ex-players had, since retiring from professional football, undergone surgery for football-related injuries.

In the U.S. many former National Football League players experience serious health problems. An editorial in *The Sunday New York Times* (2002: 22) suggested that "many former professional football players end up so debilitated that they can barely function in later life . . . degenerative arthritis is rampant . . . afflicting almost half of retired players." The results of a 1994 study commissioned by the National Football League Players Association and conducted at Ball State University revealed that two out of every three former NFL players reported diminished ability to participate in sports and other recreation during retirement and more than half had a curtailed ability to engage in physical labour (cited in Nack 2001). Moreover, injuries seemed to be getting more serious over time as indicated by the 30% increase from 1959 to the 1980s of football players who had retired because of injury.

Discussion

To date, public health strategies to promote sport and physical activity in the population have overwhelmingly assumed that the benefits of participation outweigh any potential costs associated with injury. Beyond a few studies reviewed above such as that published by Nicholl *et al.* (1991, 1994, 1995) there has not been, as yet, the development of a coherent analysis of the costs and benefits of participation and non-participation in sport, exercise and physical activity. This is a complex and important area for future research. It is important because pronouncements on what constitutes optimally increased activity levels in terms of type, duration and intensity depend on detailed assessments of both the benefits and risks for the individual in question. It is complex because opinions on what constitutes appropriate amounts and types of activity will remain in flux as long as there is insufficient evidence available to adequately guide policy makers. In sum, the promotion of physical activity needs to be informed by evidence-based strategies to develop safe participation. This will involve a clear-eyed assessment of both the benefits *and the risks* of participation.

In many ways this chapter has sounded a wake-up call. The evidence presented, when taken *in toto*, is clearly indicative that injuries sustained in sport, exercise and physical activity present a serious public health problem. Moreover, rather than merely developing reactive ways of treating injuries once they have been sustained, there is a serious need to proactively work toward *preventing* injury. Instead of allocating as many scarce resources to developing new surgical techniques for major knee injuries, there should be increased funding allocated to creating effective preventive strategies. As Janda *et al.* (1988b) have demonstrated, if factors leading to injury are identified, and if we become better able to anticipating injuries, then preventive measures can greatly diminish the severity and incidence of injury.

The various findings reported on here also show definitive gender differences in pattens of sport injury; an important issue that we must address. As consistently demonstrated in the reseach, the incidence of injury and the concomitant costs associated with those injuries are markedly higher for males than females. While boys and men are currently more susceptible to injury than girls and women, however, this may be an area of change. Females are rapidly moving into various codes of football and combat sports all of which have until recently been predominantly male preserves and the types of sports that yield higher rates of incidence of injury (White & Young 1997). Having said this, males are more likely than females to play sports associated with higher risk and to play sports in ways that more often lead to injury. With regard to the second part of that argument, White & Young (1997: 23) have suggested that:

> the way in which sport is played matters for sport injury as much as the game itself. In this regard, males are more likely than females to be socialized into ways of playing that are potentially injurious. If this pattern were challenged, the sparing of only one victim of a catastrophic sport injury would be a resounding step forward.

Research exploring the role of violent, contact, or high risk sport has associated a disregard of health with the contruction and reinforcment of a particular version of masculinity that is highly valued. Consequently, a final objective of this chapter must be to raise critical questions about the the gendered relationship between sport and health. The task remains to interrogate and challenge contemporary reverence for risky sport that leads to disproportionately high and preventable levels of incapacitation among males. With more and better-defined data at hand, transformative and transformational programmes aimed at improving the safety of sport, exercise and physical activity will be better informed and more effective.

References

Adams, S., Adrian, M., & Bayless, M. (Eds) (1987). *Catastrophic injuries in sport: Avoidance strategies.* Indianapolis, IN: Benchmark.

Bijur, P., Trumble, A., & Harel, Y. (1995). Sports and recreation injuries in U.S. children and adolescents. *Archives of Pediatric Adolescent Medicine, 149,* 1009–1016.

Bouchard, C., Shepard, R., Stephens, T., Sutton, J., & McPherson, B. (1990). *Exercise, fitness and health: A concensus of current knowledge.* Champaign, IL: Human Kinetics.

Brooks, J. (1999, June 29). Stars in ice. *Globe and Mail,* C8.

Burt, C., & Overpeck, M. (2001). Emergency visits for sport-related injuries. *Annals of Emergency Medicine, 37,* 301–308.

Centre for Health Promotion and Research (1990). *Sports injuries in Australia: Causes, costs and prevention.* Report to the National Better Health Program. Sydney: CHPR.

Chaudhary, V. (2001, Friday, January 26). Club loses 40 million pounds a year to injury. *The Guardian.*

Cole, J. (1995, July 1). Wimbledon foul underlines need to know insurance score. *The Guardian.*

Commonwealth Department of Human Services and Health (1994). *Better health outcomes for Australians. National goals, targets and strategies for better health outcomes into the next century.* Canberra: Australian Government Publsihing Service.

Conference Board of Canada (1996). *Physical activity and the cost of treating illness.* Special Report Series (No. 944S010): Canada Fitness and Lifestyle Research Institute.

Consumer Products Safety Review. (2000). Volume 4, No. 4.

Curtis, J., & Russell, S. (Eds) (1997). *Physical activity in human experience: Interdisciplinary perspectives.* Champaign, IL: Human Kinetics.

De Loes, M. (1997). Exposure data: Why are they needed? *Sports Medicine, 24,* 172–175.

Donahoe, T., & Johnson, N. (1986). *Foul play: Drug abuse in sports.* Oxford: Basil Blackwell.

Dryden, S. (1997, February 28). NHL knockout punches sideline host of players. *The Hockey News,* 2.

Egger, G. (1991). Sports injuries in Australia. Causes, costs and prevention. *Health Program Journal of Australia, 1,* 28–33.

Environics Research Group Limited (1987). *An examination of the economic costs of sport, fitness and recreation injuries in Ontario: 1986.* Report for Ontario Sports Medicine and Safety Advisory Board.

Finch, C., Cassell, E., & Stathakis, V. (1999). *The epidemiology of sport and active recreation injury in the Latrobe Valley* (Report No. 151). Melbourne: Monash University Accident Research Centre.

Finch, C., & McGrath, A. (1997). *Sportsafe Australia: A national sports safety network.* A report prepared for the Australian Sports Injury Prevention Taskforce. Canberra: Australian Sports Commission.

Finch, C., & Owen, N. (2001). Injury prevention and the promotion of physical activity: What is the nexus? *Journal of Science and Medicine in Sport, 4,* 77–87.

Fong, L. (1994). Sport-related eye injuries. *The Medical Journal of Australia, 160,* 743–750.

Gibbs, N. (1993). Injuries in professional rugby league: A three-year prospective study of the South Sydney professional rugby league football club. *American Journal of Sports Medicine, 21,* 696–700.

Goodbody, J. (1995, June 7). Injury time costs economy 405 million pounds. *The Guardian,* 7.

Guttmann, A. (1978). *From ritual to record.* New York: Columbia University Press.

Hicks, R. (1998, December). Arthritis and the professional footballer. *Football Decision,* 22–23.

Hockey, R., & Knowles, M. (2000). *Sports Injuries.* Injury Bulletin No. 59, Queensland Injury Surveillance Unit.

Hume, P., & Marshall, S. (1994). Sports injuries in New Zealand: Exploratory analyses. *New Zealand Journal of Sports Medicine, 22,* 18–22.

Impact Recherché (1993). *Sondage sur les blessures subies lors de al pratique d'activités récréatives et sportives entre Octobre 1992 et Septembre 1993.* Report prepared for la Régie de la Sécurité dans les sports de Québec and the Québec Ministry of Health and Social Services.

Janda, D. (1997). Sports injury surveillance has everything to do with sports medicine. *Sports Medicine, 24,* 169–171.

Janda, D., Hankin, F., & Wojtys, E. (1986). Softball injuries: Cost, cause, prevention. *American Family Physician, 33,* 143–144.

Janda, D., Wojtys, E., & Hankin, F. (1988a). Softball sliding injuries: A prospective study comparing standard and modified bases. *Journal of the American Medical Association, 259,* 1948–1959.

Janda, D., Wojtys, E., & Hankin, F. (1988b). Softball sliding injuries in Michigan 1986–1987. *MMWR Morbidity and Mortality Weekly Report, 37,* 169–170.

Jones, B., Cowan, D., & Knapik, J. (1994). Exercise, training and injuries. *Sports Medicine, 18,* 202–214.

Kesaniemi, Y., Danforth, E., Jensen, M., Kopelman, P., Lefebvre, P., & Reeder, R. (2001). *Dose-response issues concerning physical activity and health: An evidence-based symposium.* American College of Sports Medicine: Medicine and Science in Sport and Exercise, S351–S358.

Knees, young and old (1995, November 8). *Globe and Mail,* A16.

Koplan, J., Siscovick, D., & Goldbaum, G. (1985). The risks of exercise: A public health view of injuries and hazards. *Public Health Reports, 100,* 189–195.

Mathers, C., Vos, T., & Stevenson, C. (1999). *The burden of disease and injury in Australia.* AIHW Cat. No. PHE 17, Canberra: AIHW.

McCutcheon, T., Curtis, J., & White, P. (1997). The socio-economic distribution of sport injuries: Multivariate analyses using Canadian national data. *Sociology of Sport Journal*, *14*, 57–72.

McClaren, P. (1996). *A study of injuries sustained in sport and recreation in Ontario*. Unpublished Report for the Ontario Ministry of Citizenship, Culture and Recreation.

McKenzie, B. (1998, April 17). Making headway. *The Hockey News*, 3.

Meir, R., McDonald, K., & Russell, R. (1997). Injury consequences from participation in professional rugby league: A preliminary investigation. *British Journal of Sports Medicine*, *31*, 132–134.

Ministry of Culture, Tourism and Recreation (1993). *Injuries in sport and recreation* (Communiqué No. 6). Ottawa: Ministry of Culture, Tourism and Recreation.

Morris, J., Everitt, M., Pollard, R., & Chave, S. (1980, December 6). Vigorous exercise in leisure-time: Protection against coronary heart disease. *The Lancet*, 1207–1210.

Mueller, F., Cantu, R., & Van Camp, S. (1996). *Catastrophic injuries in high school and college sport*. Champaign, IL: Human Kinetics.

Nack, W. (2001, May 7). The wrecking yard. *Sports Illustrated*, 61–75.

New Zealand Sport Monthly (1993, April). *The pain factor*, 48–50.

Nicholl, J., Coleman, P., & Brazier, J. (1994). Health and health care costs and the benefits of exercise. *Pharmaco Economics*, *5*, 109–122.

Nicholl, J., Coleman, P., & Williams, B. (1991). *Injuries in exercise and sport: Main report*. London: Report to the Sports Council.

Nicholl, J., Coleman, P., & Williams, B. (1995). The epidemiolgy of sports and exercise-related injury in the United Kingdom. *British Journal of Sports Medicine*, *29*, 232–238.

Northern Sydney Area Health Service (1997). *New South Wales youth sports injury report*. Sydney: Northern Sydney Area Health Service.

Orchard, J., & James, T. (2001). Draft report to the Australian Cricket Board. www.users.bigpond.com/msn/johnorchard/ACB2001report.pdf.

Orthopaedics Update (2000). Press Release. www.aaos.org/wordhtml/press/sciwrit/00oupd1.htm.

Paffenbarger, R., Hyde, R., Wing, A., & Jung, D. (1993). The association of changes in physical activity level and other lifestyle characteristics with mortality among men. *New England Journal of Medicine*, *328*, 538–545.

Pain in Pro Football (2002, February 3). *Sunday New York Times* (Editorial), p. 22.

Quinney, Q., Gauvin, L., & Wall, A. (Eds) (1994). *Toward active living*. Proceedings of the International Conference on Physical Activity, Fitness and Health. Champaign, IL: Human Kinetics.

Reijnen, J., & Velthuijsen, J.-W. (1989). Economic aspects of health through sport. In: *Conference proceedings: Sports, an economic force in Europe* (pp. 76–90). Lilleshall, UK.

Royal College of Physicians (1991). *Medical aspects of exercise: Benefits and risks*. London: Royal College of Physicians.

Rutherford, G., & Miles, R. (1981). *Overview of sports-related injuries*. Washington, DC: Consumer Producer Safety Commission.

Rutherford, G., & Schroeder, T. (1998). *Sport-related injuries to persons 65 years of age and older*. Washington: U.S. Consumer Product Safety Commission.

Seward, H., Orchard, J., Hazard, H., & Collinson, D. (1995). *Football injuries in Australia*. Canberra: Australia Sports Commission.

Shoalts, D. (1996, December 2). MD urges more study of trauma to the head. *Globe and Mail*, A11.

Siscovick, D., Laporte, R., & Newman, J. (1985). The disease-specific benefits and risks of physical activity and exercise. *Public Health Reports, 100*, 180–188.

Smith, M. (1987). *Violence in Canadian amateur sport: A review of literature*. Report for the Commission of Fair Play. Ottawa, ON: Government of Canada.

Sport and Recreation Research Communiqué (1993, July). *Serious and catastrophic sport/recreational injuries*. Ottawa, ON: Ministry of Culture, Tourism and Recreation.

Sport and Recreation Research Communiqué (1996, April). *Injuries incurred by Ontario residents during participation in sport and other recreational activities*. Ottawa, ON: Ministry of Citizenship, Culture and Recreation.

Statistics Canada (1987). *General social survey*. Ottawa: Ministry of Supply and Services Canada.

Strachan, A. (1994, March 24). GMs take time to channel their energy. *Globe and Mail*, C6.

Taylor, M. (2000, March 5). Respect the slope. *National Post*, D1.

Thomson, D. (1990). *A study to determine the design of an economic cost model for the generic injury database in use by the safety leadership office: Program code and documentation*. Report by LGL Ltd. for the Sports and Fitness Branch, Ontario Ministry of Tourism and Recreation.

Thomson, D., & Richardson, D. (1989). *A study to determine the design of an economic cost component of the generic injury database in use by the safety leadership office*. Report by LGL Ltd. for the Sports and Fitness Branch, Ontario Ministry of Tourism and Recreation.

Tolpin, H., & Bentkover, J. (1986). The economic costs of sports injuries. In: P. Vinger & E. Hoerner (Eds), *Sports injuries: The unthwarted epidemic* (2nd ed., pp. 37–47). Littleton, MA: PSG Publishing.

Underwood, J. (1979). *The death of an American game: The crisis in football*. Boston, MA: Little and Brown.

University of Leicester Centre for Research in Sport and Society (1998, January). *Ludus, 3* (editorial).

U.S. Department of Health and Human Services (2000). *Healthy people 2000: National health promotion and disease prevention objectives*. Washington, DC: U.S. Department of Health and Human Services.

Van Mechelen, W. (1997). The severity of sports injuries. *Sports Medicine, 24*, 176–180.

Van Puffelen, F., Reijnen, J., & Velthuijsen, J. (1989). *Sport en gezondheid, economisch bezien*. Amsterdam: SEO.

Waddington, I. (2000). *Sport, health and drugs*. London: E and F N Spon.

Watson, W., & Ozanne-Smith, J. (1998). *The cost of injury in Victoria*. Report Number 124. Melbourne: Monash University Accident Research Center.

White, P., & Young, K. (1997). Masculinity, sport, and the injury process: A review of Canadian and international evidence. *Avante, 3*, 1–30.

Wood, L. (1993). *The impact of physical activity on disease incidence and the cost of treating illness: A model for estimation.* Unpublished report prepared for the Canadian Fitness and Lifestyle Research Institute.

Young, K. (1993). Violence, risk, and liability in male sports culture. *Sociology of Sport Journal, 10*, 373–396.

Chapter 18

The Role of the Courts in Sports Injury

Kevin Young

A Grade 13 Ontario ice hockey player participating in a high school tournament is left paralysed by an on-ice incident permissible within the rules of the game. The mid-ice check that causes the player to slide on "all fours," at high speed, into the boards and break his cervical spine is "legal" enough, but the circumstances leading up to the check are more controversial. The young man's parents take legal action: against the coach for negligent coaching practices, including requiring that he play on multiple shifts despite complaining of fatigue; against the school for participating in a tournament not sanctioned by the required governing body of the sport; against the arena for allowing a competitive collision sport to take place in a poorly maintained facility; and, against several other involved parties they perceive as culpable for their son's tragedy. After a prolonged legal investigation lasting over half a decade, a sizeable but ultimately unsatisfactory and incommensurate out-of-court settlement is reached. It does nothing to alter the fact that the young man, now in his mid-20s, will be a life-long quadriplegic.

Elsewhere, a professional soccer player's ankle is snapped badly in a career-ending tackle so gruesome to watch that even team-mates require months of counselling to come to terms with the event; the jaw of an adult rugby player is severely broken in three places when an opponent punches him, and hospitalisation is required; a 16-year old high school football lineman is paralysed when he is "speared" by an opponent's helmet; and, a young boxer is left with brain damage following a devastating blow to the head. These examples are not fictional. They are composites of real events and legal actions that occurred over the last 15 years; all but one of them resulted in sizeable pecuniary awards being paid to the "victims." Until recently, the chances of these episodes being litigated were slim; the chances today are much greater, even in cases where injuries appear to be the result of

Sporting Bodies, Damaged Selves
Research in the Sociology of Sport, Volume 2, 333–353
© 2004 Published by Elsevier Ltd.
ISSN: 1476-2854/doi:10.1016/S1476-2854(04)02018-7

actions occurring within the rules of a given sport, or the informal norms of its participants (Smith 1983).

As indicated in the Introduction to this volume, the many phases of pain and injury in sport can be understood along a continuum marked by causation and direct experience of injury as beginning points, and factors such as costs, health policy and legal outcomes as possible end points. It is to the last of these possibilities — how sports-related injury may be policed and punished in a formal sense — that this chapter now turns.

Traditionally, the courts have shown a clear reluctance to intervene in sports injury/sports violence cases. The control of on-field episodes between participants culminating in injury of one kind or another has been viewed as the jurisdiction of the world of sport itself — coaches, teams, leagues, and regional, national and international governing bodies. Statistically speaking, the courts, and especially the criminal courts, have seldom been resorted to. As such, and as a number of late 20th century studies have underlined (cf. Horrow 1980; Reasons 1992; Young 1993; Young & Wamsley 1996), sport has enjoyed relative immunity from the law, despite the routine and sometimes horrific injuries that have been inflicted.

Evidence suggests that, trans-Atlantically at least, and certainly in the USA and Canada, legal intervention into injury cases is a fairly recent phenomenon. For instance, Reasons (1992) argues that the Canadian courts became willing to hear sports injury cases in large numbers the 1970s and, speaking of the USA, Lubell (1989: 240) contends that "... the age of sports litigation was inaugurated in the mid-1960s when a New Jersey court awarded a gymnast more than $1 million in a negligence action and a California court awarded a[n injured] football player over $300,000." While Reasons and Lubell are correct to point to a late 20th century "surge" in legal actions, and Reasons is, arguably, also correct to contextualize these changes in broader social and political movements concerned with civil liberties and personal rights during a relatively counter-cultural phase of the post-war era (i.e. in the 1960s and 1970s in Canada and the USA), the implication that sports injury case law cannot be found prior to this time is not true, as may be witnessed in several substantial historical reviews, some of which trace legal cases back to the start of the 20th century (Barnes 1988; Gardiner *et al.* 1998; Grayson 1988; Moriarty *et al.* 1994; Young & Wamsley 1996).

Of course, not all sport injury episodes result in legal outcomes. Clearly, the majority do not, but evidence from a number of international contexts suggests that sport injury is increasingly being dealt with in a formally litigious way. This chapter will examine some of this evidence, raising questions of how sport injury cases become the purview of the law, what sorts of cases are involved, and the sorts of legal wrangles that arise. It also attends to the complicated matter of why, at the same time as formal charges are apparently being laid with greater frequency than ever before, prosecutions remain rare. Could it be that the relative immunity to serious legal accountability and assessment that most writers (cf. Barnes 1988; Lubell 1989; Reasons 1992; Young & Wamsley 1996) agree sport has traditionally enjoyed endures?

Smith's Typology of Player Violence and its Implications for Sports Injury Litigation

To date, sociologists have not done a good job of "typologising" or classifying sports injury. Much of its study, including the way in which it is tackled in this chapter, is subsumed under the broader rubric of sports violence, to which it clearly, but not always, relates. One of the most widely adopted typologies of player violence and, by implication, sport injury, was developed by the Canadian sociologist Michael Smith. In his 1983 book, *Violence and Sport*, Smith classified player violence into four basic categories, the first two being relatively legitimate and the last two relatively illegitimate in the eyes of both sports administrators and the law. While the typology has been summarized many times in the literature, it is so pertinent to sport injury study and to the legal discussion that follows that it is worth briefly revisiting here.

Brutal Body Contact: Brutal body contact includes what Smith called the "meat and potatoes" of our most popular sports, such as tackles, blocks, body checks, collisions, hits and jabs. Depending on the sport under scrutiny, these are all acts that can be found within the official rules of a given sport, and to which most would agree that consent is given or at the very least implied.

Borderline Violence: Borderline violence involves acts prohibited by the official rules of a given sport but that occur routinely and are more or less accepted by many people connected with the game. Examples might include: the fist fight in ice hockey; the late hit and personal foul in football; the "wandering" elbow in basketball, soccer, and road racing; the high tackle, "rake" (the violent use of cleats against skin) and scrum punch in rugby; and, the "beanball" (a pitch aimed deliberately at a batsman's head) or "knock-down" pitch in baseball. Importantly, all of these actions carry potential for causing injury as well as prompting further violence between players — the bench-clearing brawl in hockey, or retaliatory fighting in any of these other sports. Historically speaking, sanctions imposed by sports leagues and administrators for borderline violence have been notoriously light, and fines have sometimes been covered by the clubs themselves.

Quasi-Criminal Violence: Quasi-criminal violence violates the formal rules of a given sport, the law of the land and, to a significant degree, the informal norms of players. This type of violence usually results in serious injury that precipitates considerable official and public attention. Quasi-criminal violence in ice hockey may include "cheap shots," "sucker punches" or dangerous stick work, all of which can cause severe injury, and which often elicit in-house suspensions and fines.

Criminal Violence: Criminal violence includes behaviours so seriously and obviously outside of the boundaries of both the sport and wider conventions of social acceptability that they are handled as criminal from the outset. The Canadian case used by Smith is that of a Toronto teenage hockey player who, in 1973, assaulted and killed an opponent in the arena parking lot following a heated community game.

Though it has seldom been used in this connection, Smith's typology is, in my view, as resonant for sport injury study as it is for sport violence research; it clearly demonstrates how, in many (but again not all) cases, the two are mutually inclusive. The typology addresses what Ball-Rokeach (1971, 1980) would call the question of the "legitimacy of violence" — that is, the legitimation/delegitimation process with regard to what is perceived as acceptable violence and what is not. As we will see below, for example, since the late 1960s and the early 1970s era there appears to have been a shift in what is categorized as legitimate and illegitimate sports violence, no doubt prompted by shifting scales of public and legal tolerance when it comes to forms of interpersonal violence in general. Using Smith's categories, incidents considered a decade ago as quasi-criminal violence, borderline violence, or even brutal body contact are being more closely scrutinized in some quarters today and, where litigated, may be dealt with under criminal rather than civil law. But how are they being dealt with, and what stumbling blocks arise?

Litigious Sports Climates: Legal Wrangles and Contemporary Cases

At the root of historical and contemporary legal struggles regarding sports injury cases is the notion of consent. Used for centuries to exempt owners in risky work contexts from liability, the English common law notion of *volenti non fit injuria*, or voluntary assumption of risk, is based on the assumption of freedom of contract and assumes that all parties involved in a social engagement — which could include sport — share equal knowledge in all areas including such things as hazards, risks, and medical information. Given the physically forceful and risky nature of athletic contests, this means that many athletes must consent to a certain amount of physical harm done both by them and against them. Athletes such as boxers, footballers, ice hockey and rugby players, for instance, clearly *give* or *imply* consent to physically painful and even potentially disabling actions.

As essentially self-regulating organizations, much like those of doctors, lawyers and university professors, sports leagues have clearly preferred to practice their own versions of common law. This continues to include what can only be termed paths of non-action or even condonement (these are discussed below as patterns of *non-enforcement* and *covert facilitation*), in addition to responses such as warnings, fines, suspensions, and other forms of deterrence. Until the 1970s, such a process of self-regulation and accountability met more or less with legal approval (Barnes 1988: 97). Where litigated, sports violence cases typically troubled judicial experts, and their treatment and outcomes were characterised by variability and occasionally contradiction. This is ongoing.

Although much of the violence occurring in Canadian and American sport satisfies the requirements of assault set out in *Martin's Criminal Code* of Canada ("A person commits an assault when, without the consent of another person, he applies force intentionally to that other person," S. 244), it is equally clear that assault in sport is, in principle at least, distinguished by a degree of immunity from criminal liability: "It would seem clear that in common law . . . outside of sport, if actual body harm was intended or caused then the assault was unlawful" (1988: S.244). Evidence for inconsistent interpretation of legal jurisdiction over sports violence may be found in the now hundreds of investigations across North America collated in socio-legal research (Hechter 1976/1977; Horrow 1980, 1982; Reasons 1992). Many other examples remain scattered and hidden in case law annals.

In a review of litigated sports violence cases involving charges of some form of assault, Horrow (1982) details six common defences jeopardising judicial resolution in favour of the plaintiff: (i) the *battery and the problem of establishing intent defense* requires the plaintiff to prove that the injurious individual possessed the requisite *mens rea*, or harmful intent. This is especially difficult to do given that many jurors and court officers identify intimidation and pain as ordinary and acceptable dimensions of sport; (ii) the *assumption of risk defense* emphasises that players assume knowledge of ordinary game risks and dangers, but not including extraordinary risks. On a case-by-case basis, courts must thus distinguish injury in terms of foreseeable and unforeseeable risk-taking; (iii) the *consent defense* argues that players consent to all contact occurring in a game, regardless of outcome, and has historically proven to be one of the safest forms of testimony for defendants; (iv) the *provocation defense*, by contrast, is rarely taken seriously, partly because arguing that the defendant was provoked into retaliation undermines the ordinary dynamics of many sports; (v) the *involuntary reflex defense* has successfully been used to argue that assaultive players acted without malicious intent "in the heat of the game," and that professional sport contexts are conducive to loss of control anyway; and (vi) the *self-defense* argument legitimates the use of force by a defendant in situations where force is used against him or her. However, the defendant is limited, Horrow goes on to note, to use no more severe force than that used by the attacker.

This list is by no means exhaustive of all defenses available or those used, but it demonstrates the level of difficulty litigators have had separating illegal from aggressive and harmful, but nevertheless acceptable, play. Assumptions of *volenti* have become associated with most of them. Such is true in National Hockey League (NHL) case law (Reasons 1992). For example, the well-known 1969 *Regina vs. Green* case showed evidence that Ted Green of the Boston Bruins came off the boards and swiped his opponent Wayne Maki with the back of his glove. Maki retaliated by chopping Green on the head with his stick. In Horrow's (1980: 19) account, "Green sustained a serious concussion and massive hemorrhaging. After two brain operations, he regained only partial sensation and has never recovered 100%." While charges of assault were brought against both players, Green, having used a self-defense argument, was acquitted with the following assessment:

> No hockey player enters onto the ice of the National Hockey League without consenting to and without knowledge of the possibility that he is going to be hit in one of many ways once he is on the ice . . . we can come to the conclusion that this is an ordinary happening in a hockey game and that players really think nothing of it. If you go behind the net of a defenceman, particularly one who is trying to defend his zone, and you are struck in the face by that player's glove, a penalty might be called against him, but you do not really think anything of it; it is one of the types of risks one assumes (Horrow 1980: 186).

Predictably, fistfighting-related injuries in ice hockey, and in the NHL specifically, have drawn much attention publicly, academically, and legally. It has been a common court response to fight-related injuries to acquit defendants on similar grounds of consent. Horrow (1980: 186) cites the Ontario case of *R. vs. Starratt*, where the court argued that fistfighting was so frequent in the NHL as to be viewed "normal" as long as the force of the fight "does not exceed that level authorized by the other players." The significant point here is that the courts have simultaneously been willing to find aggressive athletic conduct to be outside the jurisdiction of social acceptability, but also willing to consider whether pro-aggression norms that pervade the value systems of many sport subcultures need to be factored in as mitigating factors (Smith 1983; Young 1990, 1993). *Few other social institutions enjoy this privilege.*

In brief, however hurt and injured, combatants have traditionally been understood to either express or imply consent to certain levels of force used against them, except in cases of extraordinarily savage and injurious attacks. Thus, as tolerated as sports violence and sports injury cases have been historically, their presence in tort and criminal law, coupled with what appears to be a decreasing social tolerance toward aspects of violence generally in many Western societies, has led litigators to more stringently re-evaluate certain sports offenses as excessive and unjustifiable (White 1986). Contrary to its legal conventions, *volenti* does not imply *absolute consent,* but consent *only as a matter of degree.* Absolute interpretations of *volenti* are further diluted by acts of violence causing injury occurring outside the rules of the games, or after the play has stopped, neither of which are given direct or implied consent by players. This is also true of negligent supervisory and administrative circumstances giving rise to sports injury, such as the case summarised at the outset of this chapter, and the cases summarised in the following section.

While there has been no systematic tally of litigated sports violence/injury cases involving grievances initiated by players against other players (John Barnes' book *Sport and the Law in Canada,* 1988, remains the most comprehensive and considered source in this regard), a review of the case law suggests that their numbers are growing. As White (1986: 1030–1034) has argued,

> There is a clear trend that the criminal justice systems in Canada and the United States are becoming more and more willing to control illegal violence in sports ... Canadian prosecutors have used the criminal law ... frequently against athletes accused of violently injuring fellow players. There have been more than one hundred criminal convictions for offences involving player-player violence in the last fifteen years [approximately 1970–1985].

Of the very few quantitative studies that do exist, Watson and MacLellan's Canadian study (1986) found 66 cases of player vs. player assault charges related to ice hockey injuries (including six civil suits and 60 criminal charges) between 1905 and 1982; 75% of their cases occurred in the later phase of that period, between 1972 and 1982. To date, case law indicates that charges and convictions for assault causing bodily harm are most widespread, although criminal charges of common assault, and even manslaughter and homicide, are being heard (Reasons 1992: 25).

Along with boxing, hockey appears most frequently in criminal reports, especially in Canada. Indeed, as Reasons notes, "It may be said that Canada leads the common law world in criminally prosecuting its athletes for criminal violence [and the injuries it causes]" (1992: 8). While the amateur game seems particularly cluttered with "hockey crimes," similar cases may be found at the professional level. In one of the most documented late twentieth century cases, Dino Ciccarelli of the Minnesota North Stars was convicted in an Ontario court. Among other evidence proving *mens rea*, Ciccarelli told the court that in using his stick violently, he was "probably trying to intimidate" the plaintiff (*R. vs. Ciccarelli* 1988). Although the latter was not seriously hurt, Ciccarelli was convicted on charges of common assault. Hockey observers will note that many of the issues raised in the Ciccarelli case were repeated in the first major litigated NHL case of the 21st century — the case of *Marty McSorley vs. Donald Brashear* (described below; Atkinson in press), as well as in subsequent cases of hockey "crimes."

However, prosecuting athletes for the injuries their behaviour causes is not restricted to the sport of ice hockey or to Canada. A cluster of sports have been affected, some surprising,[1] and a number of precedent-setting cases from other international contexts indicate a similar move toward legal intervention into and criminalization of sports violence/sports injury. What appear to be shifting scales of public and official tolerance have been brought into sharp relief by several highly publicised cases, such as the following:

---

[1] It is true that most sports violence/sports injury cases that become litigated occur in the "predictable" sports — that is, contact, collision and otherwise physically high-risk sports such as gridiron football, ice hockey, rugby, boxing, etc. However, some perhaps more surprising sports, such as horse racing, have also been litigated ("Jockeys Cleared of Ending Rival's Career in Fall," *The Independent*, February 2 2001: 13). Similarly, following a series of high-profile accidents in the hazardous sport of auto racing, such as the death of Canadian driver Greg Moore at the 1998 Molson Toronto Indy (*Calgary Herald*, November 1 1999: C6) and the horrifying crash of Italian Formula One driver Alex Zanardi who lost both legs in a 200 mph smash at an event in Germany in the same year (*News of the World*, February 10 2002: 64), drivers and racing officianados are asking increasingly critical questions regarding whether sponsor and fan requirements for speed meet reasonable risk and safety expectations. Perhaps the best known litigated case from the world of Formula One auto racing relates to the death of Brazilian driver Ayrton Senna. As one newspaper wrote of litigation connected to the case: "Two acquittals in the 1994 death of Formula One star Ayrton Senna were thrown out by Italy's highest court, and a new trial is expected this year for Williams' technical director Patrick Head and former team designer Adrian Newey. Senna, a three-time world champion, died when his Williams-Renault car slammed into a concrete wall during the San Marino Grand Prix. The prosecution contended a poorly modified steering column broke as the Brazilian driver entered a curve, causing him to lose control. Newey, now with the McLaren team Head, team owner Frank Williams and three race officials were accused of manslaughter but were cleared in December 1997" (*Calgary Herald*, January 29 2003: F4).

1994 (February) — The Jimmy Boni Case (European Ice Hockey): Boni, a Canadian-raised player in the Italian Hockey League, retaliated, when punched, by slashing his opponent, Miran Schrott, in the chest with his stick. Schrott fell to the ice and never regained consciousness. Initially charged with intentional homicide and facing up to 18 years in prison, Boni eventually pled guilty to the reduced charge of manslaughter, and was fined $1,800 Canadian (*Macleans*, February 28 1994: 11).

1994 (December) — The Howard Collins Case (Welsh Rugby): Rugby player Howard Collins was sentenced to up to six months in jail for stomping on an opponent's head during a game played between Welsh rugby teams Pencoed and Cardiff Institute. The head wounds suffered by his opponent, Christian Evans, required ten stitches and plastic surgery (*Calgary Herald*, December 22 1994: D2).

1995 (February) — The Eric Cantona Case (English Soccer): Manchester United's star player during the 1990s, Frenchman Eric Cantona, was charged with common assault for his "kung-fu" style assault on a taunting Crystal Palace fan during a regular Premier League game. Cantona pled guilty to the act and to injuring the fan, and was sentenced to two weeks in jail (*Calgary Herald*, March 24 1995: D3).

1995 (May) — The Duncan Ferguson Case (Scottish Soccer): Ferguson, a Scot with three previous convictions for assault, was sentenced to three months in jail for head-butting and injuring an opponent during a Scottish Premier Division game in 1994. He served 44 days in a Glasgow prison (*Toronto Star*, May 26 1995: C10; *Calgary Herald*, October 12 1995: C1).

1996 (February) — The Simon Devereux Case (English Rugby): British rugby player Devereux was found guilty on charges of grievous bodily harm and jailed for nine months by an English court for punching his opposing captain, Jamie Cowie. His jaw broken in three places, Cowie spent five nights in hospital and was forced out of the game for eight months (*The Sun*, February 23 1996: 16).

2000 (February) — The Marty McSorley Case (National Hockey League): Marty McSorley of the Boston Bruins was charged with assault after striking Vancouver Canuck Donald Brashear over the head with his stick. After crumpling to the ice and going into convulsions, Brashear recuperated fully. Judge William Kitchen in the case found McSorley guilty of assault with a weapon. McSorley received an 18-month conditional discharge at the end of which, barring any further incidents, he would not have a criminal record (*Maclean's*, October 16 2000: 17; Atkinson in press).

2001 (January) — The Ian Powell Case (Welsh Rugby): Charged with causing grievous bodily harm, Welsh rugby player Ian Powell of Gwernyfed RFC was jailed for six months for kicking an opponent, Ashley Barnett, who suffered a double fracture of the leg and had to give up the sport (*The Daily Telegraph*, April 7 2001: 7).

Additionally, an English newspaper report from 2002 compiled the following summary list of recent soccer "Challenges that Cost Dear" from that country:

> Bradford City striker Gordon Watson received £900,000 after suing defender Kevin Gray and his club Huddersfield Town over a tackle which left him out of the game for 18 months. Former Sheffield Wednesday player Ian Nolan sued after he was left with one leg shorter than the other because of a challenge by Tottenham Hotspur's Justin Edinburgh. Paul Elliott sued after his Chelsea career was ended by a collision with Dean Saunders. Saunders, who was playing for Liverpool, was acquitted of recklessness and negligence. In the 1993–1994 season, an aerial challenge between Spurs defender Gary Mabbutt and Wimbeldon's John Fashanu caused multiple fractures to Mabbutt's cheekbone and eye-socket. He did not sue but complained to the Football Association to "highlight the types of injuries that have been caused." The FA took no action as it proved impossible to conclude whether Fashanu intended harm (*Leicester Mercury*, Tuesday, July 9 2002: 3).

While, again, it is difficult to quantify the extent or frequency of these sorts of cases (this "counting" and collating work has not been done systematically), such cases suggest something of a trend, at least in certain countries, toward legal intervention into, and the criminalization of, sports violence and sports injury cases. The incidents summarised here, drawn from professional or top-level amateur sport, are examples of sports-related injuries entering the jurisdiction of either civil or criminal law in numbers that did not occur with as much regularity in earlier stages of the twentieth century. These cases represent a time span of approximately 10 years; over the same brief period, dozens of similar incidents at the amateur and recreational level, including college, high school and community sport, have resulted in criminal charges (most often of assault and assault inflicting injury), litigation, and prosecution in all of the countries named. These are not high profile cases that appear on the front pages of national newspapers or on televised news programmes; rather, they involve relatively unknown names and their coverage tends to be restricted to community and local media sources, as the following trans-Atlantic examples indicate. In a 1995 case that hardly shook the world of Canadian football, an unknown college player successfully sued an opponent for an on-field hit that left him unconscious and suffering a double fracture of the jaw and received substantial pecuniary damages (*Globe and Mail*, September 30 1995: A24). In a similarly low-key case from Great Britain, an amateur footballer was awarded £13,500 in an out-of-court settlement after having his right leg broken in a vicious tackle in a Saturday League game (*Leicester Mercury*, Tuesday, July 9 2002: 3). Indeed, even a loosely organised content analysis of the contemporary British press indicates a clearly litigious culture at all levels of rugby and soccer ("Soccer Assailant Jailed on Appeal," *The Guardian*, February 2 1994: 8; "Prop Fined £1000 for Punching Opponent," *The Times*, February 2 1997; "Footballer Sues over Tackle that Broke His Legs," *The Times*, October 14 1997: 8; "British Rugby Player Jailed for Kick," *The Independent*, April 7 2001: 13; "Rugby Player is Guilty of Assault," *Leicester Mercury*, October 29 2001: 16).

Widening the Circle of Culpability

In an earlier paper (Young 1993), I used a victimological approach to examine how sports injury results not only from that nature of athletic acts, but also from their organization (ownership, management, administration at the elite, professional and paid level) and supervision (coaching) in an often hyper-masculine culture that places disproportionate emphasis on winning at all costs and, in the professional setting, profit. While financial profit may not be a major motive for coaches/teams condoning/requiring high-risk sports practices that can cause physical harm at the non-professional level, team/school/university kudos and reputation may be. Over-training, playing while injured, and improper coaching or tackling/hitting techniques, all of which are normally avoidable (and all of which are focused on in earlier chapters of this volume), represent examples of the conventional hazards of sport settings, at all levels.

This is not groundbreaking news — people willing to tell the truth about what actually happens "inside sport" have known that these things have always characterized competitive sport cultures, some more than others. What is new, are the links that athletic participants and the courts are increasingly making between sport injury and the sorts of unreasonable circumstances that render injury possible, likely, or even inevitable. At the professional level, these sorts of complaints have been known for some time. For instance, in a revealing 1970s interview with author Studs Terkel (1974: 501), former NHL player, Eric Nesterenko, spoke of cynicism toward coaches and owners as a way of coping with workplace exploitation and risk of injury

> I have become disillusioned with the game not being the pure thing
> it was earlier in my life. I began to see the exploitation of the players

> by the owners. You realize owners don't really care for you. You're
> a piece of property. They try to get as much out of you as they can.
> I remember once I had a torn shoulder. It was well in the process
> of healing. But I knew it wasn't right yet. They brought the doctor
> in. He said, "You can play." I played and ripped it completely. I
> was laid up. So I look at the owner. He shrugs his shoulders, walks
> away. He doesn't really hate me. He's impersonal.

While many coaches and sports protagonists are irked by such allegations of callousness (Remnick 1987), others provide corroborating evidence for Nesterenko's view. In the words of George Allen, former coach and General Manager of the Washington Redskins: "... nobody is indispensable. If he can't play, we let him know he's not going to be with us" (Terkel 1974: 509).

Public revelations of such athlete exploitation first became widespread during the 1960s and 1970s with the publication of several exposés of professional sport (Bouton 1970; Meggyesy 1971; Shaw 1972), but these indictments are ongoing. More recently, while Remnick (1987: 46) speaks of "sadistic coaches treating players like dray horses," Adams *et al.* (1987: 4) discuss imprudent and suable coaching techniques, Cruise & Griffiths (1991) decry the "dog-eat-dog" business of the NHL, and Courson (1991) argues that NFL coaches might just as well write prescriptions for drugs, and steroids in particular, when they advise players to appreciably gain weight and strength in the "off season."

It is precisely these underlying dynamics of competitive sport, and in particular what I earlier called techniques of *non-enforcement* and *covert facilitation* (Young 1993: 378), that have resulted in the courts widening the circle of culpability where litigated athletic injury is concerned. Legal actions are no longer limited to grieving athletes per se; they may also extend to cases against coaches, teams, owners, referees, governing sport bodies, and even communities and municipalities as, again, witnessed in the chapter's opening vignette.

As such, in addition to player abuses causing injury, the courts are also willing to hear incidents of "vicarious liability." Specifically, should players causing injury to themselves or others be penalized when it can be shown that they have followed coaching instructions? Traditionally, cultural reverence for sport has meant that suing a coach has been considered heretical, but increasingly coaches are being named in numerous lawsuits each year (Adams *et al.* 1987: 3). Connors (1981) argues that, at the amateur level in the U.S., physical educators and coaches represent those individuals most often sued in educational settings in the United States, and similar dynamics are being experienced in the U.K. For instance, a spate of serious injuries in school-based rugby, including some resulting from collapsing scrums, have led, as one news report put it, to several schools "planning to drop rugby — partly because of the growing litigation culture over injuries" ("Public School Drops Rugby," http://news.bbc.co.uk/hi/english/education/newsid_2053000/2053233.stm).

If it can be proven that an injured player acts in accordance with his/her role requirements, that player may not be solely responsible for his/her conduct or his/her conditions. This is especially resonant, of course, where cases of younger and child athletes are concerned. Young athletes are, afterall, more likely to accept coaching advice uncritically, and be more vulnerable to potentially harmful advice coming from adults in coaching/mentoring positions. In a well known National Basketball Association case, the Los Angeles Lakers were found to be negligent when their player, Kermit Washington, punched his opponent, Rudy Tomjanovich of the Houston Rockets during a 1977 game. The punch resulted in serious injury to Tomjanovich, including "a fractured jaw, nose, and skull, severe lacerations, (and) a cerebral concussion" (Smith 1987: 12). Deemed negligent in not adequately training and supervising Washington, the Lakers were required to pay over $3 million in damages.

To date, although it is difficult to find a coach who has been charged with conspiring to assault, American and Canadian law holds anyone criminally responsible who "counsels . . . or commands another to commit a crime" (Hechter 1977: 426). This rests uneasily against the fact that coaches in football, hockey, rugby, lacrosse and other sports routinely require their players not only to overwhelm, but to ensure, often by "stretching" the rules of the sport (such as in the use of so-called "professional fouls" and the like), that their opponents are "taken out" of the game. Adams (1987) cites several cases of imprudent coaching techniques at elite amateur levels. The following, for instance, is an eminently dangerous and suable football scenario: "Coaches denied players water breaks, even on extremely hot and humid days to teach mental toughness. Football coaches employ dangerous drills such as a "suicide" drill where five to six players would tackle an unprotected lineman because he missed a block" (p. 3). The dangers inherent in tyrannical or negligent coaching regimes in (North) American football have been illuminated over the past several seasons as players have suffered, sometimes fatally, from heat stroke. As a 2002 Associated Press news story reported:

> Heat related football deaths at all levels have steadily increased, replacing direct fatal injuries as the sport's biggest on-field safety concern. Eight football players died nationwide last year because of injuries, and another three died from heat stroke . . . Twelve more deaths were by natural causes aggravated by exercise, such as a heart attack. The number of injury deaths reflected a substantial

drop since stricter rules about tackling and blocking were
enacted in the mid-1970s, when fatalities regularly reached double
digits . . . Minnesota Vikings tackle Korey Stringer collapsed during
practice July 31 and died the next day, as did Travis Stowers, a
high school player near Michigantown, Ind . . . Less than a week
earlier, Eraste Autin, an incoming freshman at the University of
Florida, died of complications of heatstroke. He collapsed at the
end of a voluntary summer conditioning session and was in a
coma for six days (http://www.newsday.com/sports/football/ny-
deaths252798612jul25.story).

Changing times and shifts in legal thinking where sport is concerned has thus
required that coaches become more legally attuned to notions of "foreseeability"
(Adams 1987: 5). Coaches, teams and game officials are increasingly required
by law to make all possible dangers or warning signs of injuries or accidents not
just known to players, but fully understood. The message is increasingly clear
— be negligent and run the risk of being sued (e.g. "Crippled Rugby Lad Sues
Ref for £1 Million: Scrums 'Were Not Safe.'" *The Sun*, April 16 2001: 15). The
way certainly seems open, then, for sports owners, administrators and authorities
to become more liable, both civilly and criminally, for the perceived negligent
treatment of players, who become hurt and injured under circumstances deemed
by the courts to represent, once again, "unreasonable" risk.

Reluctance to Prosecute

While, judged on the basis of a growing number of cases, there is clear evidence
to suggest a late twentieth century surge toward legal intervention into sports
violence/sports injury cases, the evidence for increases in criminal prosecutions is
less compelling. An early, but now outdated, attempt to account for the reluctance of
the courts to prosecute and punish sports injury/sports violence cases was offered
again by Smith (1987), who identified seven key explanations for the relative
immunity to legal sanctions of players charged with injuring opponents. According
to Smith, these reasons included the following concerns: that the courts have more
important things to do like prosecuting "real" criminals; that the leagues themselves
are in the best position to effectively control player misbehaviour; that civil law
proceedings are better suited than criminal proceedings for dealing with an injured
player's grievances; that it is unfair to prosecute an individual player while ignoring
those who may have aided, abetted or counselled; that it is unfair to prosecute a
player when the law is unclear as to what sorts of injurious acts it would define

as "unreasonable"; that it is almost impossible to reach a guilty verdict in sports violence/sports injury cases; that prosecuting athletes does little to solve the wider social causes of sports violence and injuries.

It is likely that these views will continue to reflect popular thinking in the world of sport, in the public at large, and perhaps also in the courtroom. The role of the media in "framing" sports violence/sports injury issues for the public is also noteworthy here, especially when it contributes to the view that violence and injury are ordinary, acceptable and even unavoidable features of the sports process (Ball-Rokeach & Loges 1996; Young 1986, 1990; Young & Smith 1988/1989). Despite the prevalence of these views, more punitive attitudes on the part of both sports authorities and the law seem to be emerging. A process of delegitimation of some aspects of sport that culminate in injury seems to be underway.

The following observations serve to update Smith's socio-legal explanations for the traditional reluctance of the courts to prosecute player violence to capture what may be a trend toward delegitimation:

(i) Criminologists have known for a long time that, in countries like Canada, the United States and the United Kingdom, justice systems are predisposed to policing so-called "street crime." For example, there remains in all three countries a widespread concern with youth crime and youth violence. While it may be some time before large sections of the public are willing to view athletes behaving harmfully in the same light as such "real" criminals, it seems likely that the sheer numbers of athletes being charged with assault may have affected public perceptions. Sensational media attention to sports assault cases, such as the ones listed earlier, may have served to encourage sections of the public to be more critical of sports outcomes, such as injury, especially where preventable injuries and catastrophic cases result.

(ii) The argument that "in-house" policing is the most effective means to monitor player violence and participant injury is a controversial one. It seems reasonable to argue that the leagues and clubs are in the most informed and nuanced positions to judge the magnitude of an offence relative to the rules and traditions of the game. On the other hand, we know from the criminological literature that self-regulating professional organizations entrusted with policing themselves (such as lawyers, doctors, and the police themselves) sometimes abuse that privilege by meting out only tokenist sanctions and punishments to appease public demand for "accountability." Likewise, sociological research has uncovered processes of *non-enforcement*, *covert facilitation* and *cover-ups* with respect to sports violence/injury cases (Young 1993). Moreover, we also know that there are numerous ways in which violent practices causing injury are rewarded in sport — financially, occupationally, and within the specific culture of certain sports. To my knowledge, no one has conducted a systematic study of whether in-house punishments (warnings, suspensions, fines, etc.) are increasing in sport, but impressionistic evidence suggests that this may be the case in certain contexts.

(iii) The courts have traditionally viewed civil law proceedings as more appropriate than criminal proceedings in dealing with the grievances of injured players in assault cases. Again, this approach stems from the view that a certain amount of physical damage should be expected in sport and from the previously discussed notion of *volenti non fit injuria*. While it probably remains true that most injury cases are dealt with in civil law, criminal law is also being viewed as an appropriate venue, as an already large number of cases on both sides of the Atlantic suggests.

(iv) The view that it is unfair to prosecute individual players for their *directly* injurious or otherwise negligent actions while ignoring those who may have assisted in the teaching or promotion of those acts (e.g. coaches or owners) prevails. Courts also continue to invoke the philosophy of legal individualism that tends to shift the onus of criminal responsibility from an organization (e.g. a sports team or a league) to a particular player. However, sport has already witnessed numerous precedent-setting cases where courts have decided against sports teams rather than against an individual player; this trend shows no sign of slowing down.

(v) Legal systems on both sides of the Atlantic continue to approach sports injury cases inconsistently and with great variability. Despite recent pressures on sports organizations and the courts to examine more closely, and thus define more clearly, other aspects of "risky" sports-related behaviour such as sexual harassment (Donnelly 1999) and hazing (Bryshun & Young 1999), it is probably fair to argue that among the public, sports organizations and the courts (as well as scholars), definitions of what constitutes "unreasonable" and "negligent" sports actions causing injury remain less than clear.

(vi) The argument that one should avoid sports violence/injury litigation because it is impossible to reach a guilty verdict may strike the reader as missing the point. However disagreeable one finds this logic, it is nevertheless true that the decision to litigate is often premised on the perceived chances of receiving a favourable decision in court. In this sense, it is very likely that at the level of the aggrieved player or the prosecution, courts may be avoided due to the perception that the justice system would not be sympathetic to the case. However, it is also true that many cases *have* reached the courts and *have* resulted in guilty verdicts. In other words, where sports "crimes/assaults" are concerned, there are already many precedents in law in several countries. To date, we have no record of the extent to which or rate of these cases are growing, but again anecdotal evidence seems to point in this direction — at least for Canada, England and the United States.

(vii) The argument that prosecuting injurious athletes is a "Band-Aid" solution to the problem because it does little to solve wider causes of violence is crucial. As a sociologist, and following Smith, I accept the proposition that player violence and sports-related injury are socially and culturally embedded, such that criminalizing individual cases is likely to achieve very little unless similar anti-violence/anti-injury intervention/transformation/re-education occurs elsewhere in the wider community.

In sum, this sort of socio-legal approach highlights something of a paradox on the role of the courts in sports injury — while there seems to be an increasing degree of social and legal intolerance to forms of player violence causing injury, there remains an ongoing reluctance on the part of the courts to fully sanction athletes for assault, dangerous play and for other sports "crimes" inflicting harm. In general, player violence is still defined ambiguously at best, and there remains little agreement among sports administrators and legal authorities as to the acceptable limits of aggressive, injurious, or otherwise risky sports behaviour. Also, while civil and criminal charges against athletes may be on the increase, charges are commonly commuted, and prosecutions remain rare and sentences light (Young & Wamsley 1996).

Conclusion

The primary purpose of this chapter has been to provide a review of the role of the courts in sports injury and to explore some of the legal complications that ensue as sports settings become more litigious. At the end of the 20th century, and now into the 21st century, there is increasing evidence that the courts in a number of countries are more willing to hear sport injury cases (often described as "sport violence" cases). Litigation of sport assault, or what has provocatively been tagged "sports crime" not only by critics but, fascinatingly enough, by the Government of Canada,[2] appears to be on the rise in Canada and elsewhere. What

---

[2] In response to injuries in ice hockey, including numerous paralyses, the Government of Canada released an advertisement in the late 1980s that contained a photograph of an empty hockey arena and the caption "The Scene of The Crime." The Ministry of Fitness and Amateur Sport has since allowed this particular advertising campaign to lapse, but it remains a fascinating attempt by the State to re-label and transform public thinking on the Canadian national game in light of its less-than-impressive record where player health and safety is concerned.

Michael Smith defined as "brutal body contact" and "borderline violence" over two decades ago is increasingly prompting injured athletes to step forward as private litigants to initiate not only civil, but also criminal, charges and proceedings. At the same time, non-legal forms of intervention (such as fines, suspensions, and generally closer policing practices) based on principles of deterrence are also being adopted by sports clubs, leagues and organizations. In British rugby, for instance, media reportage of such interventions is common (e.g. "Violent Players Face Clampdown," *The Guardian*, December 12 1994: 17; "Prop Banned Until 21st Century," *The Guardian*, May 10 1995: 21). But, for all of this, it would be a mistake to assume that legal intervention into sports violence and sports injury cases has been uncomplicated or homogeneous; this is clearly not true. In general, sports violence and sports injury are still defined ambiguously at best, and there remains little agreement among sports leagues and authorities as to the limits of aggressive, injurious or otherwise risky sports conduct.

Despite some high profile international sports injury cases, there is considerable evidence that the notion of *volenti non fit injuria* endures at the centre of public and legal tolerance of even the most disturbing sport injury cases. In other words, one of the main causes of the still widespread tendency to excuse and accept injury, catastrophe and even death in sport is the concept of implied consent. From this position, it comes as no great surprise that when player conduct inflicting harm becomes redefined as "assault" and is litigated, a series of commonsense rationalizations (and, as we saw earlier, readily available legal defenses) kick in to defend the violent and harmful dimensions of sport, or the violence "doer." As former England rugby "hard man," Mike Burton, proclaimed in his overly literal interpretation of the Simon Devereux incident described earlier, "Every tackle in a game of rugby is a common assault" (*The Sun*, February 23 1996: 42). It is equally clear that this sort of logic, found in both masculinist sport cultures as well as, ironically, in the institution of law itself (Atkinson in press; Young 1993; Young & Wamsley 1996) is founded on deeply gendered undercurrents that likely conflate to compromise the chances of punitive legal resolutions. Along with other factors, perhaps this explains why the growing number of charges brought against sports parties for injuring participants has not been matched by similarly stiff prosecution rates?

Where the role of the courts in sport injury is concerned, then, there are several things that we know. We know, for instance, that throughout much of the 20th century, the courts preferred not to hear sports violence and sports injury cases, "bouncing" them back to the world of sport itself to adjudicate, or reaching "acquittal" decisions quickly. On the basis of what socio-legal and criminological scholars tell us, we know that this began to change in Canada, the USA and Britain in the final third of the 20th century, and that since that time case law has grown into a voluminous body of material on both sides of the Atlantic. We know that, when litigated, the notions of voluntary assumption of risk and consent have been instrumental in judicial logic and decision-making. We know, concomitantly, that sports law is a growing professional field, and we know that what has been called a "litigation explosion" (Hans & Lofquist 1992) related to sport and its numerous compensation claims has expanded insurance costs and threatened sports programmes at many levels in many countries (e.g. "Injury Pay Out Puts Soccer on the Spot," *The Guardian*, October 15 1997:9; "£1.5 Million Injury Claim Threatens Football," *The Sunday Times*, October 12 1997:5).[3] We know that there is an apparent dissonance between the number of cases in which charges are laid and the numbers of cases actually prosecuted. We know that preliminary investigations of sports violence and sports injury case law strongly suggest that gender dynamics may be as telling once cases find their way to court as in the process of getting there in the first place (Atkinson in press; Young & Wamsley 1996). Finally, we also know that while case law has occupied sports violence scholars for some time (Barnes 1988; Grayson 1988; Smith 1983, 1987; Young 1993), the implications of this case law for better understanding *pain and injury in sport*, including the complicity of the authorities in reducing very complicated injury episodes to the nebulous concept of "consent," has not been thoroughly considered and researched. The sociological study of sport-related pain and injury may be a relatively new field of inquiry, but the more serious consideration of the role of the courts and the State in that process already seems overdue.

References

Adams, S. (1987). Liability and negligence. In: S. Adams, M. Adrian, & M. Bayless (Eds), *Catastrophic injuries in sport: Avoidance strategies* (pp. 3–11). Indianapolis, IN: Benchmark.

Adams, S., Adrian, M., & Bayless, M. (Eds) (1987). *Catastrophic injuries in sports: Avoidance strategies*. Indianapolis, IN: Benchmark.

Atkinson, M. (in press). It's still part of the game: Dangerous masculinity, crime, and victimization in professional ice hockey. In: L. Fuller (Ed.), *Sexual sport rhetoric and violence: Teaming up gender with the language of sport*. New York: Haworth Press.

Ball-Rokeach, S. (1971). The legitimation of violence. In: J. F. Short, & M. E. Wolfgang (Eds), *Collective violence* (pp. 100–111). Chicago: Aldine.

---

[3] As O'Donnell (2000: 94) writes, "The legal profession has been quick to capitalize on the misfortune of sports players who have been the subject of an accident."

Ball-Rokeach, S. (1980). Normative and deviant violence from a conflict perspective. *Social Problems, 28*, 45–62.

Ball-Rokeach, S., & Loges, W. E. (1996). Making choices: Media roles in the construction of value choices. In: C. Seligman, J. Olson, & M. Zanna (Eds), *The psychology of values: The Ontario symposium* (Vol. 8, pp. 277–298). Mahwah, NJ: Erlbaum.

Barnes, J. (1988). *Sports and the law in Canada.* Toronto: Butterworths.

Bouton, J. (1970). *Ball four: My life and hard times throwing knuckleball in the big leagues.* New York: Dell.

Bryshun, J., & Young, K. (1999). Sport-related hazing: An inquiry into male and female involvement. In: P. White, & K. Young (Eds), *Sport and gender in Canada* (pp. 269–293). Don Mills, ON: Oxford University Press.

Connors, E. T. (1981). *Educational tort liability and malpractice.* Bloomington, IN: Phi Delta Kappa.

Courson, S. (1991). *False glory.* Stamford, CT: Longmeadow.

Cruise, D., & Griffiths, A. (1991). *Net worth: Exploding the myths of pro hockey.* Toronto: Viking.

Donnelly, P. (1999). Who's fair game? Sport, sexual harassment, and abuse. In: P. White, & K. Young (Eds), *Sport and gender in Canada* (pp. 107–129). Don Mills, ON: Oxford University Press.

Gardiner, S., Felix, A., James, M., Welch, R., & O'Leary, J. (1998). *Sports law.* London: Cavendish.

Grayson, E. (1988). *Sport and the law.* London: Butterworths.

Hans, V. P., & Lofquist, W. S. (1992). Jurors' judgements of business liability in tort cases: Implications for the litigation explosion debate. *Law & Society Review, 26*(1), 85–112.

Hechter, W. (1976/1977). Criminal law and violence in sports. *Criminal Law Quarterly, 19*, 425–453.

Horrow, R. (1980). *Sports violence: The interaction between private lawmaking and the criminal law.* Arlington, VA: Carrollton Press.

Horrow, R. (1982). Violence in professional sport: Is it a part of the game? *Journal of Legislation, 9*(1), 1–15.

Lubell, A. (1989, March). Questioning the athlete's right to sue. *The Physician and Sports Medicine, 17*(3), 240–244.

Martin's Annual Criminal Code (1988). Aurora, ON: Canada Law Book.

Meggyesy, D. (1971). *Out of their League.* Berkeley, CA: Ramparts Press.

Moriarty, D., Holman, M., Brown, R., & Moriarty, M. (1994). *Canadian/American Sport, Fitness, and the Law.* Toronto: Canadian Scholars' Press Inc.

O'Donnell, E. (2000, May). Happy landings: Avoiding sport litigation. *Stadia*, 93–96.

Reasons, C. (1992). *The criminal law and sports violence: Hockey crimes.* Unpublished manuscript, University of British Columbia, Vancouver.

Remnick, D. (1987, October 5). Still on the outside. *Sports Illustrated*, 42–54.

Shaw, G. (1972). *Meat on the hoof.* New York: St. Martin's.

Smith, M. D. (1983). *Violence and sport.* Toronto: Butterworths.

Smith, M. D. (1987). *Violence in Canadian amateur sport: A review of literature*. Report for Commission for Fair Play. Ottawa: Government of Canada.

Terkel, S. (1974). *Working*. New York: Avon.

Watson, R. C., & MacLellan, J. C. (1986). Smitting to spitting: 80 years of ice hockey in the Canadian courts. *Canadian Journal of History of Sport, 17*(2), 10–27.

White, D. (1986). Sports violence as criminal assault: Development of the doctrine by Canadian criminal courts. *Duke Law Journal*, 1030–1054.

Young, K. (1986). The killing field: Themes in mass media responses to the Heysel Stadium riot. *International Review for the Sociology of Sport, 21*, 253–267.

Young, K. (1990). *Treatment of sports violence by the Canadian mass media*. Report to Sport Canada's Applied Sport Research Programme. Ottawa, Ontario.

Young, K. (1993). Violence, risk and liability in male sports culture. *Sociology of Sport Journal, 10*, 373–396.

Young, K., & Smith, M. D. (1988/1989). Mass media treatment of violence in sports and its effects. *Current Psychology: Research and Reviews, 7*, 298–312.

Young, K., & Wamsley, K. (1996). State complicity in sports assault and the gender order in twentieth century Canada: Preliminary observations. *Avante, 2*, 51–69.

About the Editor and Contributors

Edward Albert is a Professor in the Department of Sociology and Anthropology at Hofstra University in Hempstead, New York. His interests include the areas of medical sociology where he has published on issues related to AIDS and stigma and, more recently, the sociology of sport where he has looked extensively at the subculture of bicycle racing. He has published articles related to the social construction of winning, and the relationship between cooperation and competition within the cycling subculture. He has served on the editorial board of the *Sociology of Sport Journal*.

Bo J. Bernhard is an Assistant Professor of Sociology with a joint appointment in the College of Hotel Administration at the University of Nevada, Las Vegas. His research focuses on gambling and other risk-taking behaviours. He has published in the areas of gambling addiction, applications of deviance theories, and sport subcultures.

Hannah Charlesworth received an M.A. from the University of Leicester and a Ph.D. from the School of Sport and Exercise Sciences at Loughborough University, U.K. Her research interests include sports-related pain and injury, illness and gender. She is currently employed by the Institute of Youth and Sport at Loughborough University as a Research Associate.

Peter Donnelly is a Professor in the Faculty of Physical Education and Health at the University of Toronto, and Director of the Centre for Sport Policy Studies. He has served in various offices for professional organisations in the sociology of sport, including the editorship of the *Sociology of Sport Journal* (1990–1994), and President of the North American Society for the Sociology of Sport (1999–2000). He co-edited *Sport and the Sociological Imagination* (with Nancy Theberge) and *Inside Sports* (with Jay Coakley). The second edition of his collection, *Taking Sport Seriously*, was published in 2000. He is also co-author (with Jay Coakley) of the first Canadian edition of *Sports in Society: Issues and Controversies*.

James H. Frey is retired as Dean of the College of Liberal Arts and is Emeritus Professor of Sociology at the University of Nevada, Las Vegas. He is past-President of the North American Society for the Sociology of Sport and a former editor the *Journal of Sport and Social Issues*. He is the author of *Survey Research by Telephone* (Sage 1989) and co-author with Howard Nixon of a textbook on sport sociology. He has published articles and reviews on research on risk-sport, college athletics, survey research response rates, and interviewing techniques and strategies.

P. David Howe is Senior Lecturer in sport and leisure cultures in the Chelsea School at the University of Brighton, U.K. Trained as a medical anthropologist, he has published work on commercialism, pain and injury and sports medicine, and is author of *Sport, professionalism and pain: Ethnographies of injury and risk*. (Routledge 2004).

David P. Johns is Reader and Chairman of the Department of Sports Science and Physical Education at the Chinese University of Hong Kong. He gained a wide range of experiences in elite sport as an assistant coach to the Canadian Men's Gymnastic Team in 1976 and as a sport consultant to several Canadian national teams including gymnastics, wrestling and athletics. This work provided a natural access to athletes and resulted in the collection and publication of several papers related to these experiences. More recently, David's research interests have focused on school curriculum policy and practice, and the sociological and ecological factors that influence physical activity and health practices. He has lectured in the U.K., Canada, and Australia as well as Hong Kong.

Joseph A. Kotarba is Professor of Sociology at the University of Houston, Texas. He received his doctorate from the University of California, San Diego. He has conducted extensive research on chronic pain, alternative health care, wellness in the workplace, and HIV/AIDS. He is currently studying quality of life among prostate cancer patients and inner strength among persons living with HIV/AIDS. He is also writing a general theory of sports medicine as occupational health care. His most recent book is *Postmodern Existential Sociology* (co-edited with John M. Johnson, Alta Mira Press 2002).

Howard L. Nixon II is Professor of Sociology at Towson University USA. He earned his Ph.D. in Sociology from the University of Pittsburgh, and has been a faculty member and department chair at the University of Vermont, Appalachian State University and Towson University. He recently ended a nearly four-year tenure as Acting Dean of the College of Extended Programs at Towson University. He has taught, conducted research and published in sport sociology for over thirty years, and his major sports-related research interests in recent years have been cultural and social aspects of risk, pain and injury and the sociology of disability sport.

Elizabeth C. J. Pike is Senior Lecturer in the sociology of sport in the School of Sport, Exercise and Health Sciences at University College Chichester. She has been an invited speaker in several higher education institutions in the United Kingdom and elsewhere in Europe, and has presented papers on risk, pain, injury and health issues at a number of national and international conferences. These include a keynote presentation to the British Association of Chartered Physiotherapists in Sports Medicine, in addition to papers given at the Pre-Olympic Congress, the International Sociology of Sport Association conference, and various meetings of the North American Society for the Sociology of Sport. She is co-author, with Joseph Maguire, of "Injury in Women's Sport: Classifying Key Elements of 'Risk Encounters,' " in the *Sociology of Sport Journal*, 2003.

Frederick W. Preston is Professor of Sociology at the University of Nevada, Las Vegas. He is the author of introductory textbooks on sociology and social problems and has published articles on gambling behaviour and substance abuse. He is academic advisor and formerly coach to the champion UNLV college rodeo team.

Martin Roderick spent several years at the University of Leicester before moving to the University of Durham in 2004, where he is a Lecturer in Sociology. He completed his Ph.D. examining the careers of professional footballers in 2003. He has been involved in research focusing specifically on the management of injuries in professional football, and on sport for people with learning disabilities. His other interests concern the sociology of emotions and sport, and the problems of participating in sport at elite levels. He was joint author, with Dr Ivan Waddington and Graham Parker, of "Managing Injuries in Professional Football," a report for the Professional Footballers' Association.

Donald Sabo is Professor of Sociology at D'Youville College in Buffalo, New York and an Adjunct Associate Professor of Sociology at SUNY at Buffalo. He is a recognised expert on gender relations, particularly in relation to physical activity and health. He has co-authored or edited seven books, most recently *Men's Health & Illness: Gender, Power and the Body* (Sage 1995), *Masculinities, Gender Relations, and Sport* (Sage 2000), and *Prison Masculinities* (Temple University Press 2001). Don has researched gender equity struggles in middle schools, high schools, colleges, and universities. He is a trustee of the U.S.-based Women's Sports Foundation, and has worked with Human Kinetics Publishers to develop an educational video and "CD Rom"-based curriculum to help coaches integrate gender equity into school athletic programs.

Parissa Safai is a doctoral candidate in the Department of Exercise Sciences in the Faculty of Physical Education and Health at the University of Toronto. Her research interests include the political economy of health and healthcare systems, medical dominance and, more recently, risk and risk-taking in the relationship between sport and health. While still continuing research in the area of injury and pain tolerance in sport, her current interest is on the socio-historical development of the field of sport medicine in Canada, particularly within and in relation to high performance sport.

Rhonda L. Singer is Assistant Professor of Sociology at Rollins College, Winter Park, Florida, where she began working after earning her Ph.D. in Sociology from the University of Massachusetts, Amherst, in 1999. Her research includes an ethnographic study of children in a youth recreational basketball league that served as the basis for her dissertation, and her current work concerns gender issues on college campuses. Rhonda is currently developing her dissertation research for publication, including a book project and a number of articles that are under consideration.

Lone F. Thing is currently engaged in post-doctoral work as a Research Fellow in the Department of Sociology at the University of Copenhagen, Denmark. She also teaches Sociology as an External Lecturer at the Department of Public Health in Copenhagen. Her current research interests lie in the area of women's sports, especially with respect to the emotions, the body, health and pain and injury.

Ivan Waddington holds Visiting Professorships at University College Chester, at the Centre for Sports Studies, University College Dublin, and at the Norwegian University of Sport and Physical Education, Oslo. His research interests focus on the interface between sport and health. He is the senior author of a major study of club doctors and physiotherapists in English professional football clubs and is a recognised authority on doping in sport. His most recent books include *Sport, Health and Drugs* (Spon 2000), *Drugs in Sport: The Pressure to Perform* (with B. Houlihan, D. Mottram and P. Korkia, British Medical Journal Books 2002), and *Fighting Fans: Football Hooliganism as a World Phenomenon* (edited with E. Dunning, P. Murphy and A. Astrinakis, University College Dublin Press 2002).

Stephan R. Walk is Associate Professor of Kinesiology and Health Promotion at California State University, Fullerton, with degrees in both sociology and physical education and exercise science from Michigan State University. Athlete health care, the social organisation of sports medicine, and organisational sexuality are his principal research interests. He has published articles on these topics in the *Sociology of Sport Journal* and *Men and Masculinities*, as well as in book chapters in both sociology and sports medicine. His current work centres on athletes' attitudes towards risk, pain, and injury, as well as the role of team physicians in medical decision-making for athletes. Stephan is a member of the North American Society for the Sociology of Sport since 1989, and a 4-year member of the editorial board of *Sociology of Sport Journal.*

Philip White is Professor of Kinesiology and Sociology at McMaster University. In addition to contributing numerous articles and book chapters in various areas of the sociology of sport, he writes and speaks broadly on rugby development. He is also co-editor of *Sport and Gender in Canada* (Oxford University Press 1999), and has served on the editorial board of the *Sociology of Sport Journal.* He has coached rugby at the intercollegiate, provincial and national levels in Canada. As the recently appointed Chair of the Rugby Canada Coaching Committee, he is currently restructuring the coach certification system in Canada.

Kevin Young is Associate Professor of Sociology at the University of Calgary. He has published on a variety of sports-related topics such as violence, gender and subcultural identity and is the co-editor of *Sport and Gender in Canada* (Oxford University Press 1999) and *Theory, Sport & Society* (Elsevier Press 2002). He has served on the editorial boards of *International Review for the Sociology of Sport, Sociology of Sport Journal, Avante,* and *Soccer and Society,* as well as on the executive board of the North American Society for the Sociology of Sport. He is currently Vice President of the International Sociology of Sport Association.

Author Index

Subject Index